Abdominal Ultrasound

Editor

WUI K. CHONG

ULTRASOUND CLINICS

www.ultrasound.theclinics.com

Consulting Editor
VIKRAM S. DOGRA

October 2014 • Volume 9 • Number 4

ELSEVIER

1600 John F. Kennedy Boulevard • Suite 1800 • Philadelphia, Pennsylvania, 19103-2899

http://www.theclinics.com

ULTRASOUND CLINICS Volume 9, Number 4
October 2014 ISSN 1556-858X, ISBN-13: 978-0-323-32636-0

Editor: John Vassallo
Developmental Editor: Stephanie Carter

Ultrasound Clinics (ISSN 1556-858X) is published quarterly by Elsevier, Inc., 360 Park Avenue South, New York, NY 10010-1710. Months of publication are January, April, July, and October. Business and editorial offices: 1600 John F. Kennedy Boulevard, Suite 1800, Philadelphia, Pennsylvania 19103-2899. Accounting and circulation offices: 6277 Sea Harbor Drive, Orlando, FL 32887-4800. Periodicals postage paid at New York, NY, and additional mailing offices. Subscription prices are $270 per year for (US individuals), $327 per year for (US institutions), $130 per year for (US students and residents), $305 per year for (Canadian individuals), $369 per year for (Canadian institutions), $325 per year for (international individuals), $369 per year for (international institutions), and $155 per year for (Canadian and foreign students/residents). To receive student/resident rate, orders must be accompanied by name of affiliated institution, date of term, and the signature of program/residency coordinator on institution letterhead. Orders will be billed at individual rate until proof of status is received. Foreign air speed delivery is included in all Clinics subscription prices. All prices are subject to change without notice. **POSTMASTER:** Send address changes to *Ultrasound Clinics,* Elsevier Health Sciences Division, Subscription Customer Service, 3251 Riverport Lane, Maryland Heights, MO 63043. **Customer Service (orders, claims, online, change of address): Telephone: 1-800-654-2452 (U.S. and Canada); 314-447-8871 (outside U.S. and Canada). Fax: 314-447-8029. E-mail: journalscustomerservice-usa@elsevier.com (for print support); journalsonlinesupport-usa@elsevier.com (for online support).**

Reprints: For copies of 100 or more, of articles in this publication, please contact the Commercial Reprints Department, Elsevier Inc., 360 Park Avenue South, New York, NY 10010-1710. Tel.: +1-212-633-3874; Fax: +1-212-633-3820; E-mail: reprints@elsevier.com.

Contributors

CONSULTING EDITOR

VIKRAM S. DOGRA, MD
Professor of Radiology, Urology, and
Biomedical Engineering; Associate Chair for
Education and Research; Director of
Ultrasound; Department of Imaging Sciences,
University of Rochester School of Medicine,
Rochester, New York

EDITOR

WUI K. CHONG, MBBS, FRCR
Associate Professor, Department of Radiology,
University of North Carolina, Chapel Hill, North
Carolina

AUTHORS

MARK ABEL, MBBS
Clinical Research Fellow, Department of
Surgery and Cancer, Oncology Research,
Garry Weston Centre, Hammersmith Hospital,
Imperial College NHS Trust, London,
United Kingdom

SUSAN J. ACKERMAN, MD
Professor of Radiology, Medical University of
South Carolina, Charleston, South Carolina

RICHARD G. BARR, MD, PhD, FACR, FSRU
Professor of Radiology, Northeastern Ohio
Medical University, Rootstown, Ohio;
Southwoods Imaging, Youngstown, Ohio

MICHAEL D. BELAND, MD
Department of Radiology, Rhode Island
Hospital, Providence, Rhode Island

SHWETA BHATT, MD
Associate Professor, Department of Imaging
Sciences, University of Rochester School of
Medicine and Dentistry, Rochester, New York

BRIAN BOYD, MD
PGY-4 Radiology Resident, Department of
Radiology, University of North Carolina,
Chapel Hill, North Carolina

WUI K. CHONG, MBBS, FRCR
Associate Professor, Department of Radiology,
University of North Carolina, Chapel Hill, North
Carolina

MELISSA DAVIS, MD
Neuroradiology Fellow in Radiology,
University of North Carolina, Chapel Hill,
North Carolina

CORINNE DEURDULIAN, MD
Assistant Professor, Department of Radiology,
University of Southern California Keck School
of Medicine, Los Angeles, California

NICOLE FRENCH, MD
Fellow, Department of Radiology, University of
Southern California Keck School of Medicine,
Los Angeles, California

ABID IRSHAD, MBBS, MD
Professor of Radiology, Medical University of
South Carolina, Charleston, South Carolina

BARTON F. LANE, MD
Assistant Professor, Department of Diagnostic
Radiology and Nuclear Medicine, University of
Maryland School of Medicine, Baltimore,
Maryland

ELLIE R. LEE, MD
Clinical Assistant Professor, Department of
Radiology, University of North Carolina,
Chapel Hill, North Carolina

EDWARD LEEN, MD, FRCR
Professor of Radiology, Department of
Imaging, Hammersmith Hospital, Imperial
College NHS Trust, London, United Kingdom

MADELENE LEWIS, MD
Assistant Professor of Radiology, Medical
University of South Carolina, Charleston,
South Carolina

MARK E. LOCKHART, MD, MPH
Chief, Body Imaging; Professor, Department
of Radiology, University of Alabama at
Birmingham, Birmingham, Alabama

JUSTIN C. NORTH, MD
Assistant Professor, Department of
Radiological Sciences, University of Oklahoma
Health Sciences Center, Oklahoma City,
Oklahoma

KERRI L. NOVAK, MD, FRCPC
Assistant Clinical Professor, Division of
Gastroenterology, Department of Medicine,
University of Calgary, Calgary, Alberta,
Canada

JOHN S. PELLERITO, MD, FACR
Associate Professor of Radiology,
Hofstra-North Shore-Long Island Jewish
School of Medicine; Vice Chairman,
Department of Radiology, North Shore-Long
Island Jewish Health System; Director,
Peripheral Vascular Laboratory, North Shore
University Hospital, Manhasset, New York

MARGARITA V. REVZIN, MD, MS
Assistant Professor of Radiology, Department
of Diagnostic Radiology, Yale University
School of Medicine, Yale-New Haven Hospital,
New Haven, Connecticut

AMOGH SRIVASTAVA, MD
Fellow in Abdominal Imaging, Department of
Radiology, Beth Israel Deaconess Medical
Center, Harvard University, Boston,
Massachusetts

WEY CHYI TEOH, MBBS, FRCR
Clinical Research Fellow; Consultant
Radiologist, Department of Radiology, Changi
General Hospital, Singapore

JOEL P. THOMPSON, MD, MPH
Department of Imaging Sciences, University of
Rochester School of Medicine and Dentistry,
Rochester, New York

JASON M. WAGNER, MD
Assistant Professor, Department of Radiological
Sciences, University of Oklahoma Health
Sciences Center, Oklahoma City, Oklahoma

STEPHANIE R. WILSON, MD
Clinical Professor, Department of Radiology;
Division of Gastroenterology, Department of
Medicine, University of Calgary, Calgary,
Alberta, Canada

JADE J. WONG-YOU-CHEONG, MD
Professor, Department of Diagnostic Radiology
and Nuclear Medicine, University of Maryland
School of Medicine, Baltimore, Maryland

JESSICA G. ZARZOUR, MD
Assistant Professor, Department of Radiology,
University of Alabama at Birmingham,
Birmingham, Alabama

Contents

Preface: Abdominal Ultrasound xiii

Wui K. Chong

Ultrasound of the Liver and Spleen 545

Amogh Srivastava and Michael D. Beland

Ultrasound (US) imaging is a noninvasive, low-cost, and widely available modality for the evaluation of the liver and spleen. US can be performed at the bedside, allowing for rapid diagnosis and little patient preparation. Inherent in the technique is direct involvement of the patient, allowing the sonographer to interact with the patient, to ask clinically relevant questions, and to tailor the examination where possible. The liver and spleen are very amenable to ultrasound evaluation. Many diseases have varying appearances, and there may be significant overlap between benign and malignant disease.

Ultrasound of the Gallbladder and Biliary Tree: Back to Basics 567

Brian Boyd and Ellie R. Lee

 Videos of Adenomyomatosis, Intrahepatic Biliary Dilation, Gallbladder mass imaging accompany this article

Ultrasound remains the modality of choice for initial evaluation of the gallbladder and biliary tree, especially in the setting of acute right upper quadrant pain. The biliary tract is well suited to ultrasound evaluation, and although many of the imaging findings are nonspecific, when combined with clinical history, risk factors, and adjunct computed tomography or magnetic resonance imaging when indicated, it can often help to make or at least confirm the diagnosis. This article is a review of the anatomy, basic sonographic findings, and common diseases of the biliary system.

Doppler Ultrasound of the Liver, Portal Hypertension, and Transjugular Intrahepatic Portosystemic Shunts 587

Melissa Davis and Wui K. Chong

 Videos of Color Doppler scan of the liver accompany this article

Doppler ultrasound is a noninvasive and accurate modality for evaluation of the liver and liver vasculature. Its real-time capability allows rapid diagnosis in a wide range of hepatic pathology. We review hepatic doppler in normal and diseased states, including portal hypertension, congestive cardiac failure, and portal and hepatic vein obstruction. Doppler evaluation of transjugular intrahepatic portosystemic shunts (TIPS) is also included.

Contrast Evaluation of Liver Masses 605

Mark Abel, Wey Chyi Teoh, and Edward Leen

 Videos of color Doppler demonstrating feeding artery and spoke wheel configuration of an FNH, CEUS of the same FNH in the arterial phase, and typical appearance of hypervascular liver metastases on CEUS accompany this article

Contrast-enhanced ultrasound (CEUS) is an important tool in the multimodal assessment of focal liver lesions. Unlike CT and magnetic resonance contrast agents, ultrasound contrast agents are purely intravascular, allowing for dynamic visualization of macro- and microvasculature. This is a review article covering the technical considerations of ultrasound contrast imaging and its clinical application in the detection and characterization of liver masses and in the monitoring of local ablative therapy. Its limitations, pitfalls, and future prospects are also discussed.

Elastography of the Abdomen   625

Richard G. Barr

Ultrasound elastography is a new technology that determines the stiffness of tissues. There are several ultrasound elastography techniques available that can be classified into 2 groups, strain and shear wave imaging. These techniques have been shown to be able to detect and characterize lesions in multiple organs. The major application in the abdomen is noninvasive assessment of liver fibrosis. The assessment of fibrosis in chronic liver disease is pivotal for staging, prognosis, and treatment management. The characterization and detection of abdominal masses have not been as extensively investigated.

Update on the Role of Sonography in Liver Transplantation   641

Susan J. Ackerman, Abid Irshad, and Madelene Lewis

The role of ultrasonography (US) in the evaluation of liver transplants is well established and it is routinely used for pretransplantation and posttransplantation evaluation. The role of US in pretransplantation evaluation is mainly to identify any contraindication to transplantation. The major role of US in the early posttransplantation period is to evaluate any vascular or biliary complications that may require surgical intervention to save the graft. Routine US surveillance helps to identify any delayed complications of liver transplant.

Renal Ultrasound   653

Joel P. Thompson and Shweta Bhatt

Ultrasonography may be used for the detection, characterization, and follow-up of a wide variety of acute and chronic renal pathology. This article provides an overview of renal parenchymal pathology, such as renal pseudotumors, neoplasms, cystic disease, and infectious/inflammatory processes. Obstructive and nonobstructive hydronephrosis are reviewed. In addition, renovascular hypertension and vascular pathology are also covered. The objective of this article is to provide an overview of renal pathology with emphasis on the role of ultrasound in their diagnosis and follow-up evaluation.

Ultrasonography of the Renal Transplant   683

Jessica G. Zarzour and Mark E. Lockhart

Renal transplantation is the treatment of choice for patients with end-stage renal disease. Ultrasonography is often the first-line imaging modality in studying the transplanted renal allograft both in the postoperative period and for long-term follow-up. Knowledge of the imaging appearance of the normal renal transplant as well as the possible complications is of paramount importance for the radiologist. In this article, the most common complications affecting the renal transplant are reviewed, including vascular abnormalities, graft dysfunction (including the use of novel techniques), peritransplant fluid collections, nonvascular urologic complications, and concerns regarding neoplastic risks.

Sonography of the Retroperitoneum 697

Barton F. Lane and Jade J. Wong-You-Cheong

Although computed tomography (CT) and magnetic resonance (MR) imaging have largely supplanted ultrasonography for the initial diagnosis of abdominal disease, transabdominal ultrasonography remains an important imaging modality secondary to its low cost, widespread availability, and lack of ionizing radiation. Because ultrasonography is frequently the first-line imaging obtained to evaluate abdominal and retroperitoneal symptoms, it is important to recognize the appearance of common normal and pathologic conditions, and to understand the benefits and limitations of this modality. This review focuses on transabdominal imaging techniques, with limited correlation with CT and MR images where appropriate.

Ultrasonography Assessment of the Aorta and Mesenteric Arteries 723

Margarita V. Revzin and John S. Pellerito

A basic knowledge of the anatomy of the abdominal aorta and its major branches is essential for proper interpretation of sonographic findings and for understanding the pathologic disease states that affect these vessels. An understanding of relevant anatomy and hemodynamics for normal vessels as well as for multiple disease states, including abdominal aortic aneurysm, vascular stenosis, dissection, and occlusion, is important for correct diagnosis. There are various Doppler techniques, protocols, and diagnostic criteria used in the evaluation of the aorta and mesenteric arteries.

Sonography of the Bowel 751

Stephanie R. Wilson and Kerri L. Novak

 Videos of CD of Neoterminal ileum (NTI), CD of sigmoid colon, incomplete mechanical bowel obstruction, eneteroenteric fistula shown between the thick abnormal terminal ileum in cross-section, perianal fistula shown on transperineal scan, normal and perforated appendix scans accompany this article

Ultrasound (US) is a valuable modality for the evaluation of patients presenting with the so-called acute abdomen, especially those with specific right or left lower-quadrant pain. It is increasingly popular for the routine and emergency evaluation of those with inflammatory bowel disease, providing a safe and reliable method for diagnosis of disease, detection of recurrent disease following surgery, monitoring therapy, and identifying those with complications. US is safe and well tolerated and may be repeated as necessary. In this era of radiation and cost awareness, US is a valuable modality for the evaluation of the bowel.

Ultrasound of the Abdominal Wall 775

Jason M. Wagner and Justin C. North

 Videos of an inguinal fat-containing hernia enlarging with Valsalva maneuver, transverse sonography of an indirect inguinal hernia containing fluid, and transverse sonography of a direct inguinal hernia containing bowel accompany this article

Ultrasound is a highly valuable imaging modality for the abdominal wall because of its high spatial resolution, dynamic imaging capability, lower cost, and lack of ionizing radiation. Real-time sonographic evaluation, including Valsalva maneuver and upright imaging, allows diagnosis and characterization of ventral and groin hernias. Abdominal wall fluid collections, masses, vascular abnormalities, and foreign bodies are also well evaluated with ultrasound. This article reviews anatomy, sonographic technique, and common pathology of the abdominal wall.

Ultrasound-Guided Intervention in the Abdomen and Pelvis: Review from A to Z   793

Corinne Deurdulian and Nicole French

 Videos of Hydrodissection, liver biopsy-related hemorrhage, renal biopsy-related hemorrhage, and splenic biopsy accompany this article

Ultrasound guidance for invasive procedures has become a necessary and often first-line tool for procedures in the abdomen and pelvis. There are many factors that influence the success of a procedure, with an organized setup being key to optimally and efficiently perform the procedure. Risks, benefits, techniques, and complications are discussed with emphasis on common procedures. Ultrasound fusion increases the utility of ultrasound in the setting of invasive procedures.

Index   821

ULTRASOUND CLINICS

RECENT ISSUES

July 2014
Small Parts and Superficial Structures
Nirvikar Dahiya, *Editor*

April 2014
Emergency Ultrasound
Michael Blaivas and
Srikar Adhikari, *Editors*

January 2014
Oncologic Ultrasound
Vikram Dogra, *Editor*

METHOD OF PARTICIPATION

In order to claim credit, participants must complete the following:

1. Complete enrolment as indicated above.
2. Read the activity.
3. Complete the CME Test and Evaluation. Participants must achieve a score of 70% on the test. All CME Tests and Evaluations must be completed online.

CME INQUIRIES/SPECIAL NEEDS

For all CME inquiries or special needs, please contact elsevierCME@elsevier.com.

Preface
Abdominal Ultrasound

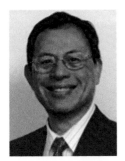

Wui K. Chong, MBBS, FRCR
Editor

Ultrasound is a unique imaging modality that can be performed quickly at the bedside with relatively compact equipment, requires little patient preparation, and has no adverse effects. This issue is dedicated to diagnostic sonography of the abdominal organs and abdominal wall, and Doppler evaluation of the abdominal vessels. It has a practical how-to-do-it focus aimed at the practicing sonographer or physician. Modern ultrasound equipment can provide exquisite imaging of the abdominal organs. Doppler plays a critical role in the evaluation of the great vessels of the abdomen, providing unique functionality for evaluating portal hypertension and hemodynamically significant arterial disease. Sonography is the first-line modality for imaging abdominal transplants, and this issue has articles dedicated to Doppler ultrasound evaluation of liver and renal allografts. Because of its real-time capability, sonography is an excellent modality for image-guided intervention. There is an article on performing basic US-guided procedures in the abdomen, and one on sonography of the abdominal wall, a structure optimally suited to ultrasound evaluation. The gastrointestinal tract, long thought to be just an impediment to visualization, can itself be beautifully evaluated with sonography, as shown by the leading expert in the field.

In recent years, technical advances in ultrasound have led to new clinical applications that have great potential in the abdomen. Contrast-enhanced ultrasound, elastography, and fusion imaging for intervention are covered in this issue. Ultrasound contrast agents and elastography in particular are major advances in noninvasive imaging of liver disease.

This issue is distinguished by a wealth of superb illustrations obtained with state-of-the-art equipment and includes a substantial number of color images. Ultrasound is a dynamic modality and we have included over 20 video clips of disease processes that are best appreciated when viewed in real-time, such as hernias. The videos are linked to the online version of the articles and can be viewed by subscribers via the Elsevier website.

I would like to thank the contributing authors, all of whom put in a tremendous amount of effort and time. Special thanks are also due to the unsung sonographers who are responsible for the many exquisite images that you see. This issue is dedicated to them.

Thanks also to the staff at Elsevier who helped make this issue possible.

Wui K. Chong, MBBS, FRCR
Department of Radiology
University of North Carolina
Chapel Hill, NC 27599-7510, USA

E-mail address:
wk_chong@med.unc.edu

Ultrasound Clin 9 (2014) xiii
http://dx.doi.org/10.1016/j.cult.2014.07.013
1556-858X/14/$ – see front matter © 2014 Published by Elsevier Inc.

Ultrasound of the Liver and Spleen

Amogh Srivastava, MD[a], Michael D. Beland, MD[b],*

KEYWORDS

• Ultrasound • Liver • Spleen

KEY POINTS

- Ultrasound is a quick, readily available, and informative first-line imaging modality for the liver and spleen.
- The liver and spleen are very amenable to ultrasound evaluation.
- Because many disease processes involving the liver and spleen can be evaluated on ultrasound, recognition of classic imaging appearances is important.
- Many diseases have varying appearances, and there may be significant overlap between benign and malignant disease.

INTRODUCTION

Ultrasound (US) imaging is a noninvasive, low-cost, and widely available modality for the evaluation of the liver and spleen. US can be performed at the bedside, allowing for rapid diagnosis and little in the way of patient preparation. Inherent in the technique is direct involvement of the patient, allowing the sonographer to interact with the patient, to ask clinically relevant questions, and to tailor the examination where possible.

LIVER

The liver lends itself to US evaluation given its location and homogeneous density, allowing for good sound transmission. However, because of the size and depth, the entire liver is often difficult to visualize. The body habitus of the patient also effects the depth of penetration with the US beam, further limiting visualization. Especially difficult areas to visualize include the subdiaphragmatic liver and the tip of the left hepatic lobe. Despite these challenges, US remains an important modality for the evaluation of the liver.

Patients should initially be placed in the left lateral decubitus position and a subcostal transducer approach should be applied. The right arm may be raised to open up and lift the rib spaces off the liver. A 3- to 5-MHz curved array transducer should be used for initial evaluation of the liver. A supine intercostal approach should also be taken to allow for complete visualization of the right hepatic lobe. Evaluation of the liver surface to assess for nodularity should be performed with a 5- to 12-MHz linear transducer. The surface is usually best evaluated in real-time because the liver surface moves with respiration. Care should be taken when evaluating surface nodularity as transducer angle and frequency can falsely create the appearance of a nodular surface.[1]

Anatomy

The liver is the largest organ in the abdomen, although the size may vary from patient to patient. The liver is located in the right upper quadrant but may extend far into the left upper quadrant and the right lower quadrant.[2] The size depends on patient sex, patient age, patient size, and alcohol consumption.[3–5] Liver size should be measured along the midclavicular line, although measuring liver size is not always standardized.[6] Most importantly, the measurement technique should be consistent

---

[a] Department of Radiology, Beth Israel Deaconess Medical Center, Harvard University, 330 Brookline Avenue, Boston, MA 02215, USA; [b] Department of Radiology, Rhode Island Hospital, 593 Eddy Street, Providence, RI 01604, USA
* Corresponding author.
E-mail address: mbeland@lifespan.org

Ultrasound Clin 9 (2014) 545–565
http://dx.doi.org/10.1016/j.cult.2014.06.001
1556-858X/14/$ – see front matter © 2014 Elsevier Inc. All rights reserved.

among patients and prior US examinations. Although size can vary, a liver length greater than 15.5 cm should be considered enlarged and indicates hepatomegaly. Extension of the right hepatic lobe below the lower pole of the right kidney has also been suggested as a sign of hepatomegaly, although this may be unreliable in patients with a Riedel lobe.[7] Additional signs of hepatomegaly include a rounded appearance to the tip of the right hepatic lobe and extension of the left lobe over the spleen.

The liver may be divided into segments delineated by the hepatic veins (**Figs. 1** and **2**). The portal vein runs within each segment. Portal and hepatic veins can be distinguished by the presence of echogenic periportal tissue and the presence of the biliary duct and hepatic artery that course within the portal triad. The ligamentum teres appears as an echogenic band that divides the medial and lateral segments of the left hepatic lobe.

Normal liver parenchyma should be homogeneous in appearance, broken only by the presence of portal triads and the hepatic veins. Diffuse liver disease, discussed later, can alter the normal echogenicity of the liver. Normal liver echogenicity can be evaluated by comparing it with renal cortex, where the liver should normally be isoechoic to slightly more echogenic than the kidney.

Diffuse Liver Disease

Several disease processes may involve the entire liver, altering the texture and echogenicity of the hepatic parenchyma while preserving the normal anatomic relationships. These liver diseases are often hard to detect given their diffuse nature.

Fatty liver

Fatty infiltration of the liver is arguably the most common cause of diffuse liver disease. Fatty liver disease or hepatic steatosis results from the

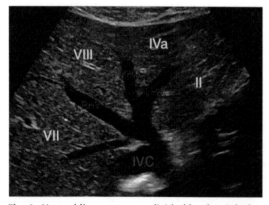

Fig. 1. Normal liver segments divided by the right hepatic vein (RHV), middle hepatic vein (MHV), and left hepatic vein (LHV), all draining into the inferior vena cava (IVC).

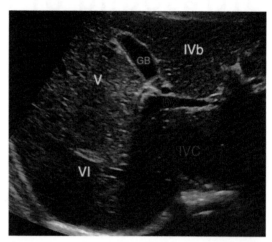

Fig. 2. Normal liver segments below the level of the portal vein (PV). Also seen is the gallbladder (GB) and the inferior vena cava (IVC).

intracellular accumulation of triglycerides within hepatocytes. Classically, hepatic steatosis has been described as a result of alcohol consumption.[8] There is another cohort of patients who are non-alcohol drinkers who develop steatosis. A large number of patients have hepatic steatosis that is not clinically significant in most cases.[9,10] However, patients can progress from hepatic steatosis to steatohepatitis and potentially cirrhosis.[10]

US is a noninvasive tool for the evaluation of fatty liver disease. Hepatic steatosis appears as diffuse, increased liver parenchymal echogenicity, a "bright liver." Normally, the liver should be isoechoic to slightly more echogenic than the renal cortex (**Fig. 3**). A more echogenic liver suggests the diagnosis of fatty liver disease. Additional findings include blurring of the normal vascular margins with increased acoustic attenuation (diminished through transmission). Glycogenosis seen in type 1 glycogen storage disease results in diffuse glycogen deposition and may have an appearance indistinguishable from hepatic steatosis.[11] Fatty infiltration may be heterogeneous and areas of fatty sparing may be seen. Fatty sparing appears hypoechoic relative to the liver parenchyma and may appear masslike or flame-shaped and has tapered margins (**Fig. 4**). Common locations for fatty sparing include along the gallbladder fossa, porta hepatis, falciform ligament, dorsal left hepatic lobe, and caudate lobe.[7] Similarly, fatty infiltration may be focal, appearing as conspicuous echogenic areas within the liver parenchyma. A useful technique in differentiating focal fatty infiltration and focal sparing is visualization of non-displaced portal triads or hepatic veins coursing through the regions (**Fig. 5**).

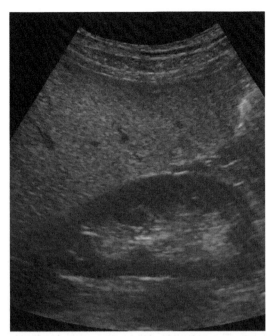

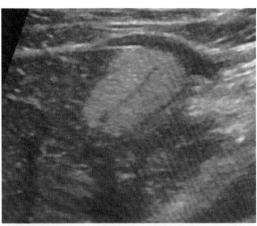

Fig. 5. Masslike echogenic focus representing focal fatty infiltration with a non-displaced hepatic vein coursing through the mass.

Fig. 3. Echogenic liver as seen in hepatic steatosis. Note the increased echogenicity of the liver parenchyma compared with the renal cortex.

Hepatitis

Hepatitis can be a result of any number of disease processes. As a result, there are no specific sonographic findings for acute hepatitis. The most commonly described finding is a "starry-night"

appearance resulting from diffuse decreased hepatic parenchymal echogenicity with increased periportal echogenicity (**Fig. 6**).[7] This pattern is not always seen in patients with acute hepatitis.[7] Another finding that may be seen in acute hepatitis is asymmetric gallbladder wall edema, predominantly involving the gallbladder wall that marginates the liver (**Fig. 7**).[7] In chronic hepatitis, the liver may develop heterogeneous increased echogenicity, likely related to fatty infiltration and developing fibrosis. In both acute and chronic hepatitis, the liver may be enlarged.[7]

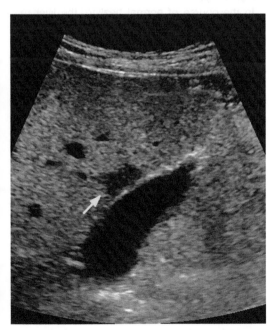

Fig. 4. Flame-shaped hypoechoic area (*arrow*) adjacent to the gallbladder fossa representing focal fatty sparing.

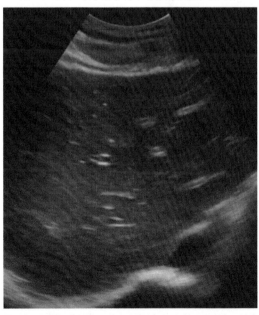

Fig. 6. Diffusely decreased hepatic echogenicity with increased periportal echogenicity representing the "starry-sky" appearance of hepatitis.

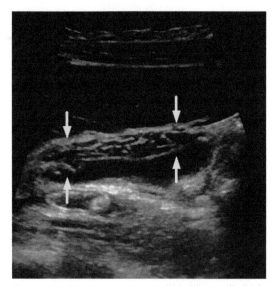

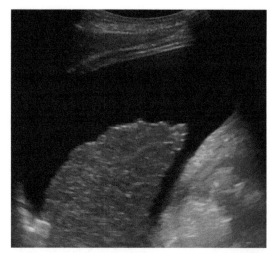

Fig. 8. Ascites in the presence of cirrhosis clearly shows liver surface nodularity.

Fig. 7. Reactive, asymmetric gallbladder wall thickening (*arrows*) from acute hepatitis along the portion of the gallbladder marginating the liver.

Cirrhosis

Hepatic cirrhosis develops as a result of chronic hepatocyte injury leading to the development of parenchymal fibrosis and regenerative nodules. On US, the liver parenchyma may have a coarsened echotexture. There may be indistinctness of the intrahepatic vasculature. These findings, however, are neither very sensitive nor specific for the diagnosis. Identification of a coarse liver echotexture is largely subjective, depending on the operator, the equipment, and the background echogenicity of the patient's liver.[12] The nodularity seen in cirrhosis can be described as macronodular or micronodular.[13] Surface nodularity may be the only finding of cirrhosis, although micronodular disease may be missed.[7] Nodules less than 3 mm are termed micronodular, whereas those larger are termed macronodular.[12] Micronodular and macronodular cirrhosis can be distinguished on US; however, this morphologic distinction does not necessarily imply a specific disease origin.[12] With time, micronodular disease can transform to macronodular disease, such as is the case with alcoholic liver disease. Evaluation of the liver surface nodularity should be performed with a high-frequency linear transducer.[12] The presence of ascites may make surface nodularity more apparent (**Fig. 8**). The normal liver surface should be a smooth echogenic line measuring less than 1 mm in thickness.[12,14] Interruption of the normal hyperechoic line is termed the "dotted-line sign" and is described as characteristic for micronodular cirrhosis.[12]

As cirrhosis progresses, the right lobe tends to be more involved than the left lobe and caudate lobe. The caudate lobe may hypertrophy to compensate for the cirrhotic right lobe.[7,15,16] The caudate-to-right-lobe ratio has been described as a highly sensitive and highly specific sign for cirrhosis.[15] However, there may be decreased sensitivity (but continued high specificity) of the caudate-to-right-lobe ratio when using US for the measurements.[16] There are also mimics of cirrhosis, described later, which slightly decrease the specificity.

In the course of normal healing, the liver may form regenerative nodules. These nodules are common but have no specific appearance on US. Nodules most commonly are in the 2- to 3-mm range. Larger nodules measuring 1 to 2 cm in diameter are rare.[13] Dysplastic nodules may also be present in cirrhotic livers and are thought to be premalignant lesions. These Dysplastic nodules also have no specific appearance on US and may be hypoechoic, isoechoic, or hyperechoic and cannot be reliably differentiated from hepatocellular carcinoma (HCC).[17,18] Isoechoic and hyperechoic regenerative nodules with a hyperechoic rim ("reverse target sign") have also been described.[19]

The classic appearance of cirrhosis on US shows decreased liver volume with hypertrophy of the left lobe and caudate lobe, a nodular liver surface, and a heterogeneous echo pattern, sometimes described as coarse. A coarse pattern can also be seen with Budd-Chiari syndrome and chronic portal venous thrombosis.[20] Pseudomyxoma peritonei may mimic a macronodular liver surface; however, this is a result of scalloping of the liver capsule from mucinous ascites rather than an intrinsic hepatic parenchymal disorder.[20,21] A pseudocirrhosis pattern with fine liver surface nodularity may be seen with treated breast cancer metastases, fulminant hepatic failure, and sarcoidosis of the liver (**Fig. 9**). Sarcoidosis may also appear as surface nodularity with granular parenchymal heterogeneity.[20]

Hepatic Masses

The differential diagnosis of hepatic masses is wide. The more common causes include infectious, neoplastic, and metastatic disease. The most common benign solid hepatic masses include cavernous hemangiomas, focal nodular hyperplasia (FNH), and adenoma. Less frequently encountered masses include lipoma and angiomyolipoma.[22] HCC is the most common malignant primary tumor of the liver. Once identified, hepatic masses need to be characterized as potentially significant lesions requiring further workup or benign lesions that require no further evaluation. A hypoechoic rim around an echogenic or isoechoic mass, a hypoechoic mass, and multiple masses are particularly worrisome signs that will require further evaluation.[22]

HCC

HCC is the most common primary liver malignancy and the most likely to occur in the setting of cirrhosis. HCC may develop in a stepwise fashion in a cirrhotic liver from a dysplastic nodule into a carcinoma. However, HCC may arise from normal liver parenchyma as well.[23] US, along with α-fetoprotein, has been used as a screening test for HCC in patients with underlying cirrhosis.[24] The accuracy of sonographic detection of HCC varies among studies.[24] In patients with severe cirrhosis, screening for HCC may be limited because of advanced fibrosis and fatty infiltration altering background echogenicity and the presence of nonneoplastic regenerative nodules. HCCs may present as single or multiple solid or infiltrative masses.[23] The appearance of HCC can also vary depending on the histology.

Three US appearances of HCC have been reported: hypoechoic, hyperechoic, and heterogeneous. Hypoechoic HCCs correspond to solid tumor with homogeneous internal architecture. These tumors tend to be small (<5 cm) in size.[22] Nonliquifactive necrosis within the tumor can give areas of hyperechogenicity leading to a heterogeneous appearance on US (**Fig. 10**). This appearance may be related to the complex structure of necrosis. Liquifactive necrosis is seen as an anechoic area with increased through transmission. HCC can undergo fatty change resulting a homogeneous hyperechoic appearance.[25,26] These fatty carcinomas may be confused with cavernous hemangiomas, discussed later, especially when they have homogeneous hyperechogenicity (**Fig. 11**).[26] A hypoechoic rim ("halo") around the mass indicates a fibrous capsule (**Fig. 12**).[23] An infiltrative margin that is irregular and indistinct may be present (**Fig. 13**). Rapid growth can result in central necrosis and a cystic appearance.[27]

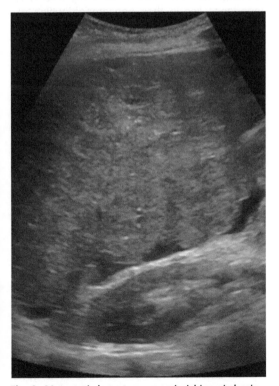

Fig. 9. Metastatic breast cancer mimicking cirrhosis.

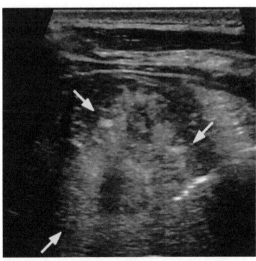

Fig. 10. Heterogeneous HCC, margins outlined by *arrows*.

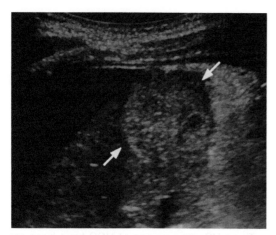

Fig. 11. Echogenic HCC, margins outlined by *arrows*.

HCC, unlike liver metastases, has a propensity for invasion into the inferior vena cava, bile ducts, hepatic veins, and portal vein.[23] Findings of venous occlusion include echogenic material within the vein, expansion of the vein, cavernous transformation, or visualization of collateral pathways. However, sonographic differentiation of bland and tumor thrombi cannot be reliably performed based solely on their gray-scale appearance.[28] Color Doppler may help in differentiating bland versus tumor thrombus. Pulsatile arterial flow on color and spectral Doppler within portal venous thrombus is diagnostic for a tumor thrombus. Lack of flow, however, does not definitively exclude the diagnosis.[28] Calcification is uncommon but has been reported.[22]

In addition to HCC, the cirrhotic liver may contain regenerative and dysplastic nodules. Regenerative nodules are benign, whereas dysplastic nodules are considered a premalignant lesion.[24,29] Dysplastic nodules may have varying

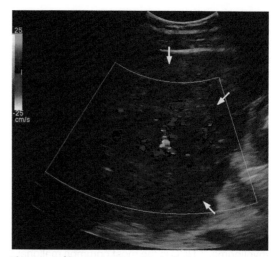

Fig. 13. Infiltrative HCC with indistinct margin outlined by *arrows*.

appearance on US and cannot be reliably differentiated from HCC. Dysplastic nodules may appear hyperechoic or hypoechoic,[18] which is especially true in livers with advanced cirrhosis.[29]

Cavernous Hemangioma

The most common benign tumors of the liver are cavernous hemangiomas. They are frequently encountered as incidental findings on routine US examinations and rarely have symptoms. Their importance lies in their appearance, which can overlap with hepatic malignancies. Typically in adulthood, hemangiomas remain stable in size; however, there have been cases of documented enlargement.[30] On US, cavernous hemangiomas are well-circumscribed, homogeneous, and uniformly hyperechoic masses that may demonstrate posterior acoustic enhancement (**Fig. 14**).[22]

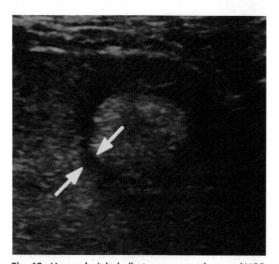

Fig. 12. Hypoechoic halo (between *arrows*) around HCC.

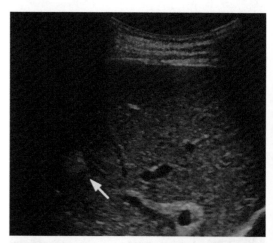

Fig. 14. Echogenic mass characteristic of a typical hemangioma, marked by an *arrow*.

However, the differential for an echogenic mass in the liver must include HCC, focal metastasis, FNH, and liver adenoma.[31] Echogenic metastases include colon cancer, choriocarcinoma, islet cell tumors, and carcinoid tumors (**Fig. 15**).[32] Because of this overlap of appearance, US alone should not be used to differentiate a hemangioma from a malignant lesion, which is especially true in older patients, patients with cirrhosis, and those with a known primary tumor. A less aggressive approach to follow-up may be considered in low-risk patients. All cavernous hemangiomas do not have the typical appearance of an echogenic mass (**Fig. 16**). Diagnosis of an atypical hemangioma may be suggested by the presence of an echogenic rim around a solid mass. However, in the setting of hepatic steatosis, the echogenic rim may be obscured.[32] Furthermore, hemangiomas may undergo thrombosis, necrosis, or growth, altering their echogenicity.[32] Hemangiomas typically show no increased blood flow on color or duplex Doppler techniques.[22]

Hepatic Cysts

Cystic lesions of the liver may represent any number of processes including congenital, infectious, or neoplastic. The appearances of many cystic lesions overlap so careful evaluation of patient history and clinical data should be performed.

Cysts in the liver can be divided into simple or complex. Simple cysts include benign congenital cysts, biliary hamartomas (von Meyenberg complexes), biliary cysts (Caroli disease), or adult polycystic liver disease. Complex cysts may be traumatic, neoplastic, or infectious. There may be atypical cystic presentations of normally noncystic tumors, such as hemangiomas or HCCs.[33]

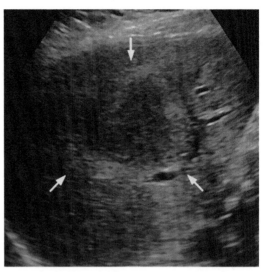

Fig. 16. Atypical hemangioma with echogenic rim and central hypoechogenicity, margins outlined by *arrows.*

Benign developmental hepatic cysts are simple cysts derived from biliary endothelium that do not communicate with the biliary system.[27] They are the second most common benign hepatic lesions after cavernous hemangiomas.[27] They may be multiple and are usually asymptomatic. On US, they have the classic appearance of a simple cyst. They are anechoic with a well-circumscribed, thin, imperceptible wall, and increased posterior acoustic enhancement (**Fig. 17**). The presence of numerous hepatic cysts may be related to autosomal-dominant polycystic kidney disease (ADPKD). Hepatic polycystic disease is seen in up to 40% of patients with ADPKD.[27] Hemorrhage

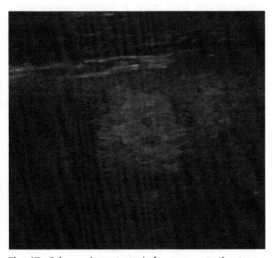

Fig. 15. Echogenic metastasis from pancreatic cancer.

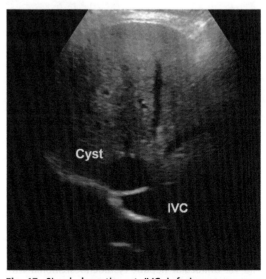

Fig. 17. Simple hepatic cyst. IVC, inferior vena cava.

into cysts is rare, although it has been reported.[34] Infection of hepatic cysts may also occur. In patients with multiple cysts as seen with ADPKD, this can prove to be a complex diagnostic and therapeutic issue. US evaluation of the liver in these cases can help identify complicated cysts; however, other imaging modalities such as positron emission tomography or In-111-labeled white blood cell scans may be more helpful in discovering the infected cyst.[35,36]

Hepatic cystadenoma and its malignant counterpart cystadenocarcinoma are cystic tumors arising from the biliary epithelium. Together, they account for less than 5% of all cystic lesions of the liver.[37] These tumors are usually large, single intrahepatic lesions, although extrahepatic involvement may occur.[38] Almost all biliary cystadenomas are multiloculated. Unilocular cystadenocarcinomas have been reported (**Fig. 18**). Multiple masses are rare. On US, they appear as well-circumscribed ovoid cystic masses with multiple internal septae (**Fig. 19**). They may be heterogeneous in appearance because of internal mucinous material, cholesterol crystals, or purulent material. Fluid-fluid levels may be seen.[38] Internal papillary projections or mural nodules may be seen in both biliary cystadenomas and cystadenocarcinomas, although they are more common in cystadenocarcinomas.[38,39] Imaging cannot reliably differentiate a cystadenoma from a cystadenocarcinoma, although the presence of thick septae with nodular and papillary projections can be suggestive.[37] Therefore, surgical resection is predominantly performed.

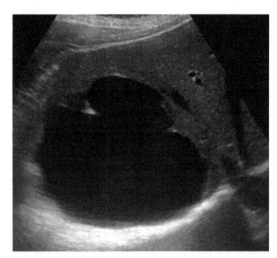

Fig. 19. Cystic mass with thin septation representing a hepatic biliary cystadenoma.

FNH

FNH is the third most common benign liver mass after hemangiomas and cysts. FNH, like cavernous hemangiomas, may be found incidentally on examination in an otherwise asymptomatic patient. Typically, a single lesion is present, although multiple lesions may occur.[22,40] Histologically, FNH represents proliferation of normal but disorganized hepatocytes. As a result, differentiating these lesions from normal hepatic parenchyma can be difficult. For this reason, FNH is sometimes termed a "stealth lesion." On US, FNH appears as a well-circumscribed isoechoic mass (**Fig. 20**). Occasionally, mass effect resulting in contour deformities on the liver capsule or displacement of adjacent vessels may occur.[22] The central scar may be difficult to visualize but when apparent shows a central hypervascular nidus, which may have a stellate appearance. Large draining vessels may be seen at the tumor margin.[40] Unfortunately, these findings may also be seen with well-differentiated HCC, requiring further evaluation in at-risk populations.

Hepatic Adenoma

Hepatic adenomas are less common than cavernous hemangiomas and FNH of the liver. They have been associated with oral contraceptive use and glycogen storage disease. These tumors may be detected incidentally in asymptomatic patients. Hepatic adenomas have a tendency to hemorrhage, causing pain, hemoperitoneum, or hemorrhagic shock in severe cases.[22] Hepatic adenomas may appear as well-circumscribed lesions containing fat or calcification, both of which could give an echogenic appearance on

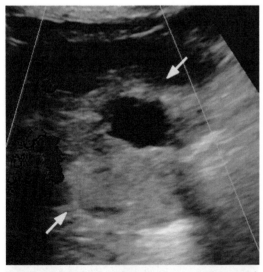

Fig. 18. Unilocular hepatic cystadenocarcinoma with thickened, nodular wall, margins outlined by *arrows*.

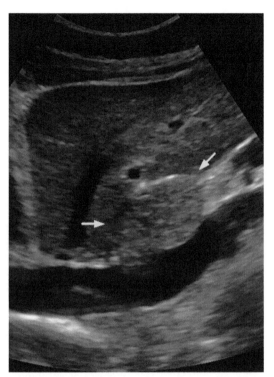

Fig. 20. FNH of the caudate lobe with echogenicity near that of the liver. The arrows mark the superior (*right*) and inferior (*left*) margins.

US (**Fig. 21**). When hemorrhage has occurred, the adenoma may appear heterogeneous with large areas of intraparenchymal hematoma. However, adenomas can be isoechoic, hyperechoic, or hypoechoic.[41] Subclassifications of adenomas have been described with varying histology and imaging appearance, most obvious on magnetic resonance imaging.[42]There is evidence to suggest

that contrast-enhanced US may help in differentiating the various subtypes.[43] Differentiating an adenoma from HCC or FNH is not possible and requires further evaluation by either additional imaging or biopsy.[44]

Metastatic Disease

The most common malignancy to involve the liver is metastatic disease. Most metastases to the liver are spread hematogenously. Lymphatic spread may occur from the stomach, pancreas, ovary, or uterus. Metastatic disease on US can present as a single lesion, although multiple lesions are much more likely. Metastatic disease can have a variety of appearances on sonography. Findings highly suggestive of metastatic disease are multiple lesions of varying sizes and masses with a hypoechoic halo. The hypoechoic halo is strongly associated with malignancy, including HCC (**Fig. 22**).[22] The hypoechoic rim represents normal compressed hepatic tissue, proliferating malignant cells, tumor fibrosis, fibrotic capsule, or vascularization. Metastatic disease to the liver may be echogenic, hypoechoic, targetoid, calcified, cystic, or diffuse. More vascular tumors (renal cell carcinoma, choriocarcinoma, carcinoid, islet cell, for example) may be more hyperechoic (**Fig. 23**).[45] Calcified metastases are most commonly mucinous adenocarcinomas. The calcifications may be small and appear as echogenic foci without distinct posterior acoustic shadowing. Cystic metastases are less common. Rapidly growing hypervascular tumors may show central necrosis or cystic degeneration. Examples include sarcoma, melanoma, neuroendocrine, and carcinoid tumors.[22,27] Diffuse, infiltrative metastatic disease, which is difficult to see on US except as

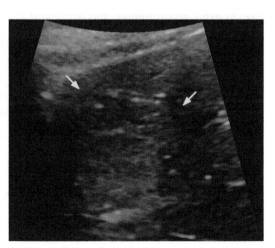

Fig. 21. Slightly echogenic liver mass representing a hepatic adenoma, margins outlined by *arrows*.

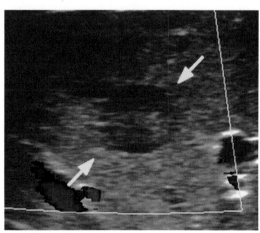

Fig. 22. Subtle hypoechoic halo seen with breast cancer metastasis, margins outlined by *arrows*.

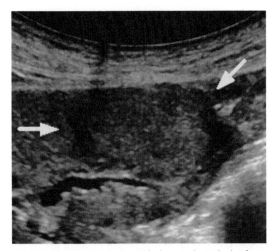

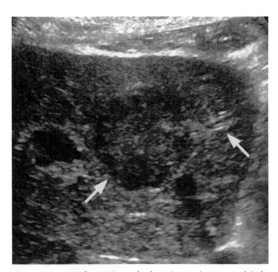

Fig. 23. Echogenic mass with hypoechoic halo from metastatic neuroendocrine tumor, margins outlined by *arrows.*

Fig. 25. Intrahepatic cholangiocarcinoma (*right arrow*) with dilation of a peripheral intrahepatic biliary duct (*left arrow*).

disorganization of the hepatic parenchyma, may be seen with breast cancer, lung cancer, and melanoma (**Fig. 24**).[22]

Cholangiocarcinoma

Cholangiocarcinoma is a rare primary malignant neoplasm of the bile ducts. Intrahepatic cholangiocarcinomas are classified as peripheral or hilar.[46] Intrahepatic cholangiocarcinomas have been described to have 3 morphologic appearances: mass forming, periductal infiltrating, and intraductal. The mass-forming morphology is the most common.[47] Growth patterns of cholangiocarcinomas have been described as exophytic, infiltrative, polypoid, or a combination of these.[48,49]

Mass-forming cholangiocarcinomas are morphologically homogeneous and have a well-defined, although irregular, margin (**Fig. 25**). As

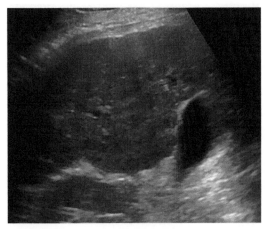

Fig. 24. Diffuse breast cancer metastases to the liver mimicking cirrhosis.

the mass enlarges, it may take on a more heterogeneous appearance.[46] On sonography, these may have a hypoechoic rim, which represents proliferating tumor cells or compressed liver parenchyma.[47] Although cholangiocarcinoma is most commonly associated with peripheral biliary ductal dilatation due to obstruction, HCC and metastases may also cause biliary obstruction.[46,50] Satellite nodules may be present. In addition, hyperechoic foci with acoustic shadowing may be present that correspond to calcifications.[51]

Periductal infiltrating cholangiocarcinomas are characterized by growth along the bile ducts. Small tumors appear as solid masses centered in the bile duct. Larger tumors encircle and grow along the bile duct. The lumen may appear as an echogenic line parallel to the long access of the tumor. In extrahepatic tumors, this echogenic line has been described as the "middle echo sign."[49]

Intraductal cholangiocarcinomas grow slowly and have a relatively favorable prognosis. Imaging features include duct ectasia with or without a polypoid of papillary intraductal mass.[47,49]

Dilation of the intrahepatic ducts with normal caliber of the extraheptic ducts suggests the presence of a hilar cholangiocarcinoma. These masses may be small and not apparent on US. However, US is still important in evaluation of the patency of the portal vein.[52]

The differentiation of cholangiocarcinoma from HCC or metastatic disease is not possible.[46] Additional imaging and histologic correlation are required to confirm the diagnosis. Unlike HCC, cirrhosis is not associated with a higher rate of cholangiocarcinoma.[46] Cholangiocarcinoma has been associated with *Clonorchis sinensis* (liver fluke) infection.[53] Additional risk factors include hepatolithiasis, recurrent pyogenic cholangitis, ingestion of nitrosamine compounds, choledochal cyst, biliary hamartoma, and primary sclerosing cholangitis.[47,49]

Characteristic radiologic findings seen in clonorchis infection associated with cholangiocarcinoma include diffuse, uniform dilation of the intrahepatic bile ducts. The parasite may be seen as a nonshadowing echogenic focus or cast within the bile duct. Flukes are easier to see in the gallbladder, where they may be shown to move.[54] Thickening of the bile ducts may also been seen.

In recurrent pyogenic cholangitis, the liver fluke is thought to act as a nidus or cause strictures, allowing for intrahepatic bile duct stone formation that predisposes to biliary stasis, bacterial overgrowth, and recurrent infection. Sonography shows intrahepatic ductal dilation with echogenic, shadowing foci representing hepatoliths. The biliary dilation may be segmental.[49]

Hepatic Abscess

Imaging is important in the diagnosis of hepatic infection; however, the imaging appearance can be nonspecific and mimic hepatic cysts or necrotic tumors. Hepatic abscesses are most commonly pyogenic or amebic.

Pyogenic hepatic abscesses may be solitary or multiple, have no sex predilection, and may have a varied clinical presentation. The most common organisms are gut flora, anaerobic or aerobic, the most common being *Escherichia coli*. On histology, abscesses may have a thickened rind merging into normal liver tissue and can have a varying level of central necrosis and debris.[55] This histologic appearance mirrors the US appearance.

Pyogenic hepatic abscesses can be classified as either microabscesses (<2 cm) or macroabscesses (>2 cm). On US, microabscesses appear as discrete hypoechoic nodules or areas of altered liver echogenicity. Enhancement through transmission is variable but usually not a prominent finding.[55] Large pyogenic abscesses may demonstrate a variety of appearances depending on the stage of necrosis (**Fig. 26**). Abscesses may appear focally echogenic, diffusely echogenic, contain fluid-debris levels, or be hypoechoic.[56] Subacute and chronic abscesses may have an echogenic wall. A thin peripheral halo has also been described. Gas within large abscesses causes linear, echogenic foci.[56]

Amebic abscess of the liver is the most common extraintestinal complication of amebiasis. Amebic liver infection is most common in India, Africa,

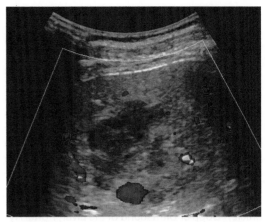

Fig. 26. Pyogenic hepatic abscess seen as a predominantly hypoechoic mass.

Far East, and Central and South America. Compared with pyogenic liver abscesses, patients with amebic abscesses appear more acutely ill. Amebic abscesses may be difficult to differentiate from pyogenic abscesses in some patients. At US, amebic abscesses are hypoechoic and may have low-level internal echoes. There may be an absence of significant wall echoes. The lesions are typically round or oval and located near the liver capsule.[55,57] Amebic abscesses have variable posterior acoustic enhancement, which is not as intense as the gallbladder.[57] Small abscesses may be more echogenic compared with larger lesions.[58]

Hydatid disease caused by *Echinococcus granulosus* is more common in the Mediterranean basin and sheep-herding areas. Histologically, the hyatid cyst is composed of multiple layers with internal cysts and daughter cysts. Peripheral calcifications may be present. US findings are variable but these lesions may range from cystic to solid. Internally, wavy bands of delaminated endocyst have been described ("water-lily sign").[35]

Hydatid disease as result of *Echinococcus multilocularis* is endemic in the upper Midwest region of the United States, Alaska, Canada, Japan, central Europe, and parts of Russia. Compared with the unilocular disease caused by *E granulosus*, the disease caused by *E multilocularis*, as its name suggests, is multilocular. This organism produces multiple alveolar cysts ranging from 1 to 10 mm in size. On sonography, these cysts show a "hailstorm" appearance characterized by multiple echogenic nodules with irregular and indistinct margins. This appearance represents heterogeneous stroma containing vesicles, nonliquifactive necrosis, host tissue, and microcalcifications.[59,60]

Schistosoma infection begins in the bowel lumen. Schistosomes lay eggs within the bowel, which embolize into the liver via the portal vein. The eggs themselves do not survive and may calcify. The eggs can elicit an inflammatory reaction resulting in a granulomatous response, fibrosis, and perisinusoidal hypertension. Chronic infection can lead to cirrhosis and HCC. US evaluation of acute infection does not significantly contribute to diagnosis. The characteristic changes related to infection are seen years after initial inoculation. Typical US features include an irregular liver surface, a mosaic liver pattern with echogenic septae outlining areas of normal-appearing liver parenchyma[61] (*"for more on schistosomiasis including images, see page 594 in the article,* "Doppler Ultrasound of the Liver, Portal Hypertension, and Transjugular Intrahepatic Portosystemic Shunts" *by Davis and Chong"*).

Disseminated fungal diseases are most common in immunosuppressed patients. Fungal microabscesses may affect the liver, spleen, and occasionally, the kidney. Most disseminated infections are caused by *Candida albicans*, although other species have also been implicated.[55] Four US patterns of hepatic involvement have been described. The first is a "wheel-within-a-wheel" pattern, which consists of a central hypoechoic area of necrosis surrounded by an echogenic rim of inflammatory cells, which in turn is surrounded by a thin hypoechoic rim resulting from fibrosis. The second pattern is a "bull's-eye" pattern consisting of a central echogenic focus with hypoechoic rim. The third pattern is a hypoechoic nodule, which is the most common but least specific. The last pattern is an echogenic focus with varying degrees of increased posterior acoustic shadowing. This last pattern is seen late in the course of the disease. The first 2 patterns are more often seen in previously neutropenic patients whose neutrophil counts have returned to normal.[62]

Biliary Hamartoma

Biliary hamartomas, also known as von Meyenburg complexes, are rare, focal disordered collections of bile ducts surrounded by fibrous stroma.[43] They are congenital lesions caused by failure of embryonic involution. The bile ducts can be of varying caliber with extreme dilation leading to a cystic appearance.[63] These lesions are benign but are clinically important because they can mimic metastatic disease, microabscesses, lymphoma, and leukemia.[64] Biliary hamartomas are associated with autosomal-dominant polycystic kidney disease, polycystic liver disease, Caroli disease, and congenital hepatic fibrosis. When they are multiple, biliary hamartomas can mimic metastatic disease.[65]

On sonography, biliary hamartomas appear as small (<10 mm) hyperechoic and hypoechoic

lesions (**Fig. 27**). The small, hyperechoic lesions are a conglomerate of small cysts. Reverberation in the cysts can cause comet-tail echoes.[64] They may be scattered throughout the liver and are relatively uniform in size.[63]

Lymphoma

Lymphoma involving the liver is almost always related to extranodal disease rather than primary disease. Extranodal lymphoma is seen in approximately 40% of patients with lymphoma. Extranodal disease is more common with non-Hodgkin lymphoma, particularly higher-grade disease. The most common locations involved are the spleen, liver, and gastrointestinal tract.[66] AIDS-related and posttransplant lymphoproliferative disorder are also highly associated with extranodal involvement.[66] Diffuse large B cell, follicular, Mantle cell, lymphoblastic, Burkitt, and mucosa-associated lymphoid tissue lymphoma are also likely to involve extranodal sites.

Hepatosplenic lymphoma is usually diffuse with hypoechoic nodules that show variable posterior acoustic enhancement. The lesions may be anechoic and mimic fluid collections (**Fig. 28**).[67] Less common are hyperechoic lesions or hypoechoic lesions with a central hyperechoic focus. The diffuse or infiltrative form of the disease can result in patchy, irregular periportal infiltrates. These lesions may be indistinguishable from metastatic disease on US.[66,68] There may be associated hepatomegaly.

Primary hepatic lymphoma is rare but the US appearance is similar to hepatic involvement of other types of lymphoma. Primary lymphoma of the liver is most commonly of the diffuse large B-cell histology.[68] Sonography may show hypoechoic or anechoic lesions, although the overall appearance is nonspecific.[69]

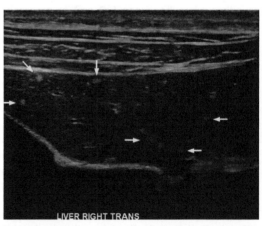

LIVER RIGHT TRANS

Fig. 27. Multiple small echogenic foci representing biliary hamartomas, marked by *arrows*.

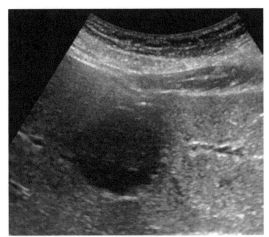

Fig. 28. Markedly hypoechoic mass typical of lymphoma.

Hepatic Trauma

The liver is the second most commonly injured organ in the abdomen after the spleen. The most common cause of liver injury is from blunt abdominal trauma.[70] Injuries to solid organs, such as the liver, may be seen on US as alterations of the normal parenchymal architecture.[71] Fresh hemorrhage has been shown to be echogenic; however, it can take on a heterogeneous appearance.[71,72] Old hematomas can appear anechoic.[73] Focal parenchymal lacerations may appear anechoic, hypoechoic, or hyperechoic (**Fig. 29**). More extensive parenchymal lacerations can take on a more heterogeneous appearance with loss of the normal parenchymal architecture.[74] However, US remains less sensitive than CT for the evaluation of solid organ injury.[74]

SPLEEN

As with the liver, the spleen lends itself to US evaluation given its relatively superficial location in the left upper abdomen. The most common indications for evaluation of the spleen include size, diagnosis of masses, evaluation for the cause of left upper quadrant pain, evaluation of the splenic vessels, and portal hypertension.

Anatomy

The spleen is normally located in the left upper quadrant, intraperitoneal and deep to the left 9 to 11 ribs. The spleen has a normal trapezoidal appearance with a crescent shape on US. The primary blood supply is from the splenic artery, which arises from the celiac axis. The splenic artery at the splenic hilum branches and can become tortuous with age. Normal splenic parenchyma is slightly

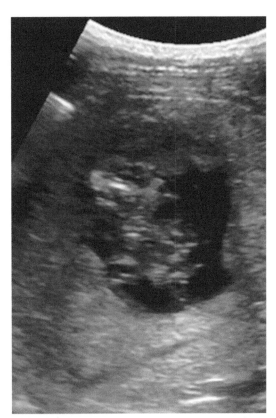

Fig. 29. Heterogeneous parenchymal hematoma from liver laceration.

more echogenic than the liver and always more echogenic than the normal kidney (**Fig. 30**).[75]

Evaluation of normal spleen size is difficult given the large distribution in splenic size dependent on patient demographics. A single US examination for splenic size may not be useful.[76] Normal splenic size has been described as ranging from 12 to

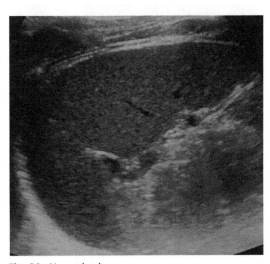

Fig. 30. Normal spleen.

14 cm in adults.[76] Tall athletes have been shown to have larger spleens.[77] In addition to increased size, a bulging of the normal splenic shape and rounding of the poles may be seen with splenomegaly (**Fig. 31**).

The accessory spleen is a very common normal variant that is found in 10% to 25% of all patients. The most common location is below the lower pole of the spleen. Accessory spleens should be differentiated from lymph nodes, pancreatic tail masses, adrenal glands, and neoplasms. They can usually be distinguished from other masses by their echogenicity similar to that of the adjacent spleen (**Fig. 32**). A heat-damaged tagged red blood cell scan can be performed to confirm the diagnosis if clinically necessary.

Polysplenia is uncommon and associated with left-sided heterotaxy. Asplenia is associated with right-sided heterotaxy. However, some patients with either heterotaxy syndrome can have a single spleen. The spleens in either case are located on the same side as the stomach, owing to the embryologic origin of the spleen from the dorsal mesogastrium.[78]

Technique

Patients should be supine or in the right lateral decubitus position for evaluation of the spleen. The location of the spleen can vary widely with respiration. Deep inhalation can displace the spleen inferiorly below the ribs, making visualization easier. Deep inspiration should only be used in the supine position because deep inspiration in the right lateral decubitus position can cause the spleen to fall away medially and out of the optimal field of view as well as interpose the hyperinflated left lung between the spleen and abdominal wall.

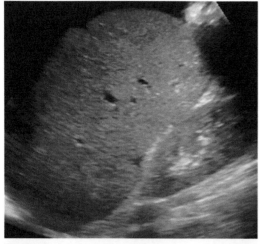

Fig. 31. Increased splenic length, bulging of the normal shape, and rounding of the poles seen in splenomegaly.

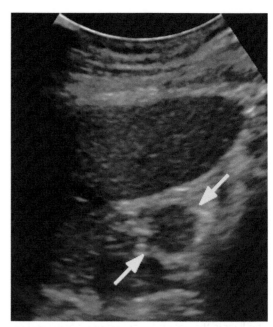

Fig. 32. Accessory spleen at the splenic hilum. Note the similar echotexture compared with the spleen (between two *arrows*).

This deep inspiration requires patient cooperation, making US evaluation of the spleen in a noncooperative patient more difficult. An intercostal approach can also be taken. A curved array 3- to 5-MHz transducer should be used for evaluation of the spleen.

Splenic Trauma

Trauma to the spleen is usually a result of blunt trauma. Splenic trauma can result in parenchymal laceration with or without involvement of the splenic capsule. Traumatic splenic fissures may be hypoechoic or hyperechoic with respect to splenic parenchyma (**Fig. 33**). However, splenic lacerations may be occult on US and only seen at surgery.[74] Violation of the splenic capsule can result in hemoperitoneum. Free perisplenic fluid in a trauma patient suggests the presence of a splenic laceration regardless of a discretely visualized splenic laceration. A hyperacute hematoma may appear hypoechoic, although few patients present during this time (**Figs. 34** and **35**). As clot forms, parenchymal or subcapsular hematomas begin to appear hyperechoic (**Fig. 36**).[75] As the hematoma organizes, it can take on a more heterogeneous appearance. Doppler US is useful in identifying splenic pseudoaneurysm in trauma.[79]

Splenic Infarction

Splenic infarction may result in patients with myeloproliferative syndrome, hemolytic anemia,

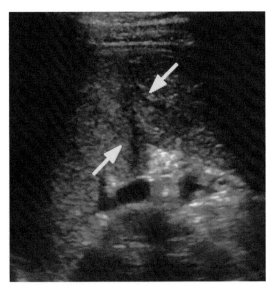

Fig. 33. Splenic fissure from trauma seen as a hypoechoic line between two *arrows*.

Epstein-Barr virus (EBV) infection, and sepsis. Clinically, patients present with left upper quadrant pain in the acute setting. Various processes affect the appearance of the spleen related to infarction, including edema, hemorrhage, fibrosis, and necrosis.

Approximately 24 hours after therapeutic embolization of the splenic artery, splenic infarcts have been described as hypoechoic, well-demarcated triangular lesions appearing on US with the base at the splenic capsule and the apex pointed centrally.[80,81] Splenic infarcts serve as fertile ground

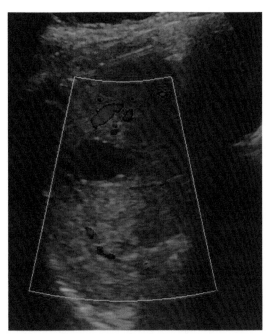

Fig. 35. Hypoechoic splenic hematoma.

for superinfection, which can be a potentially fatal complication.[80] Subcapsular hemorrhage is another complication of splenic infarct.[75] Abscesses in the spleen, described more in detail later, are important to keep in the differential diagnosis, although they have some distinguishing features. On serial examinations, infarcts become more hyperechoic due to fibrosis and scarring, although they retain their triangular shape (**Figs. 37** and **38**).[80]

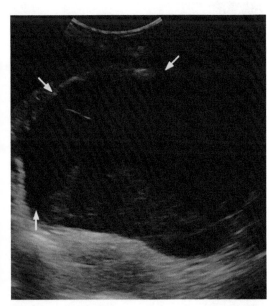

Fig. 34. Hypoechoic acute subcapsular splenic hematoma, margins outlined by *arrows*.

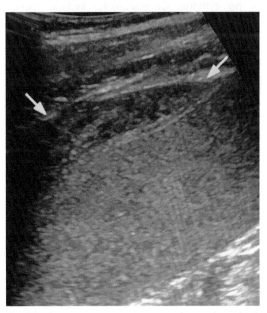

Fig. 36. Heterogeneous subacute subcapsular splenic hematoma, margins outlined by *arrows*.

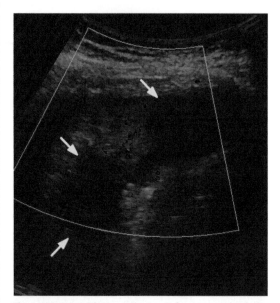

Fig. 37. Hypoechoic splenic infarcts marked by *arrows*.

Splenic Cysts

Splenic cysts are often divided into nonparasitic versus parasitic (*Echinococcus sp, Taenia solium*) causes. Nonparasitic cysts may be congenital or neoplastic. Congenital cysts include primary, dermoid, and epidermoid cysts.[75,82]

Primary (congenital) splenic cysts have a true epithelial lining and may be solitary or multiple. They typically do not cause symptoms, but when they do, it is a result of enlargement from trauma or hemorrhage. Complications include hemorrhage, infection, and rupture. On sonography, splenic cysts are round, hypoechoic, or anechoic, with a smooth, thin wall and increased posterior acoustic enhancement. Infection or hemorrhage can result in echogenic internal debris. Peripheral calcifications may also be present (**Figs. 39 and 40**).[82]

Splenic Hamartoma

A splenic hamartoma is a rare, benign lesion of the spleen. Hamartomas are usually less than 3 cm in size but may be larger. Most patients are asymptomatic, and the lesion is discovered incidentally.[82] US shows a sharply demarcated solid mass. The internal echotexture may be heterogeneous to more echogenic than the remainder of the spleen. The mass may contain internal echogenic foci representing small calcifications. Doppler imaging demonstrates a hypervascular lesion with radial blood flow signal.[82]

Splenic Abscess

Splenic abscesses may occur with splenic infarcts and may also be hypoechoic but can be distinguished by their ill-defined border, the presence of central necrosis and debris, and a thick and irregular wall. Echogenic foci within the abscess may present necrotic debris or gas.[80] Gram-negative bacteria are the most common organisms associated with splenic abscesses and are more likely to produce multiple abscesses. Color Doppler imaging may show hypervascularity in the abscess capsule, although early in abscess formation this may not be present.[78]

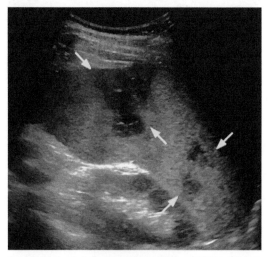

Fig. 38. Splenic infarcts in the setting of EBV infection and splenomegaly, marked by *arrows*.

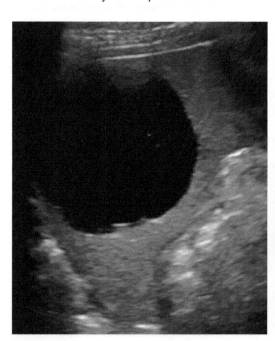

Fig. 39. Simple splenic epithelial cyst.

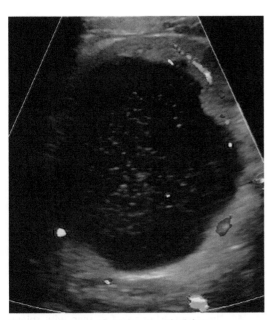

Fig. 40. Splenic epithelial cyst with debris.

Fungal abscesses of the spleen are predominantly seen in patients with immunosuppression. Candida species are the most common organism and frequently also involve the liver. Splenomegaly may be the initial sonographic findings but focal lesions begin to appear as the patient's granulocyte count increases. The patterns described earlier ("wheel-within-a-wheel," "bull's-eye," multiple echogenic foci with varying posterior acoustic enhancement) seen in the liver can also be seen in the spleen.[62]

Hydatid cysts secondary to *Echinococcus* species occur more commonly in the liver (60%–70%) than in the spleen (3%).[78] Sonographically, hydatid cysts appear as homogeneous, anechoic cysts. Daughter cysts, internal debris, and peripheral calcification can be seen.[78] The "water-lily" sign caused by separation of the membranes or the presence of a daughter cyst and the "cyst-within-a-cyst" appearance may also be seen.[82]

Splenic Hemangioma

Splenic hemangiomas are the most common benign tumor of the spleen. They are typically asymptomatic but may cause spontaneous rupture when located at the capsule.[83] Splenic hemangiomas have 2 histologic appearances that can be differentiated on US. A cavernous hemangioma has a mixed echogenic or hypoechoic appearance and may contain cystic spaces and small calcifications. A capillary hemangioma is hyperechoic with a sharply defined margin

(**Fig. 41**). The cavernous histology is more common.[75]

Splenic Lymphoma

Lymphoma involving the spleen may be primary or secondary. Primary lymphoma of the spleen represents approximately 1% of all lymphoma. Hodgkin and non-Hodgkin lymphoma involve the spleen secondarily in 30% to 40% of patients. The sonographic appearance depends on the pattern of lymphomatous involvement. Four patterns have been described: diffuse, multiple small nodules, large nodules, or bulky disease. Sonographically, lymphomatous masses are anechoic to hypoechoic in appearance, although echogenic masses with a hypoechoic rim may be seen ("target sign") (**Figs. 42 and 43**).[75,78]

Splenic Metastatic Disease

Splenic metastases usually appear hypoechoic, although on occasion may be hyperechoic. Central necrosis can result in an inhomogeneous appearance with central hypoechogenicity. Mucinous tumors may calcify. Isolated metastatic disease to the spleen is rare, and splenic metastases usually occur in the setting of widespread metastases. Metastases may become cystic as central necrosis occurs.[75] The most common metastases are lung, stomach, pancreas, liver, and colon, in decreasing order.[78]

Splenic Sarcoidosis

Sarcoidosis is a granulomatous disease that can involve multiple organ systems, most commonly the lung. Patients with sarcoidosis of the liver and spleen may present with hepatosplenomegaly

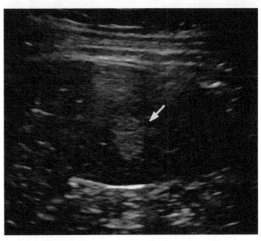

Fig. 41. Echogenic mass typical of a splenic hemangioma, marked by an *arrow*.

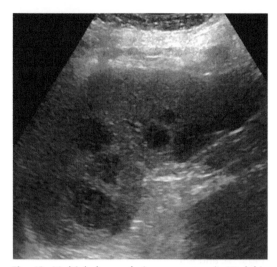

Fig. 42. Multiple hypoechoic masses seen in Hodgkin lymphoma of the spleen.

or nodular disease. Sonographically, the granulomas associated with sarcoidosis are hypoechoic.[78] Hepatosplenomegaly is the most common presentation in patients with sarcoidosis. On US, in addition to enlargement of the liver and spleen, the organ parenchyma may take on a diffuse increased homogeneous or heterogeneous echogenicity.[78,84] Nodular disease is typically innumerable and diffusely involving the liver or spleen. The nodules may range from 0.1 to 3 cm in size. Calcification of the nodules may occur.[84] A mimic of calcifications can be seen in splenic siderosis in the setting of splenic iron deposition with innumerable hyperechoic foci (**Fig. 44**).

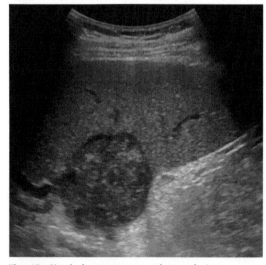

Fig. 43. Single heterogeneous, hypoechoic mass representing B-cell lymphoma of the spleen.

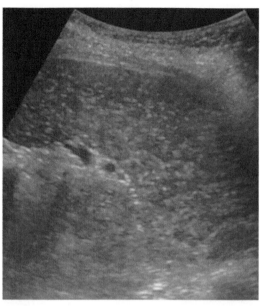

Fig. 44. Numerous echogenic foci seen with splenic siderosis.

REFERENCES

1. Chong WK, Shah MS. Sonography of right upper quadrant pain. Ultrasound Clin 2008;3(1):121–38.
2. Kudo M. Reidel's lobe of the liver and its clinical implication [editorial]. Intern Med 2000;39(2):87–8.
3. Niederau C, Sonnenberg A, Muller JE, et al. Sonographic measurements of the normal liver, spleen, pancreas, and portal vein. Radiology 1983;149(2):537–40.
4. Kratzer W, Fritz V, Mason RA, et al. Factors affecting liver size: a sonographic survey of 2080 subjects. J Ultrasound Med 2003;22(11):1155–61.
5. Wolf DC. Chapter 94: evaluation of the size, shape, and consistency of the liver. In: Walker HK, Hall WD, Hurst JW, editors. Clinical methods: the history, physical, and laboratory examinations. 3rd edition. Boston: Butterworths; 1990. Available at: http://www.ncbi.nlm.nih.gov/books/NBK421/.
6. Gosink BB, Leymaster CE. Ultrasonic determination of hepatomegaly. J Clin Ultrasound 1981;9(1):37–44.
7. Tchelepi H, Ralls PW, Radin R, et al. Sonography of diffuse liver disease. J Ultrasound Med 2002;21(9):1023–32 [quiz: 1033–4].
8. Joy D, Thava VR, Scott BB. Diagnosis of fatty liver disease: is biopsy necessary? Eur J Gastroenterol Hepatol 2003;15(5):539–43.
9. Boyce CJ, Pickhardt PJ, Kim DH, et al. Hepatic steatosis (fatty liver disease) in asymptomatic adults identified by unenhanced low-dose CT. AJR Am J Roentgenol 2010;194(3):623–8.

10. Lall CG, Aisen AM, Bansal N, et al. Nonalcoholic fatty liver disease. AJR Am J Roentgenol 2008; 190(4):993–1002.

11. Pozzato C, Botta A, Melgara C, et al. Sonographic findings in type I glycogen storage disease. J Clin Ultrasound 2001;29(8):456–61.

12. Di Lelio A, Cestari C, Lomazzi A, et al. Cirrhosis: diagnosis with sonographic study of the liver surface. Radiology 1989;172(2):389–92.

13. Freeman MP, Vick CW, Taylor KJ, et al. Regenerating nodules in cirrhosis: sonographic appearance with anatomic correlation. AJR Am J Roentgenol 1986; 146(3):533–6.

14. Simonovsky V. The diagnosis of cirrhosis by high resolution ultrasound of the liver surface. Br J Radiol 1999;72(853):29–34.

15. Harbin WP, Robert NJ, Ferrucci JT Jr. Diagnosis of cirrhosis based on regional changes in hepatic morphology: a radiological and pathological analysis. Radiology 1980;135(2):273–83.

16. Giorgio A, Amoroso P, Lettieri G, et al. Cirrhosis: value of caudate to right lobe ratio in diagnosis with US. Radiology 1986;161(2):443–5.

17. Lim JH. Dysplastic nodules in liver cirrhosis: detection with triple phase helical dynamic CT. Br J Radiol 2004;77(923):911–6.

18. Lim JH, Choi BI. Dysplastic nodules in liver cirrhosis: imaging. Abdom Imaging 2002;27(2):117–28.

19. Kraus GJ, Schedlbauer P, Lax S, et al. The reverse target sign in liver disease: a potential ultrasound feature in cirrhotic liver nodules characterization. Br J Radiol 2005;78(928):355–7.

20. Jha P, Poder L, Wang ZJ, et al. Radiologic mimics of cirrhosis. AJR Am J Roentgenol 2010;194(4): 993–9.

21. Lipson JA, Qayyum A, Avrin DE, et al. CT and MRI of hepatic contour abnormalities. AJR Am J Roentgenol 2005;184(1):75–81.

22. Kim TK, Jang H-J, Wilson SR. Hepatic neoplasms: features on grayscale and contrast enhanced ultrasound. Ultrasound Clin 2007;2(3):333–54.

23. Kim TK, Jang HJ, Wilson SR. Imaging diagnosis of hepatocellular carcinoma with differentiation from other pathology. Clin Liver Dis 2005;9(2):253–79.

24. Bennett GL, Krinsky GA, Abitbol RJ, et al. Sonographic detection of hepatocellular carcinoma and dysplastic nodules in cirrhosis: correlation of pretransplantation sonography and liver explant pathology in 200 patients. AJR Am J Roentgenol 2002;179(1):75–80.

25. Tanaka S, Kitamura T, Imaoka S, et al. Hepatocellular carcinoma: sonographic and histologic correlation. AJR Am J Roentgenol 1983;140(4):701–7.

26. Yoshikawa J, Matsui O, Takashima T, et al. Fatty metamorphosis in hepatocellular carcinoma: radiologic features in 10 cases. AJR Am J Roentgenol 1988;151(4):717–20.

27. Vachha B, Sun MR, Siewert B, et al. Cystic lesions of the liver. AJR Am J Roentgenol 2011;196(4): W355–66.

28. Tanaka K, Numata K, Okazaki H, et al. Diagnosis of portal vein thrombosis in patients with hepatocellular carcinoma: efficacy of color doppler sonography compared with angiography. AJR Am J Roentgenol 1993;160(6):1279–83.

29. Kim CK, Lim JH, Lee WJ. Detection of hepatocellular carcinomas and dysplastic nodules in cirrhotic liver: accuracy of ultrasonography in transplant patients. J Ultrasound Med 2001;20(2):99–104.

30. Nghiem HV, Bogost GA, Ryan JA, et al. Cavernous hemangiomas of the liver: enlargement over time. AJR Am J Roentgenol 1997;169(1):137–40.

31. Bree RL, Schwab RE, Neiman HL. Solitary echogenic spot in the liver: is it diagnostic of a hemangioma? AJR Am J Roentgenol 1983;140(1):41–5.

32. Moody AR, Wilson SR. Atypical hepatic hemangioma: a suggestive sonographic morphology. Radiology 1993;188(2):413–7.

33. Del Poggio P, Buonocore M. Cystic tumors of the liver: a practical approach. World J Gastroenterol 2008;14(23):3616–20.

34. Hagiwara A, Inoue Y, Shutoh T, et al. Haemorrhagic hepatic cyst: a differential diagnosis of cystic tumour. Br J Radiol 2001;74(879):270–2.

35. Sallee M, Rafat C, Zahar JR, et al. Cyst infections in patients with autosomal dominant polycystic kidney disease. Clin J Am Soc Nephrol 2009;4(7):1183–9.

36. Jouret F, Lhommel R, Devuyst O, et al. Diagnosis of cyst infection in patients with autosomal dominant polycystic kidney disease: attributes and limitations of the current modalities. Nephrol Dial Transplant 2012;27(10):3746–51.

37. Teoh AY, Ng SS, Lee KF, et al. Biliary cystadenoma and other complicated cystic lesions of the liver: diagnostic and therapeutic challenges. World J Surg 2006;30(8):1560–6.

38. Choi BI, Lim JH, Han MC, et al. Biliary cystadenoma and cystadenocarcinoma: CT and sonographic findings. Radiology 1989;171(1):57–61.

39. Forrest ME, Cho KJ, Shields JJ, et al. Biliary cystadenomas: sonographic-angiographic-pathologic correlations. AJR Am J Roentgenol 1980;135(4):723–7.

40. Buetow PC, Pantongrag-Brown L, Buck JL, et al. Focal nodular hyperplasia of the liver: radiologic-pathologic correlation. Radiographics 1996;16(2):369–88.

41. Welch TJ, Sheedy PF, Johnson CM, et al. Radiographic characteristics of benign liver tumors: focal nodular hyperplasia and hepatic adenoma. Radiographics 1985;5(4):673–82.

42. Katabathina VS, Menias CO, Shanbhogue AK, et al. Genetics and imaging of hepatocellular adenomas: 2011 update. Radiographics 2011;31(6):1529–43.

43. Laumonier H, Cailliez H, Balabaud C, et al. Role of contrast-enhanced sonography in differentiation of

subtypes of hepatocellular adenoma: correlation with MRI findings. AJR Am J Roentgenol 2012; 199(2):341–8.

44. Hung CH, Changchien CS, Lu SN, et al. Sonographic features of hepatic adenomas with pathologic correlation. Abdom Imaging 2001;26(5):500–6.

45. Jang HJ, Kim TK, Wilson SR. Imaging of malignant liver masses: characterization and detection. Ultrasound Q 2006;22(1):19–29.

46. Colli A, Cocciolo M, Mumoli N, et al. Peripheral intrahepatic cholangiocarcinoma: ultrasound findings and differential diagnosis from hepatocellular carcinoma. Eur J Ultrasound 1998;7(2):93–9.

47. Chung YE, Kim MJ, Park YN, et al. Varying appearances of cholangiocarcinoma: radiologic-pathologic correlation. Radiographics 2009;29(3):683–700.

48. Robledo R, Muro A, Prieto ML. Extrahepatic bile duct carcinoma: US characteristics and accuracy in demonstration of tumors. Radiology 1996; 198(3):869–73.

49. Lee WJ, Lim HK, Jang KM, et al. Radiologic spectrum of cholangiocarcinoma: emphasis on unusual manifestations and differential diagnoses. Radiographics 2001;21(Spec No):S97–116.

50. Jhaveri KS, Halankar J, Aguirre D, et al. Intrahepatic bile duct dilatation due to liver metastases from colorectal carcinoma. AJR Am J Roentgenol 2009;193(3):752–6.

51. Soyer P, Bluemke DA, Reichle R, et al. Imaging of intrahepatic cholangiocarcinoma: 1. Peripheral cholangiocarcinoma. AJR Am J Roentgenol 1995; 165(6):1427–31.

52. Soyer P, Bluemke DA, Reichle R, et al. Imaging of intrahepatic cholangiocarcinoma: 2. Hilar cholangiocarcinoma. AJR Am J Roentgenol 1995;165(6): 1433–6.

53. Choi BI, Han JK, Hong ST, et al. Clonorchiasis and cholangiocarcinoma: etiologic relationship and imaging diagnosis. Clin Microbiol Rev 2004;17(3): 540–52 [table of contents].

54. Lim JH. Radiologic findings of clonorchiasis. AJR Am J Roentgenol 1990;155(5):1001–8.

55. Mortele KJ, Segatto E, Ros PR. The infected liver: radiologic-pathologic correlation. Radiographics 2004;24(4):937–55.

56. Subramanyam BR, Balthazar EJ, Raghavendra BN, et al. Ultrasound analysis of solid-appearing abscesses. Radiology 1983;146(2):487–91.

57. Ralls PW, Meyers HI, Lapin SA, et al. Gray-scale ultrasonography of hepatic amoebic abscesses. Radiology 1979;132(1):125–9.

58. Sukov RJ, Cohen LJ, Sample WF. Sonography of hepatic amebic abscesses. AJR Am J Roentgenol 1980;134(5):911–5.

59. Czermak BV, Unsinn KM, Gotwald T, et al. Echinococcus multilocularis revisited. AJR Am J Roentgenol 2001;176(5):1207–12.

60. Didier D, Weiler S, Rohmer P, et al. Hepatic alveolar echinococcosis: correlative US and CT study. Radiology 1985;154(1):179–86.

61. Cheung H, Lai YM, Loke TK, et al. The imaging diagnosis of hepatic schistosomiasis japonicum sequelae. Clin Radiol 1996;51(1):51–5.

62. Pastakia B, Shawker T, Thaler M, et al. Hepatosplenic candidiasis: wheels within wheels. Radiology 1988;166(2):417–21.

63. Lev-Toaff AS, Bach AM, Wechsler RJ, et al. The radiologic and pathologic spectrum of biliary hamartomas. AJR Am J Roentgenol 1995;165(2):309–13.

64. Zheng RQ, Kudo M, Onda H, et al. Imaging findings of biliary hamartomas (von Meyenburg complexes). J Med Ultrason 2005;32(4):205–12.

65. Eisenberg D, Hurwitz L, Yu AC. CT and sonography of multiple bile-duct hamartomas simulating malignant liver disease (case report). AJR Am J Roentgenol 1986;147(2):279–80.

66. Lee WK, Lau EW, Duddalwar VA, et al. Abdominal manifestations of extranodal lymphoma: spectrum of imaging findings. AJR Am J Roentgenol 2008; 191(1):198–206.

67. Rizzi EB, Schinina V, Cristofaro M, et al. Non-hodgkin's lymphoma of the liver in patients with AIDS: sonographic, CT, and MRI findings. J Clin Ultrasound 2001;29(3):125–9.

68. Appelbaum L, Lederman R, Agid R, et al. Hepatic lymphoma: an imaging approach with emphasis on image-guided needle biopsy. Isr Med Assoc J 2005;7(1):19–22.

69. Avlonitis VS, Linos D. Primary hepatic lymphoma: a review. Eur J Surg 1999;165(8):725–9.

70. Khan AN, Chandramohan M. Liver trauma imaging. 2013. Available at: http://emedicine.medscape.com/article/370508-overview. Accessed May 1, 2014.

71. Richards JR, Schleper NH, Woo BD, et al. Sonographic assessment of blunt abdominal trauma: a 4-year prospective study. J Clin Ultrasound 2002; 30(2):59–67.

72. vanSonnenberg E, Simeone JF, Mueller PR, et al. Sonographic appearance of hematoma in liver, spleen, and kidney: a clinical, pathologic, and animal study. Radiology 1983;147(2):507–10.

73. Wicks JD, Silver TM, Bree RL. Gray scale features of hematomas: an ultrasonic spectrum. AJR Am J Roentgenol 1978;131(6):977–80.

74. McKenney KL, Nunez DB, McKenney MG, et al. Sonography as the primary screening technique for blunt abdominal trauma: experience with 899 patients. AJR Am J Roentgenol 1998;170:979–85.

75. Benter T, Kluhs L, Teichgraber U. Sonography of the spleen. J Ultrasound Med 2011;30(9):1281–93.

76. Hosey RG, Mattacola CG, Kriss V, et al. Ultrasound assessment of spleen size in collegiate athletes. Br J Sports Med 2006;40(3):251–4 [discussion: 251–4].

77. Spielmann AL, DeLong DM, Kliewer MA. Sonographic evaluation of spleen size in tall healthy athletes. AJR Am J Roentgenol 2005;184(1):45–9.

78. Sutherland T, Temple F, Hennessy O, et al. Abdomen's forgotten organ: sonography and CT of focal splenic lesions. J Med Imaging Radiat Oncol 2010; 54(2):120–8.

79. Saad NEA, Saad WEA, Davies MG, et al. Pseudoaneurysms and the role of minimally invasive techniques in their management. Radiographics 2005; 25(Suppl 1):S173–89.

80. Weingarten MJ, Fakhry J, McCarthy J, et al. Sonography after splenic embolization: the wedge-shaped acute infarct. AJR Am J Roentgenol 1984;142(5): 957–9.

81. Goerg C, Schwerk WB. Splenic infarction: sonographic patterns, diagnosis, follow-up, and complications. Radiology 1990;174(3 Pt 1):803–7.

82. Giovagnoni A, Giorgi C, Goteri G. Tumours of the spleen. Cancer Imaging 2005;5:73–7.

83. Willcox TM, Speer RW, Schlinkert RT, et al. Hemangioma of the spleen: presentation, diagnosis, and management. J Gastrointest Surg 2000;4(6):611–3.

84. Warshauer DM, Lee JK. Imaging manifestations of abdominal sarcoidosis. AJR Am J Roentgenol 2004;182(1):15–28.

Ultrasound of the Gallbladder and Biliary Tree: Back to Basics

 CrossMark

Brian Boyd, MD*, Ellie R. Lee, MD

KEYWORDS

- Bile duct • Portal vein • Cholecystitis • Intrahepatic duct • Common bile duct

KEY POINTS

- Ultrasound is the modality of choice and is well suited for the initial evaluation of the gallbladder and biliary tree.
- Ultrasound imaging benefits include lower cost, faster acquisition time, portability, and the advantage of being a dynamic examination.
- Although ultrasound may be the initial modality that identifies biliary tract malignancy, cross-sectional imaging with computed tomography and MR imaging will be required to evaluate the extent of disease.
- Sonographic findings in the biliary system are often nonspecific, but when combined with clinical history, these can often help to determine the diagnosis.

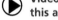 Videos of Adenomyomatosis, Intrahepatic Biliary Dilation, Gallbladder mass imaging accompany this article at http://www.ultrasound.theclinics.com/

INTRODUCTION

Ultrasound is the initial imaging modality of choice to evaluate the biliary tract. Because acute gallbladder disease is a common cause of right upper quadrant pain and cholecystectomy remains one of the most common abdominal surgeries performed, ultrasound imaging of the gallbladder and biliary tree accounts for a significant portion of the volume in many radiology practices. Although MR imaging, more specifically magnetic resonance cholangiopancreatography (MRCP), and computed tomography (CT) scans are being increasingly ordered as part of the diagnostic workup, ultrasound remains the workhorse modality for initial imaging. Ultrasound imaging benefits include lower cost, faster acquisition time, portability, and the advantage of being a dynamic examination.

The structure and location of the gallbladder and bile ducts lends itself to ultrasound evaluation. The fluid-filled nature of the gallbladder and bile ducts provides a natural contrast resolution from the surrounding organs in the upper abdomen.[1] In addition, the liver typically functions as a solid tissue acoustic window through which the biliary system can be visualized.

The primary goal of this article is to review the fundamentals of gallbladder and biliary imaging as it pertains to the diagnostic radiologist. The basic anatomy, normal measurements, common diseases, and pertinent ultrasound findings of the biliary tract are also reviewed.

The authors have nothing to disclose.
Department of Radiology, University of North Carolina, 2107 Old Clinic Bldg, Chapel Hill, NC 27599-7510, USA
* Corresponding author.
E-mail address: bboyd@unch.unc.edu

Ultrasound Clin 9 (2014) 567–586
http://dx.doi.org/10.1016/j.cult.2014.07.009

GALLBLADDER ANATOMY

- Ovoid, anechoic viscus
- Lies along posterior liver surface and interlobar fissure
- Three parts: neck, body, fundus
- Wall thickness less than 3 mm
- Less than 10 cm in length and 5 cm in diameter

The gallbladder is an ovoid, hollow viscus normally filled with simple fluid (bile) and therefore predominantly anechoic on ultrasound when distended (**Fig. 1**). The gallbladder wall is thin, smooth, and relatively hyperechoic, measuring less than 3 mm in thickness in a normal, fasting patient.[2] The gallbladder typically lies along the inferior surface of the liver between the left and right lobes, but can vary in orientation from patient to patient.

The gallbladder is divided into 3 main parts: fundus, body, and neck (see **Fig. 1A**). Unlike the stomach, the fundus is the distal most aspect of the gallbladder. The body lies between the neck and the fundus with the neck being the most proximal aspect of the gallbladder, leading into the cystic duct. The neck is a potential site for stones to become impacted, which can lead to cystic duct obstruction and acute cholecystitis (**Fig. 2**).

The gallbladder varies in shape, size, and contour from one normal patient to another. The normal size of the gallbladder should be less than 10 cm in length from neck to fundus and less than 5 cm in diameter at the widest point of the body (see **Fig. 1**). Prominent folds can be noted in the normal gallbladder. A common variation in shape caused by such a fold is the phrygian cap (**Fig. 3**); this is caused by a prominent fold at the junction of the body and fundus. Stones can

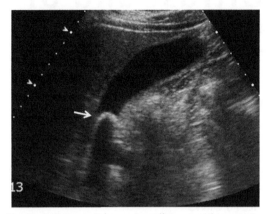

Fig. 2. Gallstone. Echogenic gallstone with posterior shadowing located in the gallbladder neck (*solid arrow*).

settle in this folded portion with no clinical significance.

BILIARY TREE ANATOMY

- Component of the portal triad
- Divided into intra- and extrahepatic ducts
- Right/left hepatic ducts less than 2 mm in diameter
- Normal common bile duct less than 7 mm in diameter, varies with age and cholecystectomy

The bile ducts can be separated into 2 major categories: intrahepatic and extrahepatic. The intrahepatic biliary ducts are one of the components that form the portal triad. The portal triad is a complex of a bile duct, portal vein, and hepatic artery that branches together throughout the liver (**Fig. 4**). Because there is no consistent orientation

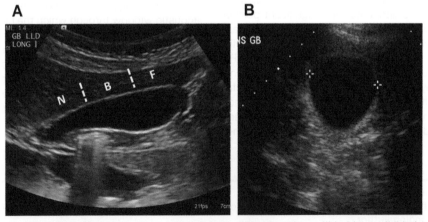

Fig. 1. Normal gallbladder. (*A*) Longitudinal view of the gallbladder. The gallbladder is divided into 3 parts: fundus (F), body (B), and neck (N). Normal gallbladder length less than 10 cm. (*B*) Transverse view of the gallbladder. Normal gallbladder diameter less than 5 cm (*cursors*).

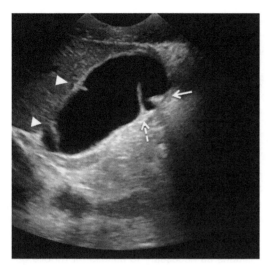

Fig. 3. Phrygian cap. Prominent fold at the junction of the gallbladder body and fundus (*dashed arrow*). Note a shadowing stone within this folded portion (*solid arrow*). Additional folds are seen in the body and neck (*arrowheads*).

of the bile ducts relative to the other 2 vascular structures, color and/or spectral Doppler can be used to distinguish the bile ducts from the adjacent vessels.

The intrahepatic ducts tend to follow the same branching pattern as the other structures of the portal triad, separating into the right and left hepatic lobes along the Couinaud segmental anatomy of the liver. The right-lobe intrahepatic ducts typically divide into anterior and posterior branches that

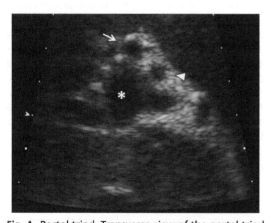

Fig. 4. Portal triad. Transverse view of the portal triad in the porta hepatis consists of the portal vein (*asterisk*), common bile duct (*solid arrow*), and hepatic artery (*arrowhead*). Also, referred to as the "Mickey Mouse" appearance with the portal vein as the head and the common bile duct and the hepatic artery as the ears.

drain liver segments V/VIII and VI/VII, respectively. The left-lobe intrahepatic ducts typically divide between the medial segments IVa and IVb and lateral segments II and III. The segmental and lobar branches coalesce centrally to form the right and left hepatic ducts. There are several recognized variations in the pattern described earlier, but this is the most common.[3,4]

The right and left hepatic ducts are centrally located in the porta hepatis and normally measure less than 2 mm in diameter. The more peripheral intrahepatic ducts are considered abnormal if they can be visualized or if they are greater than or equal to one-half the diameter of the adjacent portal vein (**Fig. 5**).[5]

The right and left hepatic ducts join to form the common hepatic duct, the beginning of the extrahepatic biliary tree. This duct is later joined by the cystic duct to form the common bile duct. The location of the common hepatic duct and cystic duct confluence can vary, and the cystic duct is often not well visualized on ultrasound. The site where the right hepatic artery crosses the common bile duct, most often to the posterior, can be used as an approximation of this demarcation when the cystic duct is not visualized.

The definition of common bile duct dilatation is not a simple issue. A review of the literature shows a variety of "normal" values with a general consensus that a common bile duct diameter equal or greater than 7 mm is abnormal and warrants further investigation (**Fig. 6**).[6–8] There is considerable controversy over the impact of age and cholecystectomy on the normal common bile duct diameter.

One of the more recent studies included a thorough review of the literature, in addition to providing novel research, that concluded that increasing age and cholecystectomy does result in common bile duct dilatation. The age at which this dilatation becomes significant is approximately 70 years, but even in normal patients older than 70 years of age with an intact gallbladder, the diameter did not exceed 7.6 mm.[8] Therefore, the common bile duct should be considered dilated if it is equal to or greater than 8 mm in an individual older than the age of 70 years.

In a patient who has undergone prior cholecystectomy, common bile duct diameter is equally, if not more, variable than with increasing age alone and can be seen up to 1 cm.[8] The dilatation can extend into the common hepatic duct, but generally not into the intrahepatic ducts. In the postcholecystectomy patient, comparison with prior examinations is essential in differentiating a stable, expected finding versus a new, possibly pathologic biliary dilatation.

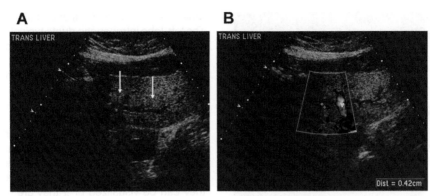

Fig. 5. Dilated intrahepatic bile ducts. (*A*) Transverse view of the left hepatic lobe demonstrates mild intrahepatic biliary dilatation (*arrows*). (*B*) Color Doppler imaging of the liver is useful in differentiating portal vein (V) from bile duct (*cursors*).

ULTRASOUND TECHNIQUE

- Fasted patient, 4 to 6 hours
- Transverse and longitudinal planes
- Patient positioning to assess for mobility and/or layering
- Sonographic Murphy sign

An important factor in gallbladder and biliary ultrasound is the fasting status of the patient. The gallbladder is typically scanned after 4 to 6 hours of fasting to avoid gallbladder contraction. If a patient has not fasted for at least 4 hours before the examination, the gallbladder can be anywhere along the spectrum of distended to contracted and findings such as gallbladder wall thickening, gallstones, and gallbladder sludge cannot be reliably assessed (**Fig. 7**). If the gallbladder is contracted due to a postprandial state, the examination should be delayed or rescheduled for a time when the patient can be adequately fasted.

The gallbladder should be imaged in both transverse and longitudinal planes with different patient

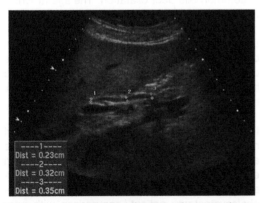

Fig. 6. Normal common bile duct. The normal common bile duct measures less than 7 mm in diameter (*cursors*). Notice the consistent size along the entire length of the duct.

positions as necessary to assess for mobile gallstones or layering sludge. Examination of the gallbladder is initially performed in the supine position. Other maneuvers are routinely used including right and left decubitus, prone, and upright standing positions.

A technique that deserves specific attention is the sonographic Murphy sign. The original Murphy sign was described by Dr John B. Murphy as a physical examination maneuver to differentiate gallbladder pathology from other causes of abdominal pain many years before the advent of ultrasound. His description involved elicitation of pronounced pain by hooking a finger beneath the right costal margin, asking the patient to take a deep breath, and then striking that finger forcibly down with the other hand eliciting severe pain.[9]

The sonographic Murphy sign is a simple adaptation of this original description that takes advantage of the real-time ability to confirm placement of the transducer directly over the gallbladder. The transducer is held firmly in place as the patient is asked to take a deep breath. The sign is considered positive if the patient admits to intense focal pain at the site of the transducer. Patients may evidence this pain by abruptly ceasing inspiration. Absence of a sonographic Murphy sign may be seen in the setting of recent analgesic administration or altered mental status.

GALLSTONES

- Common finding
- Major risk factor for acute cholecystitis
- Highly echogenic with dense posterior shadow
- Wall-echo-shadow (WES) sign

Cholelithiasis is a common finding in the symptomatic as well as the asymptomatic patient. Risk factors for developing gallstones include

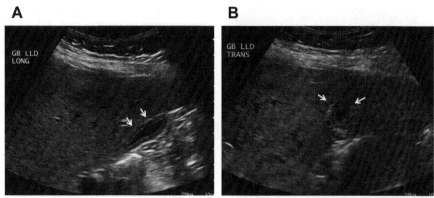

Fig. 7. Contracted gallbladder. (*A*) Longitudinal view of the right upper quadrant demonstrates a contracted gallbladder (*arrows*) with an echogenic inner mucosal layer and hypoechoic outer muscular layer. (*B*) Transverse view of the right upper quadrant demonstrates apparent wall thickening due to underdistention (*arrows*). This patient was rescheduled and instructed on the appropriate fasting time before the examination (4–6 hours). **Fig. 1** demonstrates a normally distended gallbladder on the repeat examination.

obesity, increased age, female gender, pregnancy, and diabetes.[1] Although asymptomatic cholelithiasis is not a disease that requires immediate intervention, it is generally accepted as the major risk factor for developing biliary colic or acute cholecystitis.

Gallstones are most often primarily composed of cholesterol, but in patients with a history of a chronic hemolytic process, pigmented stones can be seen. Regardless of their composition, gallstones have high acoustic impedance and appear highly echogenic (**Fig. 8**). Gallstones greater than 4 mm in size will likely cause posterior acoustic shadowing.[10] Also, the mobility of the gallstones is important to demonstrate to distinguish them from other entities, such as polyp, tumefactive sludge or tumor.

When a gallbladder is filled with multiple gallstones or a single large gallstone, the question can arise as to whether there is air or calcium in the gallbladder wall itself. This question can be answered by looking for the WES sign. When a gallbladder is filled with stones, the echogenic gallbladder wall (W) is still visible as a distinct structure due to a thin layer of hypoechoic bile overlying the brightly echogenic surface of the gallstones (E), which is then followed by posterior shadowing (S) from the stones, hence WES (**Fig. 9**).

In the instance of porcelain gallbladder or emphysematous cholecystitis, the calcium or air within the gallbladder wall disrupts the normal, thin appearance of the wall and therefore only one echogenic line and posterior shadowing will be visualized. Differentiation of cholelithiasis from emphysematous cholecystitis and porcelain gallbladder is important given the implications of the latter 2 processes.

BILIARY SLUDGE

Biliary sludge is a mixture of particulate matter that precipitates in bile.[11] Risk factors for the formation of sludge include rapid weight loss, pregnancy, critical illness, and prolonged total parenteral

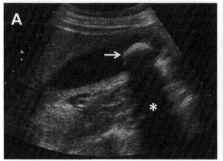
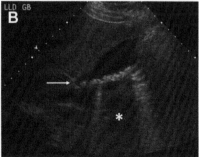

Fig. 8. Gallstones. (*A*) Single, large gallstone in the gallbladder fundus (*solid arrow*). (*B*) Multiple small stones in the gallbladder body and neck (*solid arrow*). Note the bright echogenic signal of the stones with homogeneous posterior shadowing in both images (*asterisk*).

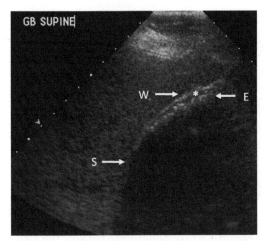

Fig. 9. Wall-echo-shadow (WES) sign. Longitudinal image of the gallbladder demonstrates an echogenic curvilinear line representing the gallbladder wall (W), thin layer of hypoechoic bile (*asterisk*) and echogenic stone surface (E) with homogeneous posterior shadowing (S).

nutrition.[11–13] Although the composition would suggest a precursor to gallstone formation, the incidence of cholelithiasis in patients with known biliary sludge is approximately 5% to 15%.[11] Sludge typically appears as an amorphous, dependently layering echogenicity within the gallbladder that moves with changes in patient positioning and does not demonstrate posterior shadowing (**Fig. 10**).

Occasionally, biliary sludge will form into globular "sludge balls", called tumefactive sludge, that can adhere to the gallbladder wall, raising the question of a polyp or tumor. These sludge balls will not shadow, regardless of size, which differentiates them from gallstones greater than

4 mm in size that typically shadow or polyps that demonstrate blood flow (**Fig. 11**). Imaging the patient in more than one additional position, applying color or spectral Doppler, or repeating the examination at a later date will often help to differentiate a sludge ball from a polyp or tumor.

CHOLECYSTITIS

- Most often caused by gallstones
- Acalculous cholecystitis typically seen in critically ill patients
- Complicated cholecystitis: gangrenous, emphysematous, perforation

Cholecystitis is defined as inflammation of the gallbladder. It is divided into calculous and acalculous cholecystitis depending on whether gallstones are present. Of these 2, calculous cholecystitis accounts for 90% to 95% of cases.[14] Calculous cholecystitis can be further subdivided into acute and chronic cholecystitis.

Acute cholecystitis is typically caused by gallstones lodged in the gallbladder neck or cystic duct. This obstruction can lead to gallbladder distention and inflammatory changes in the gallbladder wall, which may eventually lead to ischemia, superinfection, and necrosis of the gallbladder wall. The findings classically associated with the diagnosis of acute cholecystitis include gallbladder wall thickening (>3 mm), a positive sonographic Murphy sign, gallbladder distention, gallbladder wall hyperemia, and pericholecystic fluid (**Fig. 12**). The presence of stones, a positive sonographic Murphy sign, and wall thickening were originally found to have the highest positive and negative predictive values.[15] Although subsequent studies have challenged the validity of the sonographic Murphy sign, the overall sensitivity

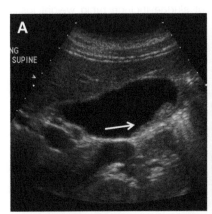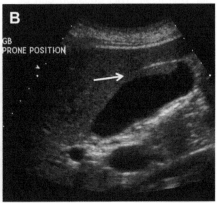

Fig. 10. Gallbladder sludge. Amorphous, nonshadowing echogenic material within the gallbladder lumen that moves freely and usually assumes a dependent position (*solid arrows*) as seen on the supine (*A*) and prone (*B*) images.

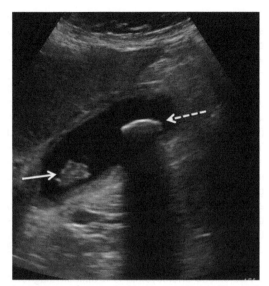

Fig. 11. Tumefactive sludge or "sludge ball". Globular, echogenic lesion within the gallbladder lumen (*solid arrow*) that does not demonstrate posterior shadowing. On color Doppler, no internal vascularity was seen. In addition, the sludge ball demonstrated mobility. A shadowing echogenic gallstone is also seen (*dashed arrow*) and provides an excellent comparison in the different appearances of the 2 entities.

and specificity of these 3 "primary" signs along with the other "secondary" signs fall into the 80% to 90% range.[16–18]

Complications associated with acute cholecystitis are rare, accounting for less than 1% to 2% of cases, but the morbidity and mortality are high.[19,20] Risk factors generally associated with elevated complication rates include diabetes, male gender, Hispanic descent, and cardiovascular disease.[19,20] Some of these complications can be identified by specific sonographic features.

Gangrenous cholecystitis is defined as necrosis within the gallbladder wall. It can result from severe or prolonged inflammation or infections. There is an association with diabetes. Older studies suggested that echogenic striations within the gallbladder wall were an indicator of necrosis.[16,21] Some of these studies also suggested that absence of the sonographic Murphy sign should raise the suspicion of necrosis related to denervation of the nervous supply to the gallbladder.[16] However, recent studies have shown that a markedly thickened gallbladder wall, in the range of 7 mm for gangrenous versus 4 mm for uncomplicated acute cholecystitis, and a white blood cell count greater than 15K ($\times$109/L) should raise the concern for this complication.[19,22] Although difficult to delineate from stones and sludge, sloughing of the gallbladder wall as well as the presence of thrombus in the lumen of the gallbladder, seen as irregular bands of echogenic material, can be seen in gangrenous cholecystitis (**Fig. 13**).

Perforation of the gallbladder can be associated with prolonged cholecystitis, but can also be seen in the setting of trauma. Findings that may suggest perforation include a focal defect in the gallbladder wall, loss of the normal ovoid gallbladder shape, which may suggest decompression, and complex fluid collections adjacent to the gallbladder suggesting abscess (**Fig. 14**).

Emphysematous cholecystitis is rare and caused by rapidly progressing infection of the gallbladder with a gas-forming organism. In addition to the typical findings of acute cholecystitis, gas is seen within the gallbladder wall and lumen, which appears as irregular or small round echogenic foci that demonstrate a heterogeneous posterior shadowing, as opposed to the homogeneous posterior shadowing caused by stones

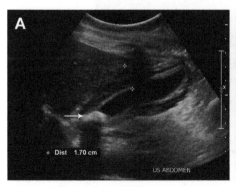
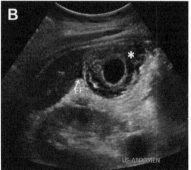

Fig. 12. Acute cholecystitis. (*A*) Longitudinal view. Large shadowing stone in the gallbladder neck (*arrow*) with markedly edematous gallbladder wall thickening (*cursors*). (*B*) Transverse view of the gallbladder demonstrates marked edematous wall thickening (*asterisk*) and trace pericholecystic fluid (FF). The patient presented with right upper quadrant pain and exhibited a positive sonographic Murphy sign.

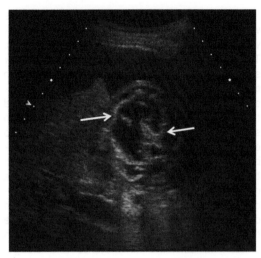

Fig. 13. Gangrenous cholecystitis. Sloughing of the gallbladder wall is identified, indicating necrosis, as evidenced by the linear echogenicities (*solid arrows*) within the gallbladder lumen. A cirrhotic liver is partially visualized and ascites is present (not directly related to the cholecystitis).

(Fig. 15). However, air within the wall can mimic a stone-filled gallbladder. CT can be considered to confirm the presence of air in the gallbladder wall. Pneumobilia can also be seen with emphysematous cholecystitis.

Chronic calculous cholecystitis is associated with gallstones and chronic inflammation and leads to gallbladder wall thickening and fibrosis (Fig. 16). The primary contribution of ultrasound in the workup is identifying the presence of gallstones in the absence of any other additional findings to suggest acute cholecystitis, such as gallbladder distention, sonographic Murphy sign, and hyperemia. Gallbladder wall hyperemia has been specifically suggested as a way to differentiate acute from chronic cholecystitis, although it can be seen in normal patients and is accentuated by a contracted gallbladder.[23–25]

Acalculous cholecystitis is a difficult diagnosis to establish and is more a diagnosis of exclusion. The patient population in which it is seen is fairly specific. It is most often associated with patients

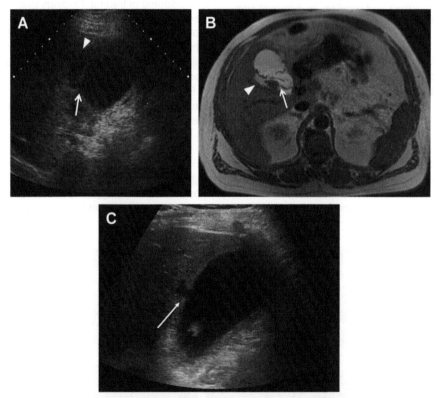

Fig. 14. Perforated gallbladder. (A) Transverse image of the gallbladder demonstrating a defect in the wall (*solid arrow*) as well as pericholecystic fluid (*arrowhead*). (B) T1-weighted axial MR image confirms the findings from the ultrasound (*solid arrow*: perforation; *arrowhead*: pericholecystic fluid). Note that the gallbladder wall is thickened. Additional findings, not seen on these images, supported the diagnosis of acute cholecystitis with rupture. (C) Another ultrasound image of gallbladder perforation. A focal defect is identified in the gallbladder wall (*arrow*).

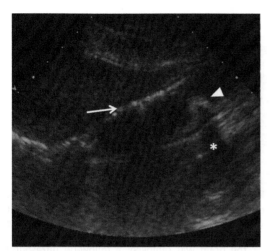

Fig. 15. Emphysematous cholecystitis. Air within the gallbladder wall (*solid arrow*) appears as a single curvilinear echogenicity with heterogeneous, "dirty" posterior shadowing. Contrast this with the dense posterior shadowing (*asterisk*) from the gallstone (*arrowhead*).

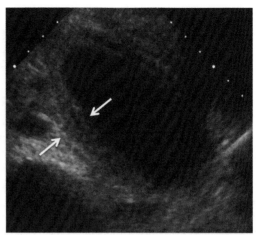

Fig. 17. Acalculous cholecystitis. The gallbladder wall is markedly thickened (*arrows*). No stones were present and the bile ducts were not dilated. Sludge was not seen in this case, but can be present. The patient had been in the intensive care unit for 30 days for an unrelated illness and was noted to have an increasing bilirubin level without clinical evidence to suggest another cause. Cholescintigraphy confirmed the diagnosis.

who are critically ill, have sustained significant burns or trauma, or receive prolonged parenteral nutrition.[12] Sonographic findings are similar to that of acute cholecystitis, which include gallbladder distention, gallbladder wall thickening, pericholecystic fluid, positive sonographic Murphy sign, and often biliary sludge, but in the absence of stones (**Fig. 17**). Assessment of a sonographic Murphy sign in this patient population is often difficult.

Xanthogranulomatous cholecystitis is a rare form of chronic inflammation. Sonographic findings for this diagnosis include hypoechoic nodules and

bands within the gallbladder wall. These are felt to represent the collections of lipid laden macrophages that define this disease pathologically.[26,27]

INTERVENTIONAL COMPLICATIONS

Common interventions associated with the biliary tract include cholecystectomy, cholecystostomy, cholangiostomy, sphincterotomy, and biliary stent placement. Each of these procedures can result in injury to the gallbladder and/or the biliary tree. The 3 major complications include bile leak/biloma, hemorrhage, and abscess. These complications appear as diffuse or focal fluid collections with varying degrees of echogenicity and heterogeneity depending on the exact cause and chronicity (**Fig. 18**). Biloma can be differentiated with the use of cholescintigraphy or cholangiography.

GALLBLADDER WALL THICKENING AND PORCELAIN GALLBLADDER

Gallbladder wall thickening is one of the major findings associated with most forms of cholecystitis. By itself, however, it is very nonspecific. A thickened gallbladder wall can be the result of many other nonbiliary tract disease processes including congestive heart failure, renal failure, hypoalbuminemia, and acute hepatitis (**Fig. 19**).[28,29] In addition, many intrinsic biliary diseases cause

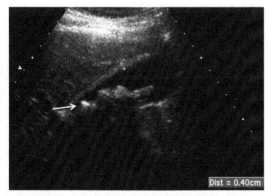

Fig. 16. Chronic cholecystitis. Mildly thickened gallbladder wall (*cursors*) and gallstones (*solid arrow*). Patient had no additional findings to suggest acute cholecystitis, including a negative sonographic Murphy sign.

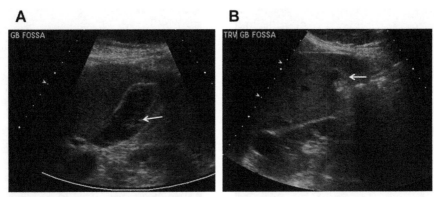

Fig. 18. Gallbladder fossa hematoma. (*A*) Patient was several days status post-cholecystectomy with persistent right upper quadrant pain. A complex collection in the gallbladder fossa is heterogeneous with a retractile appearance of the central echogenic focus (*arrow*), typical of hematoma. A drain was placed for concern of developing abscess, but confirmed aseptic hematoma. (*B*) After the drain was removed, a follow-up ultrasound demonstrated near complete resolution of the fluid collection (*arrow*).

gallbladder wall thickening as noted throughout this article. This is an important fact to keep in mind if the solitary abnormality on ultrasound is gallbladder wall thickening.

Porcelain gallbladder is calcification in the wall of the gallbladder, associated with gallstone disease and chronic cholecystitis. Sonographic appearance may vary from an interrupted thin to thick echogenic line within the gallbladder wall with posterior shadowing (**Fig. 20**). Porcelain gallbladder can be difficult to differentiate with a stone-filled gallbladder and CT can be considered for further evaluation. Porcelain gallbladder is associated with a high rate of gallbladder malignancy, and although recent studies have disputed the rate of association, prophylactic resection is still recommended.[30,31]

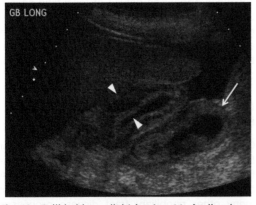

Fig. 19. Gallbladder wall thickening. Markedly edematous, thickened gallbladder wall (*arrowheads*) secondary to hypoproteinemia. Note the wall thickening of the adjacent bowel loop (*solid arrow*) and ascites.

GALLBLADDER POLYPS AND ADENOMYOMATOSIS

Polypoid lesions of the gallbladder can represent several different entities. Overall, cholesterol polyps are the most common cause (Video 1), but additional considerations include adherent stones or sludge balls, thrombus, adenomas, adenomyomas, inflammatory polyps, or tumors. These lesions are nonshadowing, nonmobile, and typically characterized by size alone (**Fig. 21**). The most recent studies have found that polyps less than 7 mm in size are unlikely to be neoplastic in nature and do not warrant imaging follow-up.[32–34] Ultrasound imaging follow-up is recommended for polyps above this cut off. Polyps greater than 1 cm are considered higher risk for malignancy and resection is recommended. However, a recent study showed a low risk of malignancy in polyps less than 2 cm in size and suggested that surgery may not be immediately required in younger (<50 years), asymptomatic patients.[33]

Adenomyomatosis is a benign process that occurs in the gallbladder wall. There are 3 morphologic types: generalized, segmental (annular), and localized.[35] This process is caused by hyperplasia of the epithelial and muscular layers of the gallbladder wall and causes invaginations along the inner gallbladder wall to form. These are known as Rokitansky-Aschoff sinuses and can accumulate bile, sludge, and cholesterol crystals. An often associated pathologic condition, called cholesterolosis, involves only accumulation of cholesterol crystals in macrophages within the gallbladder wall. The sonographic appearance of adenomyomatosis is that of diffuse, focal, or segmental wall thickening with multiple intramural echogenic foci that can cause posterior ring-down or comet tail

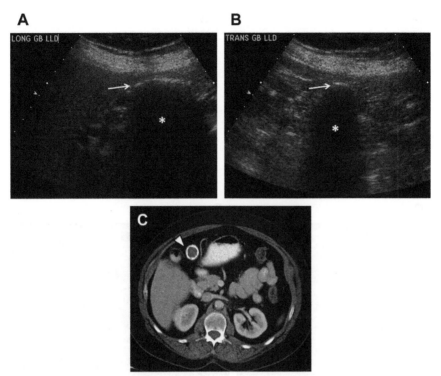

Fig. 20. Porcelain gallbladder. (*A*) Longitudinal and (*B*) transverse views of the gallbladder demonstrate curvilinear echogenicity in the gallbladder wall (*arrow*) with posterior acoustic shadowing (*asterisk*). (*C*) CT confirmation of calcification in the gallbladder wall (*arrowhead*).

reverberation artifact (**Fig. 22**). Cholesterolosis can have a similar appearance, but without wall thickening. Intramural cystic spaces or diverticula may also be seen with adenomyomatosis.

BILIARY OBSTRUCTION

Obstruction of the biliary system can be identified sonographically by identifying dilated intra- and extrahepatic bile ducts (**Fig. 23**, Video 2). This disease process can be divided into 3 major categories: stone-related, inflammatory/infectious, and neoplastic. Biliary obstruction due to stones is the most common of the 3 categories.

CHOLEDOCHOLITHIASIS

- Low overall incidence, but significant morbidity/mortality
- Low sensitivity, high operator dependence for identification on ultrasound
- Decreased conspicuity compared to gallstones
- Mirizzi syndrome and other rare complications of chronic impaction
- Pneumobilia

Choledocholithiasis is defined as stones within the bile ducts. If the stones form within the ducts, it is termed primary and if the stones originated from the gallbladder, it is termed secondary. The incidence of stones in the common bile duct varies somewhere between 5% and 15% in patients undergoing cholecystectomy, with approximately 5% of patients being asymptomatic.[36] There is increased morbidity and mortality associated with the sequelae of common duct obstruction, such as cholangitis and pancreatitis.

Although the biliary system is well evaluated overall through the use of ultrasound, its sensitivity for identifying common duct stones is low and operator dependent with a wide range of reported values between 20% and 80%.[37,38] The specificity, however, is higher and slightly less variable with reported values between 60% and 100%. Given these numbers and variability, MRCP is increasingly used in patients with suspected common bile duct stones. MRCP demonstrates a more consistent, higher sensitivity and specificity, which results in a greater level of diagnostic confidence.[36,37,39] It can help identify the specific patients who would benefit from therapeutic endoscopic retrograde cholangiopancreatography.

Stones within the common bile duct are similar in sonographic appearance to stones within the gallbladder. They appear as round, highly echogenic foci with posterior shadowing (**Fig. 24**). The

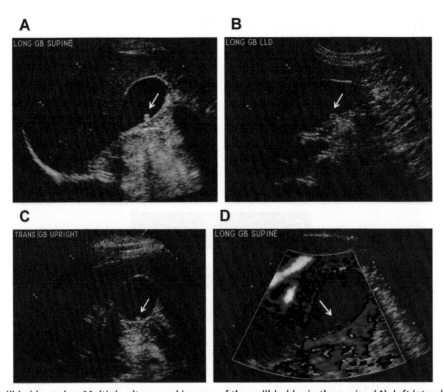

Fig. 21. Gallbladder polyp. Multiple ultrasound images of the gallbladder in the supine (A), left lateral decubitus (B), and upright (C) views from the same patient demonstrating an echogenic, nonshadowing polypoid lesion on the posterior gallbladder wall (arrow). The lesion does not demonstrate mobility with changes in patient position. (D) Power Doppler images of the gallbladder polyp demonstrate a vascular stalk within the lesion (arrow).

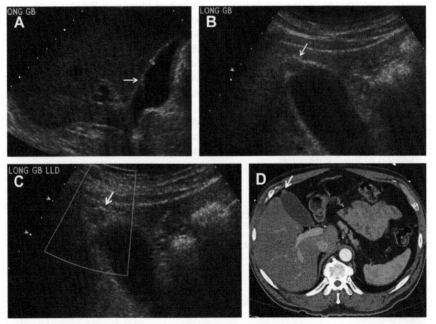

Fig. 22. Adenomyomatosis. (A) Focal area of subtle gallbladder wall thickening with tiny internal echogenic focus causing ring-down artifact, typical of adenomyomatosis (arrow). (B) More prominent focal wall thickening at the gallbladder fundus (arrow) that does not demonstrate vascularity on color Doppler (C). (D) CT image of this same patient demonstrates the soft tissue density of the focal adenomyomatosis in the gallbladder fundus (arrow).

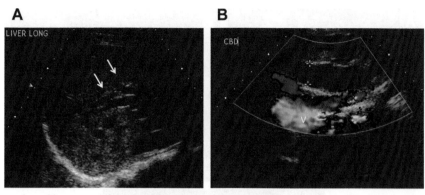

Fig. 23. Biliary duct dilatation. (*A*) Severe intrahepatic biliary dilatation (*arrows*). (*B*) Marked dilatation of the common bile duct (*cursors*). The portal vein (V) and common bile duct are nearly equal in diameter.

only difference is the decreased conspicuity of common duct stones secondary to a relative lack of surrounding bile as compared with stones within the gallbladder. Many common bile duct stones are located in the distal common bile duct near the ampulla of Vater. However, bowel gas in this region further limits evaluation. These factors likely contribute to the low overall sensitivity and high operator dependence in identifying common duct stones.

Mirizzi syndrome occurs when there is compression or obstruction of the common hepatic or common bile duct from an impacted stone in the gallbladder neck or cystic duct. This syndrome is rare in developed Western countries with an annual incidence of less than 1%.[40] Mirizzi syndrome can lead to formation of an erosive fistula between the gallbladder or cystic duct and adjacent structures like the common bile duct, liver, or duodenum. Sonographic findings include the appearance of acute or chronic cholecystitis with biliary duct dilatation.

Pneumobilia is air within the biliary tree; this can be seen rarely with the erosive complications leading to fistula formation from the gallbladder and

bile ducts to the adjacent bowel, but is more commonly associated with biliary or surgical procedures such as sphincterotomy, biliary enteric anastomosis, or biliary stent placement. Pneumobilia can also arise from air in the gallbladder caused by emphysematous cholecystitis.

Pneumobilia characteristically appears as bright, highly echogenic foci within the bile ducts (**Fig. 25**). The air can be coalescent and appear linear in appearance. Posterior shadowing from pneumobilia, in contradistinction to that from gallstones, is described as heterogeneous due to the incomplete and irregular reflection of sound waves. The most unique finding in pneumobilia is visualizing the echogenic air bubbles moving through the bile ducts on real-time imaging.

INFLAMMATORY AND INFECTIOUS BILIARY OBSTRUCTION

- Acute bacterial cholangitis is the most common infectious cause in the United States.
- Recurrent pyogenic cholangitis is more common in East Asia.

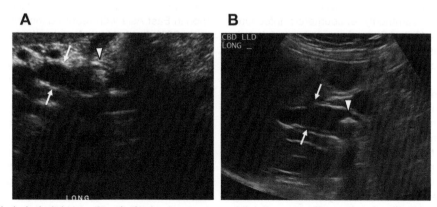

Fig. 24. Choledocholithiasis. (*A*, *B*) Shadowing common bile duct stone (*arrowhead*) with ductal dilatation (*arrows*).

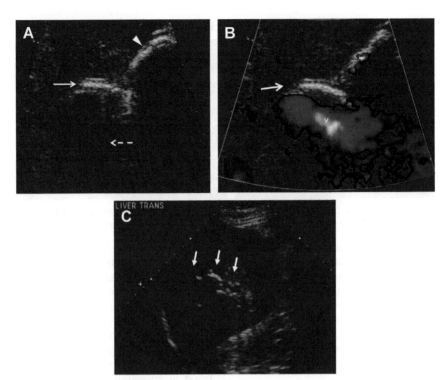

Fig. 25. Pneumobilia. (*A*) Air within the common bile duct. Bright linear echogenic focus in the common bile duct (*arrow*) causing heterogeneous posterior shadowing as well as ring-down artifact (*dashed arrow*). Bowel gas within the duodenum is also seen (*arrowhead*). (*B*) Color Doppler image confirms air is within the common bile duct (*arrow*), adjacent to the main portal vein (*V*). (*C*) Branching echogenic structures with faint acoustic shadowing identified in the liver (*arrows*), indicating air within the intrahepatic ducts. Note that the echogenic foci are more central in the liver as opposed to portal venous gas, which tends to be more peripheral in location.

- Human immunodeficiency virus (HIV) cholangiopathy and primary sclerosing cholangitis (PSC) have a similar appearance on US.
- Hemobilia

Inflammatory causes of biliary obstruction include infectious and noninfectious causes. The ultrasound findings of inflammatory obstruction are often nonspecific because they can be seen with many of the various distinct clinical entities.

The most commonly encountered infectious cause in the United States is acute bacterial cholangitis. This disease entity, classically associated with Charcot triad—fever, right upper quadrant pain, and jaundice—is a medical emergency. This cause is most commonly associated with common bile duct stones in more than 80% of cases.[41] The most common organisms are gram-negative enteric bacteria. Imaging findings include biliary ductal dilatation, circumferential bile duct wall thickening, and choledocholithiasis (**Fig. 26**). These findings are not specific and are common among the other inflammatory causes of biliary obstruction. A finding more specific to acute bacterial cholangitis are hepatic abscesses, although

these may not be present. Ultrasound can visualize these as vague hypoechoic lesions within the liver once they develop central liquefactive necrosis. CT and MR imaging are helpful adjuncts in evaluating for this sequela.

Stones can form directly in the biliary ducts and result in chronic biliary obstruction, stasis, and recurrent inflammation. Known as primary hepatolithiasis, recurrent pyogenic cholangitis, or oriental cholangiohepatitis, this disease process is common in East Asia with reported incidence rates of up to 20%, but in North America the incidence remains low.[42,43] Sonographic findings include biliary ductal dilatation containing sludge and stones within one or more segments of the liver. Longstanding stasis and inflammation often leads to severe atrophy and cirrhosis of the affected segment. In addition, there is an increased risk of cholangiocarcinoma.

HIV cholangiopathy could be considered a subset of both acute bacterial and sclerosing cholangitis; this can be associated with opportunistic infections, such as cryptosporidium or cytomegalovirus in patients with advanced disease. Sonographic findings include findings of biliary ductal

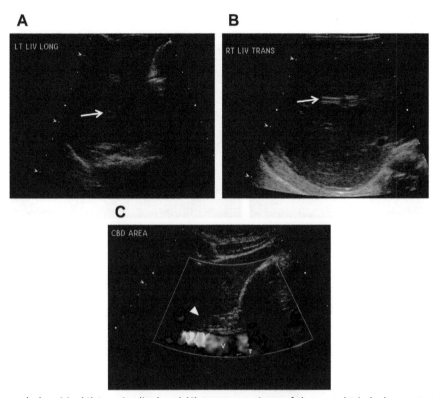

Fig. 26. Acute cholangitis. (*A*) Longitudinal and (*B*) transverse views of the portal triads demonstrate increased echogenicity about the portal triads and the "double barrel" appearance of the portal vein and enlarged adjacent bile duct (*arrow*). The wall of the bile duct demonstrates circumferential thickening. (*C*) Color Doppler image at the level of the porta hepatis showing the markedly thickened common bile duct wall (*arrowhead*), which is also dilated. Portal vein (V). This patient presented with fever, right upper quadrant pain, and jaundice (Charcot triad).

dilatation and wall thickening.[44] The ductal dilatation is irregular demonstrating areas of focal dilatation and stricture as in PSC. The papilla of Vater is typically inflamed and can be seen as an echogenic nodule in the distal common bile duct.[45]

The final infectious cause that will be discussed is ascariasis, a parasitic roundworm. This entity, like recurrent pyogenic cholangitis, is exceedingly rare in the United States compared to other parts of the world. Of the 1.4 billion cases globally, only approximately 4 million are diagnosed in the United States and many of these individuals are immigrants from endemic regions.[46] The worm migrates from the small bowel into the biliary tree through the ampulla of Vater causing biliary obstruction. The imaging finding most specific to this cause is that of the worm itself. The appearance is similar to that of a biliary stent: a tubular structure composed of parallel echogenic lines within the bile ducts. The lack of a history of stent placement as well as other clinical risk factors such as immigration from an endemic region and young age should raise the suspicion for ascariasis.[46]

The overriding pathophysiology in noninfectious inflammatory biliary obstruction is chronic inflammation that leads to fibrosis and scarring. This process can be secondary to a variety of causes such as AIDS, prior surgery or trauma, choledocholithiasis, and ischemia. Biliary sclerosis has also been related to immunoglobulin G4–related systemic disease. If the cause of the inflammation cannot be identified, the process is considered to be idiopathic and is known as PSC.

PSC affects the entire biliary tree. It has a strong association with inflammatory bowel disease and occurs more frequently in men. The characteristic sonographic features of PSC are irregular, circumferential bile duct wall thickening and an overall beaded appearance of the biliary tree as a result of alternating areas of focal stricture and dilatation (**Fig. 27**). Associated findings can include choledocholithiasis and hepatic cirrhosis. Depending on the severity of cirrhosis, additional findings of portal hypertension can also be present. PSC is a common risk factor for developing cholangiocarcinoma.

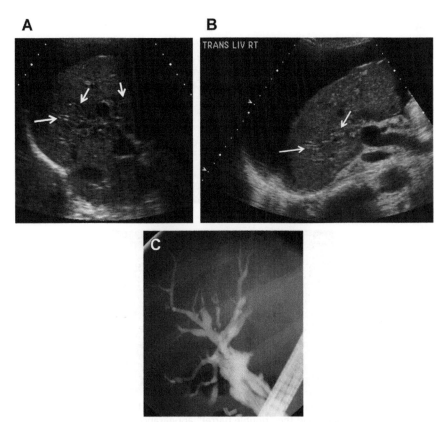

Fig. 27. PSC. (*A, B*) Ultrasound images demonstrate dilated intrahepatic bile ducts (*arrows*) that have thickened walls and an irregular beaded appearance. Findings related to the chronic sequela of PSC are seen, including cirrhosis and ascites. (*C*) An endoscopic retrograde cholangiopancreatography (ERCP) image demonstrates dilatation, stricturing, and beading of the intrahepatic bile ducts.

Hemobilia is often associated with many of the disease entities described earlier. This disorder is commonly due to iatrogenic biliary trauma related to biliary procedures and liver biopsies and can also occur spontaneously in patients on anticoagulation, underlying coagulopathy, or vascular malformations. Blood within the biliary system is similar in appearance to hemorrhage and thrombus elsewhere in the body. Depending on the acuity of the bleeding, the blood could be primarily hypoechoic with low-level echoes (acute hemorrhage) or heterogeneously echogenic with areas of retraction (chronic thrombus).

BILIARY TRACT MALIGNANCIES

- Primary gallbladder carcinoma makes up 98% of gallbladder malignancy
- Cholangiocarcinoma classified by location within the biliary tree
- Ultrasound alone is usually inadequate to diagnose cholangiocarcinoma; additional imaging is required

Neoplasms that cause biliary obstruction can either be extrinsic or intrinsic. Extrinsic neoplasms include pancreatic, duodenal (particularly ampullary), and regional metastatic disease and can involve the bile duct. The characteristic appearance of a malignant stricture is an abrupt caliber change from a proximally dilated bile duct to a stenotic or often nonvisualized distal bile duct. Ultrasound is generally not the optimum modality to identify and fully evaluate the primary tumor and extent of disease, so an additional modality, such as CT or MR imaging, is required to complete the workup.

The incidence of intrinsic biliary tract malignancies has increased in recent years, with an estimated 9810 new cases in 2012, not accounting for intrahepatic ductal malignancies, which are reported together with primary hepatic cancer.[47] Although this incidence is lower in comparison with the other major cancers such as colon, breast, and prostate, biliary cancers are highly fatal due to the typically advanced stage at the time of presentation.

Cholangiocarcinoma is the primary malignancy of the biliary tree. It is associated with recurrent biliary tract infections and chronic inflammatory conditions, most notably PSC. It is more common in older patients with a peak incidence in the 8th decade of life.[1] Cholangiocarcinoma is classified by its location along the biliary tree. The most common location is in the perihilar region (Klatskin tumor), followed by distal bile ducts and finally intrahepatic[48] [see "Liver and Spleen" by Drs Srivastava and Beland in this issue for more on intrahepatic cholangiocarcinoma]. Sonographic findings are nonspecific and include biliary dilatation, thickening of the bile duct walls, which can be diffuse or focal, and intrahepatic masses that follow the normal branching of the biliary tree (Fig. 28).

Gallbladder carcinoma, primarily adenocarcinoma, accounts for 98% of all gallbladder malignancies.[49] It is more common in women by 3:1 and occurs more frequently in older patients with an average age at presentation of 72 years.[49]

Gallbladder carcinoma presents most frequently as an irregular mass that replaces the gallbladder, often blending into the background liver. It can also present as diffuse irregular gallbladder wall thickening or as a focal polypoid mass that demonstrates internal vascularity (Fig. 29, Video 3). Calcification can be present within the gallbladder wall, within the tumor, or coexistent gallstones may be present.

Although ultrasound may be the initial modality that raises the suspicion of biliary tract malignancy, CT or MR imaging will generally be required to evaluate the extent of disease.

CHOLEDOCHAL CYSTS

Congenital cystic dilatation of the biliary tree is most commonly seen in individuals of East Asian descent.[50,51] The Todani classification system breaks the cysts down by appearance (Table 1).[52] The Type I cysts are the most common and defined as typically diffuse or focal segmental

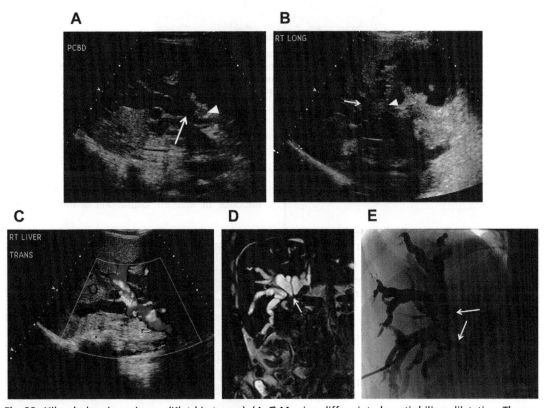

Fig. 28. Hilar cholangiocarcinoma (Klatskin tumor). (A–C) Massive, diffuse intrahepatic biliary dilatation. The central intrahepatic bile ducts come to an abrupt end (arrow) at the site of a vague, isoechoic mass at the hilum (arrowhead), adjacent to the main portal vein (V). T2-weighted axial MR image (D) and fluoroscopic spot image from a percutaneous cholangiogram (E) further demonstrate the characteristic malignant stricture (arrows) and massive proximal intrahepatic biliary dilatation. The patient was inoperable and nodularity along the gallbladder raised the suspicion of gallbladder carcinoma, but brushings from the ERCP confirmed cholangiocarcinoma.

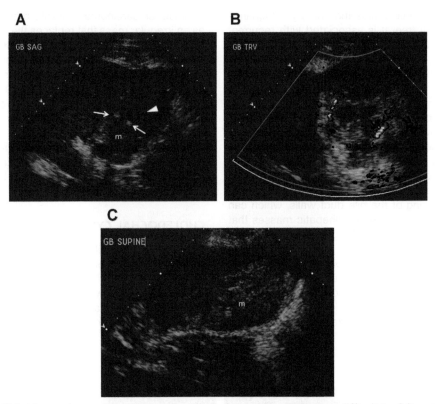

Fig. 29. Gallbladder carcinoma. (*A*) Invasive mass (M) replacing the gallbladder, difficult to delineate from the adjacent liver. Central hypoechoic region represents necrosis (*arrowhead*). Internal calcifications (*arrows*). (*B*) Color Doppler image of the same patient demonstrates the internal vascularity of the mass. (*C*) Different patient. Heterogeneous mass (M) filling the gallbladder lumen. Pathology confirmed gallbladder carcinoma.

dilatation of the common bile duct (**Fig. 30**). Type II cysts are true diverticula of the common bile duct. Type III cysts, choledochoceles, are dilatation limited to the intraduodenal segment of the common bile duct. Type IVa cysts appear as multiple saccular or fusiform dilatations of the intra- and

Table 1
Choledochal cysts

Type I (most common)	Diffuse or focal dilatation of the common bile duct (CBD)
Type II	Diverticulum of the CBD
Type III	Choledochocele—localized fusiform dilatation of the distal CBD
Type IVa	Multiple dilatations of the intra- and extrahepatic ducts
Type IVb	Multiple dilatations of the extrahepatic duct
Type V	Caroli disease—multiple dilatations of the intrahepatic ducts

Data from Todani T, Watanabe Y, Narusue M, et al. Congenital bile duct cysts: classification, operative procedures, and review of thirty-seven cases including cancer arising from choledochal cyst. Am J Surg 1977;134(2): 263–9; with permission.

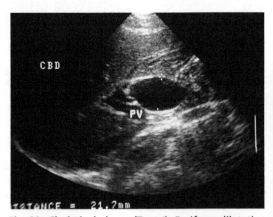

Fig. 30. Choledochal cyst (Type I). Fusiform dilatation of the common bile duct (*cursors*). PV, portal vein. (*Courtesy of* D. Warshauer, MD, Chapel Hill, NC.)

extrahepatic ducts. Type IVb cysts are multiple saccular or fusiform dilatations of only the extrahepatic ducts. There is an associated risk of cholangiocarcinoma.

Type V cysts, also known as Caroli disease, represent a pathogenesis that is different from the other choledochal cysts. The appearance of Type V cysts is similar to that of Type IV, but the multiple saccular and fusiform dilatations are isolated to the intrahepatic ducts.

SUMMARY

Ultrasound has been and will continue to be the modality of choice for initial evaluation of the gallbladder and biliary tree. This is due to its low cost, fast acquisition time, and portability as well as diagnostic accuracy with regards to the most common indication for evaluation, right upper quadrant pain. Although many of the sonographic findings for other diseases along the biliary tract are nonspecific, when combined with clinical history, risk factors, and adjunct CT and MR imaging when indicated, it can often help to make or at least confirm the diagnosis.

SUPPLEMENTARY DATA

Supplementary data related to this article can be found online at http://dx.doi.org/10.1016/j.cult. 2014.07.009.

REFERENCES

1. Rumack CM, Wilson SR, Charboneau JW. Diagnostic ultrasound. 3rd edition. St Louis (MO): Elsevier Mosby; 2004.
2. Handler SJ. Ultrasound of gallbladder wall thickening and its relation to cholecystitis. AJR Am J Roentgenol 1979;132(4):581–5.
3. Puente SG, Bannura GC. Radiological anatomy of the biliary tract: variations and congenital abnormalities. World J Surg 1983;7(2):271–6.
4. Russell E, Yrizzary JM, Montalvo BM, et al. Left hepatic duct anatomy: implications. Radiology 1990; 174(2):353–6.
5. Bressler EL, Rubin JM, McCracken S. Sonographic parallel channel sign: a reappraisal. Radiology 1987;164(2):343–6.
6. Parulekar SG. Ultrasound evaluation of common bile duct size. Radiology 1979;133(3 Pt 1):703–7.
7. Bowie JD. What is the upper limit of normal for the common bile duct on ultrasound: how much do you want it to be? Am J Gastroenterol 2000; 95(4):897–900.
8. Benjaminov F, Leichtman G, Naftali T, et al. Effects of age and cholecystectomy on common bile duct

9. diameter as measured by endoscopic ultrasonography. Surg Endosc 2013;27(1):303–7.
9. Murphy JB, Hospital M. Surgical clinics of John B. Chicago: Murphy at Mercy Hospital; 1913.
10. Good LI, Edell SL, Soloway RD, et al. Ultrasonic properties of gallstones. Effect of stone size and composition. Gastroenterology 1979;77(2):258–63.
11. Ko CW, Sekijima JH, Lee SP. Biliary sludge. Ann Intern Med 1999;130(4 Pt 1):301–11.
12. Ko CW, Lee SP. Gastrointestinal disorders of the critically ill. Biliary sludge and cholecystitis. Best Pract Res Clin Gastroenterol 2003;17(3):383–96.
13. Ko CW, Beresford SA, Schulte SJ, et al. Incidence, natural history, and risk factors for biliary sludge and stones during pregnancy. Hepatology 2005; 41(2):359–65.
14. Krishnan M, Middleton WD. Ultrasonographic evaluation of right upper quadrant pain in emergency departments. Ultrasound Clin 2011;6(2):149–61.
15. Ralls PW, Colletti PM, Lapin SA, et al. Real-time sonography in suspected acute cholecystitis. Prospective evaluation of primary and secondary signs. Radiology 1985;155(3):767–71.
16. Simeone JF, Brink JA, Mueller PR, et al. The sonographic diagnosis of acute gangrenous cholecystitis: importance of the Murphy sign. AJR Am J Roentgenol 1989;152(2):289–90.
17. Bree RL. Further observations on the usefulness of the sonographic Murphy sign in the evaluation of suspected acute cholecystitis. J Clin Ultrasound 1995;23(3):169–72.
18. Shea JA, Berlin JA, Escarce JJ, et al. Revised estimates of diagnostic test sensitivity and specificity in suspected biliary tract disease. Arch Intern Med 1994;154(22):2573–81.
19. Fagan SP, Awad SS, Rahwan K, et al. Prognostic factors for the development of gangrenous cholecystitis. Am J Surg 2003;186(5):481–5.
20. Stefanidis D, Sirinek KR, Bingener J. Gallbladder perforation: risk factors and outcome. J Surg Res 2006;131(2):204–8.
21. Teefey SA, Baron RL, Bigler SA. Sonography of the gallbladder: significance of striated (layered) thickening of the gallbladder wall. AJR Am J Roentgenol 1991;156(5):945–7.
22. Teefey SA, Dahiya N, Middleton WD, et al. Acute cholecystitis: do sonographic findings and WBC count predict gangrenous changes? AJR Am J Roentgenol 2013;200(2):363–9.
23. Soyer P, Brouland JP, Boudiaf M, et al. Color velocity imaging and power Doppler sonography of the gallbladder wall: a new look at sonographic diagnosis of acute cholecystitis. AJR Am J Roentgenol 1998;171(1):183–8.
24. Tessler FN, Tublin ME. Blood flow in healthy gallbladder walls on color and power Doppler sonography: effect of wall thickness and

gallbladder volume. AJR Am J Roentgenol 1999; 173(5):1247–9.

25. Draghi F, Ferrozzi G, Calliada F, et al. Power Doppler ultrasound of gallbladder wall vascularization in inflammation: clinical implications. Eur Radiol 2000;10(10):1587–90.

26. Parra JA, Acinas O, Bueno J, et al. Xanthogranulomatous cholecystitis: clinical, sonographic, and CT findings in 26 patients. AJR Am J Roentgenol 2000;174(4):979–83.

27. Shetty GS, Abbey P, Prabhu SM, et al. Xanthogranulomatous cholecystitis: sonographic and CT features and differentiation from gallbladder carcinoma: a pictorial essay. Jpn J Radiol 2012;30(6):480–5.

28. Juttner HU, Ralls PW, Quinn MF, et al. Thickening of the gallbladder wall in acute hepatitis: ultrasound demonstration. Radiology 1982;142(2):465–6.

29. Suk KT, Kim CH, Baik SK, et al. Gallbladder wall thickening in patients with acute hepatitis. J Clin Ultrasound 2009;37(3):144–8.

30. Opatrny L. Porcelain gallbladder. CMAJ 2002; 166(7):933.

31. Stephen AE, Berger DL. Carcinoma in the porcelain gallbladder: a relationship revisited. Surgery 2001;129(6):699–703.

32. Corwin MT, Siewert B, Sheiman RG, et al. Incidentally detected gallbladder polyps: is follow-up necessary?–long-term clinical and US analysis of 346 patients. Radiology 2011;258(1):277–82.

33. Donald G, Sunjaya D, Donahue T, et al. Polyp on ultrasound: now what? The association between gallbladder polyps and cancer. Am Surg 2013;79(10):1005–8.

34. Ito H, Hann LE, D'Angelica M, et al. Polypoid lesions of the gallbladder: diagnosis and followup. J Am Coll Surg 2009;208(4):570–5.

35. Nguyen MS, Voci S. Adenomyomatosis. Ultrasound Q 2013;29(3):215–7.

36. Topal B, Van de Moortel M, Fieuws S, et al. The value of magnetic resonance cholangiopancreatography in predicting common bile duct stones in patients with gallstone disease. Br J Surg 2003;90(1):42–7.

37. Varghese JC, Liddell RP, Farrell MA, et al. The diagnostic accuracy of magnetic resonance cholangiopancreatography and ultrasound compared with direct cholangiography in the detection of choledocholithiasis. Clin Radiol 1999;54(9):604–14.

38. Mandelia A, Gupta AK, Verma DK, et al. The Value of magnetic resonance cholangio-pancreatography

(MRCP) in the detection of choledocholithiasis. J Clin Diagn Res 2013;7(9):1941–5.

39. Wong HP, Chiu YL, Shiu BH, et al. Preoperative MRCP to detect choledocholithiasis in acute calculous cholecystitis. J Hepatobiliary Pancreat Sci 2012;19(4):458–64.

40. Beltran MA. Mirizzi syndrome: history, current knowledge and proposal of a simplified classification. World J Gastroenterol 2012;18(34):4639–50.

41. Csendes A, Diaz JC, Burdiles P, et al. Risk factors and classification of acute suppurative cholangitis. Br J Surg 1992;79(7):655–8.

42. Tabrizian P, Jibara G, Shrager B, et al. Hepatic resection for primary hepatolithiasis: a single-center Western experience. J Am Coll Surg 2012;215(5):622–6.

43. Liu CL, Fan ST, Wong J. Primary biliary stones: diagnosis and management. World J Surg 1998; 22(11):1162–6.

44. Tonolini M, Bianco R. HIV-related/AIDS cholangiopathy: pictorial review with emphasis on MRCP findings and differential diagnosis. Clin Imaging 2013; 37(2):219–26.

45. Da Silva F, Boudghene F, Lecomte I, et al. Sonography in AIDS-related cholangitis: prevalence and cause of an echogenic nodule in the distal end of the common bile duct. AJR Am J Roentgenol 1993;160(6):1205–7.

46. Khuroo MS. Ascariasis. Gastroenterol Clin North Am 1996;25(3):553–77.

47. Siegel R, Naishadham D, Jemal A. Cancer statistics, 2012. CA Cancer J Clin 2012;62(1):10–29.

48. Nakeeb A, Pitt HA, Sohn TA, et al. Cholangiocarcinoma. A spectrum of intrahepatic, perihilar, and distal tumors. Ann Surg 1996;224(4):463–73 [discussion: 473–5].

49. Levy AD, Murakata LA, Rohrmann CA Jr. Gallbladder carcinoma: radiologic-pathologic correlation. Radiographics 2001;21(2):295–314 [questionnaire: 549–55].

50. Sato M, Ishida H, Konno K, et al. Choledochal cyst due to anomalous pancreatobiliary junction in the adult: sonographic findings. Abdom Imaging 2001;26(4):395–400.

51. de Vries JS, de Vries S, Aronson DC, et al. Choledochal cysts: age of presentation, symptoms, and late complications related to Todani's classification. J Pediatr Surg 2002;37(11):1568–73.

52. Todani T, Watanabe Y, Narusue M, et al. Congenital bile duct cysts: classification, operative procedures, and review of thirty-seven cases including cancer arising from choledochal cyst. Am J Surg 1977;134(2):263–9.

Doppler Ultrasound of the Liver, Portal Hypertension, and Transjugular Intrahepatic Portosystemic Shunts

Melissa Davis, MD, Wui K. Chong, MBBS, FRCR*

KEYWORDS

- Doppler ultrasound • Portal hypertension • Portal vein thrombosis • Budd-Chiari syndrome
- Right heart failure • TIPS

KEY POINTS

- Doppler ultrasound is more than 90% accurate for diagnosing portal and hepatic vein thrombosis and is the screening modality for evaluating transjugular intrahepatic portosystemic shunt patency.
- Doppler findings in portal vein stenosis include turbulence, high velocity at the site of stenosis, and poststenotic dilatation.
- Portal venous thrombosis results from stagnant flow due to portal hypertension, neoplasms, or inflammation in organs drained by the portal circulation, such as the pancreas, and hypercoagulable states may cause portal venous thrombus.
- Normal portal venous flow is always unidirectional (hepatopetal or toward the liver). Normal hepatic venous flow has forward and reversed components.
- Ultrasound can accurately diagnose portal hypertension. Portal hypertension leads to reduction in hepatopetal portal venous flow, and diversion of blood into porto-systemic collaterals, changes that can be detected with Doppler.

 Videos of Color Doppler scan of the liver accompany this article at http://www.ultrasound.theclinics.com/

INTRODUCTION

Doppler ultrasound is the first-line modality for imaging a wide range of liver disease. It is quick, can be performed portably, and has no adverse effects. Flow velocity and direction in the hepatic arteries, hepatic veins, and portal and splenic veins are evaluated. It is the study of choice for evaluating portal hypertension. Color (and power) Doppler ultrasound is more than 90% accurate for diagnosing portal and hepatic vein thrombosis.[1]

Liver disease, vascular obstruction, or congestive heart failure leads to alterations in hemodynamics that can be detected with hepatic Doppler ultrasound. In this article, we review normal hepatic waveforms and how they are altered in the setting of portal hypertension, congestive cardiac failure, and portal vein pathology. We also discuss the

Disclosure: None.
Radiology, University of North Carolina, 101 Manning Drive, Chapel Hill, NC 27599-7510, USA
* Corresponding author.
E-mail address: wk_chong@med.unc.edu

Ultrasound Clin 9 (2014) 587–604
http://dx.doi.org/10.1016/j.cult.2014.07.001

evaluation of and potential complications involving transjugular intrahepatic portosystemic shunts (TIPS).

DOPPLER ULTRASOUND TECHNIQUE

The Doppler Effect is the change in frequency of a reflected wave from a moving object. An increase in frequency is seen if the object is moving toward the observer, whereas a decrease in frequency occurs if the source is moving away. Frequency shift translates into blood velocity, allowing depiction of flow in the hepatic vasculature.[2]

A 2-MHz to 5-MHz probe is typically used for evaluating the hepatic vasculature. A lower frequency can be used in larger patients to increase penetration. The left lobe of the liver is evaluated through a subcostal approach. The right lobe can also be evaluated subcostally or by an intercostal approach, with the patient in the right anterior oblique position.

In patients with portal hypertension, the following should be assessed:

- Echotexture of the liver parenchyma for signs of cirrhosis and masses. The contour of the liver is evaluated for nodularity. This is best seen by using a linear high-frequency transducer focused on the liver surface.
- Patency and flow direction in the hepatic artery, and portal, splenic, and superior mesenteric and hepatic veins.
- Size of the hepatic artery, portal vein, and hepatic veins.
- Doppler waveforms from the right, left, and main portal veins, and right, middle, and left hepatic veins. Angle-corrected velocities are obtained from the main portal vein.
- Spleen size (longitudinal diameter and/or cross-sectional area).
- Presence or absence of porto-systemic collateral vessels.
- Presence or absence of ascites.
- Assessment of respiratory variation of the diameter of splenic vein and superior mesenteric vein (SMV).

Flow in the portal venous system may be slow or stagnant in portal hypertension. Doppler parameters should therefore be optimized to detect small frequency shifts. A small velocity range, setting the focal zone to the level of the portal vein, using a small Doppler angle and color box, minimizing the wall filter, and reducing the distance from transducer to the portal vein as much as possible will increase sensitivity to slow flow.

HEPATIC ARTERIES

Approximately 25% of the liver's blood supply comes from the proper hepatic artery.[3] The proper hepatic artery courses left of the bile duct and anterior to the portal vein, dividing into the left and right hepatic arteries in the hepatic hilum. At the hilum, the hepatic artery is posterior to the common hepatic duct.

The normal hepatic artery has a low-resistance waveform with forward flow throughout the cardiac cycle. The normal hepatic artery resistive index is 0.5 to 0.7 (**Fig. 1**). Velocities within the hepatic artery range between 30 and 60 cm/s[2].

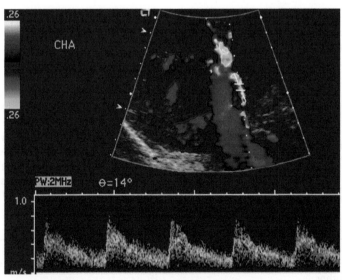

Fig. 1. Normal common hepatic artery spectral Doppler evaluation. The hepatic artery is the multicolored vessel over which the Doppler cursor is placed. The portal vein (*red*) lies adjacent. The hepatic artery has a low-resistance waveform with forward flow throughout the cardiac cycle.

The resistive index of the hepatic artery ranges between 0.5 and 0.7. A high-resistance waveform is nonspecific, but can be found in advanced cirrhosis, severe parenchymal liver disease, hepatic congestion, hepatic venous obstruction, or diffuse microvascular disease (**Fig. 2**). A high-resistance waveform also can be found in a healthy postprandial individual or in advanced age. A low-resistance waveform can be seen if there is a proximal stenosis in the celiac or common hepatic arteries or at the site of the hepatic artery anastomosis in a transplant (**Fig. 3**). It also may be found in advanced cirrhosis or in arteriovenous shunting.

A normal artery has a narrow range of velocities at any particular point, causing the Doppler spectrum to appear as a line with a clear space beneath. Spectral broadening is a term used to describe widening of the spectral bandwidth due to increase in the velocity range. The spectral window is consequently obliterated. A broad spectral window is a sign of turbulent flow, and is found distal to a stenosis.

A tardus-parvus (late and low) waveform is a low-amplitude arterial waveform with a prolonged systolic rise. It implies a proximal stenosis in the hepatic artery (see **Fig. 3**). The acceleration time is prolonged (>80 ms) and the acceleration index or slope of the systolic rise is reduced. It is associated with a low resistive index (<0.5).[4]

PORTAL VENOUS SYSTEM

The portal venous system drains the gastrointestinal tract, pancreas, spleen, and biliary tree. It empties via the main portal vein, which supplies 70% of the blood flow to the liver.[3] Blood from the hepatic artery and portal vein flows through the hepatic sinusoids, and empties into the central vein of each lobule. The central veins coalesce into the hepatic veins, which drain into the inferior vena cava. Portal hypertension results if there is obstruction at any point in this process.

The main portal vein is formed by the union of the superior mesenteric and splenic veins. This vessel courses posterior to the common bile duct and proper hepatic artery to divide into the left and right portal veins at the hepatic hilum. The normal portal vein is less than 13 mm in diameter. The normal portal vein flow is hepatopetal, with a velocity of 20 to 33 cm per second, but there is considerable variation in the peak velocity in a healthy population. Transmitted cardiac pulsation causes the portal vein to have a mildly pulsatile waveform, but unlike the hepatic veins, flow is never retrograde at any point in the cardiac cycle (**Fig. 4**). Portal vein velocity increases postprandially and in the supine position. Flow in the extrahepatic portal vein is laminar, but helical flow can be seen as it enters the porta hepatis (**Fig. 5**). When flow is helical, it can be confused with slow or retrograde flow. Although it can be a normal finding, helical flow is more frequently associated with portal hypertension, after liver transplantation, or following TIPS placement.[5]

Portal Vein Gas

Portal venous gas is associated with bowel ischemia, inflammation (including appendicitis and diverticulitis), and sepsis. It is also seen in benign conditions, such as intestinal pneumatosis or after endoscopy. Gas appears as intraluminal strongly echogenic foci that move with the blood (**Fig. 6**). It generates a characteristic "spiky" artifact on the Doppler spectrum consisting of intermittent strong signals that extend over the baseline, superimposed on the normal venous waveform.

PORTAL VEIN STENOSIS

Portal vein stenosis can be caused by pancreatic enlargement by tumor or inflammation encroaching on the vein, postsurgical stenosis, or anastomotic stenosis in a patient after transplantation. Doppler findings in portal vein stenosis include turbulent, poststenotic flow on color Doppler imaging and poststenotic dilatation on gray-scale ultrasound. Spectral Doppler imaging shows elevated peak systolic velocity (**Fig. 7**).

Congestive Cardiac Failure

As in the hepatic veins, in congestive heart failure increased cardiac pulsatility is transmitted to the

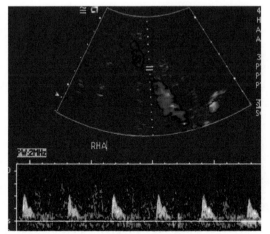

Fig. 2. Right hepatic artery showing a high-resistance waveform. There is no flow in diastole.

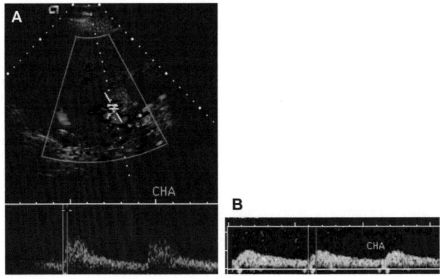

Fig. 3. (A) Normal common hepatic artery waveform and (B) tardus-parvus waveform. Note that the tardus par-vus waveform has a prolonged acceleration time (marked by the *white* and *green vertical lines*) compared with the normal waveform.

portal veins. This causes a characteristic Doppler waveform with accentuated pulsatility and cyclical retrograde flow. This waveform also is seen in tricuspid regurgitation and hypervolemic states, such as hereditary hemorrhagic telangiectasia.

Portal Hypertension

Normal portal vein pressures range from 5 to 10 mm Hg. Portal vein hypertension is defined as venous pressure higher than 10 mm Hg.[5] Portal hypertension is usually a sequel of chronic liver disease, but can occur in fulminant liver failure.

Doppler ultrasound is highly accurate for evalu-ating sequelae of portal hypertension and

identifying the cause. The liver is evaluated for the presence of cirrhosis. A cirrhotic liver has a nodular contour and heterogeneous echotexture. The liver may be large in the early stages of cirrhosis, but it is small in advanced cirrhosis. If cirrhosis is present, splenomegaly is a strong indi-cator of portal hypertension. The spleen is consid-ered enlarged if the maximum longitudinal diameter is greater than 12 cm or maximum cross-sectional area is greater than 45 cm.[6]

In portal hypertension, the diameter of the portal vein increases and velocity falls (Fig. 8). Portal vein diameter increases to 1.3 cm or greater.[7,8] Normal portal vein velocity is 20 to 30 cm per sec-ond and low velocities are a specific indicator of

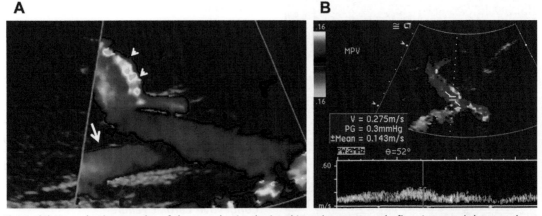

Fig. 4. (A) Normal color Doppler of the portal vein, depicted in red, as antegrade flow is toward the transducer. The IVC (*arrow*) is in blue, and the hepatic artery (*arrowheads*) lies superficial to the portal vein. (B) Normal spec-tral Doppler demonstrates gentle pulsatility with antegrade flow throughout the cardiac cycle.

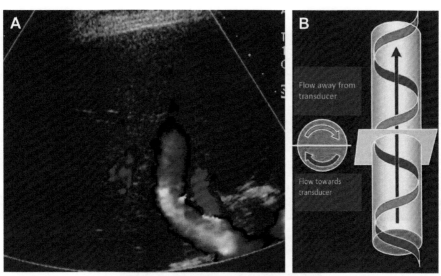

Fig. 5. (A) Color Doppler of helical portal venous flow at the hepatic hilum. Flow is antegrade, but appears as alternating red and blue spiral bands (B). This appearance should not be confused with hepatofugal flow.

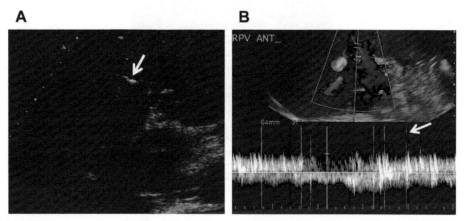

Fig. 6. (A) Portal vein gas. Strongly echogenic linear shadowing foci (arrow) in the portal vein. (B) Bidirectional spike artifacts on Doppler spectrum (arrow).

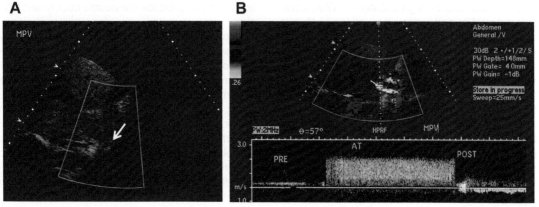

Fig. 7. (A) Gray-scale ultrasound demonstrates focal stenosis in the portal vein (arrow) and post stenotic dilatation. (B) Spectral Doppler imaging demonstrates a velocity step-up of greater than 3:1 when comparing poststenosis with prestenosis velocity.

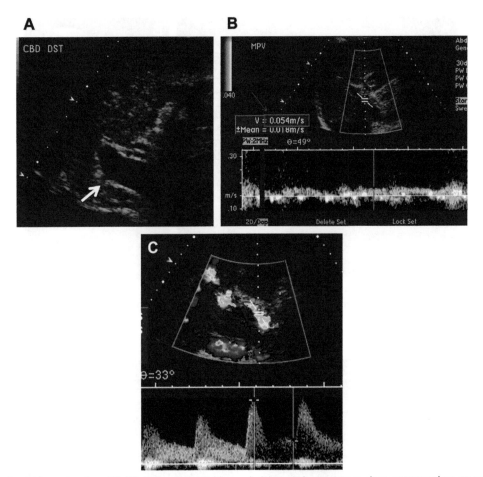

Fig. 8. Portal hypertension. (*A*) Dilated portal vein (*arrow*). (*B*) Doppler spectrum demonstrates slow, to-and-fro flow in the portal vein with a maximum velocity of 5.4 cm/s. (*C*) Hypertrophied hepatic artery in portal hypertension. The hepatic artery is the multicolored vessel superficial to the portal vein (*red*). Doppler spectrum confirms arterial waveform.

portal hypertension. However, normal portal vein velocities can sometimes be found in the presence of portal hypertension if the portal circulation is decompressed through collaterals. With worsening portal hypertension, flow slows until it is almost stagnant with barely perceptible movement forward or reverse (to and fro flow, **Fig. 8B**). Slow to and fro flow can be mistaken for thrombosis. Distinguishing slow flow from thrombus can be optimized by using the appropriate Doppler settings, such as a low wall filter. Eventually flow reverses (hepatofugal) and hepatofugal flow is a sign of severe portal vein hypertension (**Fig. 9**). Portal hypertension is associated with increased hepatic and splenic artery resistance (measured by Resistive or Pulsatility Index).There is increased flow in the hepatic artery in portal hypertension and the artery may become enlarged. This is presumably a compensatory response to reduction in portal venous flow. The enlarged

hepatic artery is apparent on color Doppler (see **Fig. 8C**). On the gray-scale image, dilated hepatic artery branches may be mistaken for biliary dilatation, as it can produce the double duct or shotgun sign.

Hepato-renal syndrome is renal insufficiency caused by arterial vasoconstriction due to activation of the renin-angiotensin-aldosterone catecholamine pathways in the setting of portal hypertension.[9] An increase in renal artery Resistive Index to greater than 0.70 is associated with development of hepato-renal syndrome.[10]

Cirrhosis causes the liver to become less compliant. It becomes less responsive to cardiac pulsation and as a result the hepatic vein waveform flattens. There is loss of respiratory variation in the caliber of the SMV and splenic veins (**Box 1**).

The causes of portal hypertension can be classified into intrahepatic, prehepatic, and posthepatic based on the location of the obstruction.

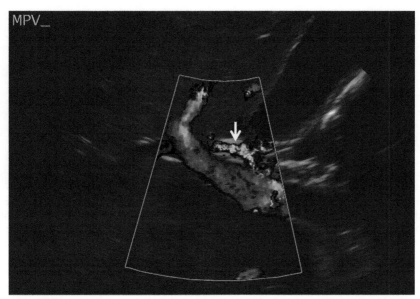

Fig. 9. Hepatopetal portal vein flow, shown in blue indicative of the most severe stage of portal hypertension. It is also seen in fulminant hepatic failure. The multicolored vessel (*arrow*) superficial to the portal vein is the hepatic artery.

Prehepatic portal hypertension is obstruction at the level of the portal vein and its branches. Causes include portal vein thrombosis, stenosis, or extrinsic compression. Schistosomiasis causes obstruction at the presinusoidal level. Worldwide, it is one of the commonest causes of portal hypertension. Schistosomiasis is a parasitic infection caused by the *Schistosoma* trematode, several species of which affect the gastrointestinal tract.[11]

Schistosoma mansoni is found in Africa, the Middle East, the Caribbean, and South America. *Schistosoma japonicum* and *Schistosoma mekongi* are found in Asia. In intestinal schistosomiasis, the worm resides in the mesenteric venules. It releases eggs that are carried within the portal circulation where they lodge in the portal venules. The eggs incite a granulomatous inflammatory reaction, leading to periportal fibrosis and obstruction to portal flow. This periportal fibrosis has a magnetic resonance appearance of a tortoise shell. On ultrasound, this fibrosis can be seen as increased periportal echogenicity (**Fig. 10**).[12] Other causes of presinusoidal obstruction are hepatic fibrosis and sarcoidosis.

In developed countries, most cases of portal hypertension are due to *intrahepatic* disease, of which cirrhosis is the commonest. Cirrhosis leads to bridging fibrosis that causes increased resistance to flow in the hepatic sinusoids. It is a major cause of morbidity and mortality in the United States. Hepatitis C virus leads to cirrhosis in up to 80% of those infected and along with alcohol, is the commonest cause of cirrhosis in the United States.[13] The virus is bloodborne and highly associated with intravenous drug use.[14–16] Nonalcoholic fatty liver disease is the fastest growing cause in the United States. It has a high association with obesity and hypertriglyceridemia. Fat deposition within the hepatocytes cause inflammation and fibrosis, which can eventually lead to cirrhosis.

Box 1
Sonographic features of portal hypertension

- Initially there is slow (<20 cm/s) hepatopetal flow in the MPV; stagnant and hepatofugal flow is seen with progression.
- Enlarged hepatic artery
- Enlarged portal vein greater than 1.3 cm
- Splenomegaly: greater than 12 cm longitudinal diameter or greater than 45 cm² maximum cross-sectional area
- Ascites
- Varices: gastroesophageal, splenic
- Portosystemic collaterals: recanalized umbilical vein, coronary vein
- Monophasic waveforms in the hepatic veins
- Increased resistive index in hepatic and splenic arteries

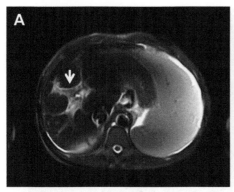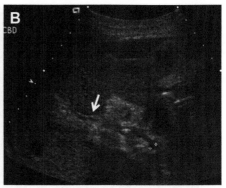

Fig. 10. Hepatic schistosomiasis. (A) Magnetic resonance image, T2-weighted half-Fourier acquisition single-shot turbo spin-echo sequence showing high signal bands (*arrow*) in the liver representing periportal fibrosis (called the tortoiseshell liver), and splenomegaly. (B) Periportal echogenic band caused by fibrosis (*arrow*) surrounds stenosed portal vein (calipers).

Primary biliary cirrhosis is an autoimmune disease characterized by the progressive destruction of biliary ducts. Over time there is a toxic build-up of bile material within the liver that leads to hepatic scarring, fibrosis, and eventually cirrhosis.[17]

Posthepatic portal hypertension is caused by obstruction at the level of the hepatic veins (Budd-Chiari syndrome) or the inferior vena cava (IVC).

Portal vein thrombosis

Stagnant portal venous flow from portal hypertension can cause portal vein thrombosis. Thrombosis also may result from neoplasms that obstruct portal venous flow, such as pancreatic carcinoma and cholangiocarcinoma. Inflammation in organs drained by the portal circulation, such as acute pancreatitis or diverticulitis, and hypercoagulable states may cause portal venous thrombus. The latter conditions include dehydration, prothrombotic states, myoproliferative disorders, and the oral contraceptive pill. Thrombus due to hepatocellular carcinoma (HCC) is unusual. HCC has a predilection for directly invading the portal veins, thus creating a thrombus composed of tumor rather than clot.

On gray-scale imaging, acute thrombus may appear as a filling defect within the vein lumen (**Fig. 11**). The thrombus may partially or completely occlude the lumen. In acute thrombosis, the thrombus is hypoechoic and the vein appears enlarged.[4] The thrombus is visible only as a filling defect with color or Power Doppler imaging. Retrograde filling of the portal vein branches from collateral vessels may be seen (**Fig. 12**).

As the thrombus fibroses, it becomes more echogenic and the vein may appear normal or small in caliber (**Fig. 13**). Cavernous transformation is the formation of collateral venous channels secondary to portal vein thrombus. These appear as tortuous hypoechoic vessels traveling within the echogenic bed of the thrombosed portal vein

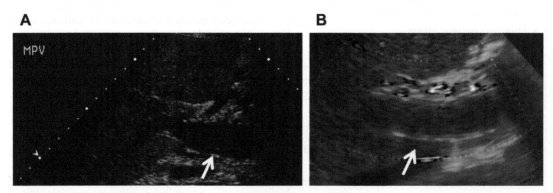

Fig. 11. (A) Visible thrombus (*arrow*) in the portal vein on a gray-scale image in the main portal vein. (B) It is more common for acute thrombus to be anechoic. In this patient, it is only visible as absence of flow on color Doppler (*arrow*). Flow is seen in the hepatic artery superficial to the portal vein.

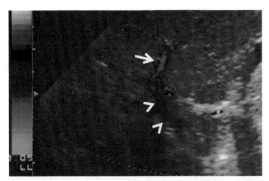

Fig. 12. Retrograde filling (*arrow*) of the left portal vein in a patient with thrombus in the main portal vein (*arrowheads*).

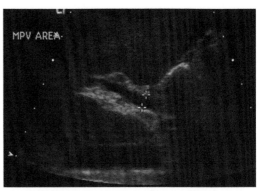

Fig. 13. In chronic portal vein thrombosis, the portal vein wall is thickened and the lumen (marked by calipers) is narrowed.

(**Fig. 14**). The venous nature of these vessels is confirmed with Doppler.

Tumor thrombus from hepatocellular carcinoma propagates fugally from peripheral portal veins closest to the tumor into the main vein (Video 1). The thrombus is characterized by having its own blood supply, which sometimes can be seen as vessels with arterial waveforms running within the thrombus (**Fig. 15**).

Varices occur at the sites of portosystemic communication. The recanalized umbilical vein arises from the left portal vein and runs in the falciform ligament inferiorly toward the umbilicus (Video 2). It then joins with systemic epigastric veins at the level of the umbilicus. It appears as a vessel with hepatofugal flow running inferiorly immediately deep to the abdominal wall (**Fig. 16**).

The coronary or left gastric vein is another route of portosystemic communication. It normally empties into the portal or splenic veins near their confluence. Its flow is reversed and the vein enlarges in portal hypertension. Varices develop where the coronary vein communicates with the systemic distal esophageal veins around the gastroesophageal junction. These are best seen posterior to the left lobe of the liver on the sagittal, midline images as tortuous tubular structures with venous flow. Another portosystemic pathway lies in the splenorenal ligament. Splenorenal varices appear as tortuous veins in the splenic hilum that can be seen to drain directly into the left renal vein (**Fig. 17**).

HEPATIC VEINS

There are 3 main hepatic veins (right, middle, and left), supplemented by a variable number of accessory veins. These converge onto the IVC on the posterior surface of the liver (**Fig. 18**). A common variant is to see the middle and left hepatic veins join before draining, as a common trunk, into the IVC.

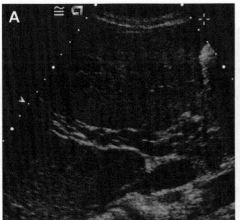
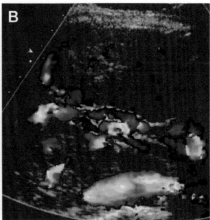

Fig. 14. Cavernous transformation. (*A*) Gray-scale images and (*B*) color Doppler images showing the portal vein replaced by tortuous collateral vessels.

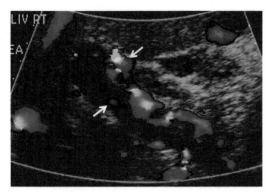

Fig. 15. Tumor thrombus. Sagittal view of main portal vein showing thrombus with internal flow (*arrow*). Hepatic artery (*yellow arrow*) is seen anterior to the thrombosed portal vein.

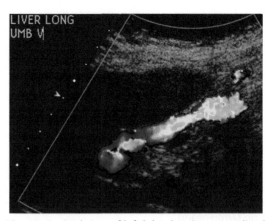

Fig. 16. Sagittal view of left lobe showing recanalized umbilical vein with hepatofugal flow toward the umbilicus.

The hepatic veins drain posteriorly into the IVC, so antegrade flow in the hepatic veins is away from the transducer (below the baseline on the Doppler spectrum). The hepatic venous waveform is triphasic, with 2 antegrade and 1 retrograde wave during each cardiac cycle. The end of atrial systole is followed by accelerating antegrade flow into the empty right atrium (S-wave). As the right atrium fills, flow is impeded and velocity is reduced. The opening of the tricuspid valve results in a rise in antegrade flow (the D-wave). When the right atrium contracts, blood is propelled forward into the right ventricle and backward into the hepatic veins, leading to the third phase: the retrograde A-wave (**Fig. 19**).[2] Note that the antegrade components (the S and D waves) are larger than the A-wave.

Change with Respiration

In addition to cardiac phasicity, the hepatic venous waveform is affected by respiration. Forward flow increases during inspiration due to negative intrathoracic pressure and is reduced during Valsalva or expiration.

Right heart failure
Right heart failure due to myocardial disease or fluid overload leads to changes in the hepatic vein waveform. The normally small A-wave becomes larger and may approach the S and D waves in amplitude (**Fig. 20**). If the tricuspid valve remains competent, the "S" and "D" waves keep their normal configuration. In tricuspid regurgitation, the S-wave disappears and becomes part of the A-wave.[4] The IVC and hepatic veins will appear enlarged. In severe cases A-wave hyperpulsatility is transmitted to the portal vein, which will show reversal of flow during the A wave (Video 3).

In cirrhosis, reduced compliance can cause a monophasic waveform in the hepatic veins (**Fig. 21**).

A

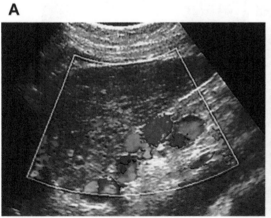

B

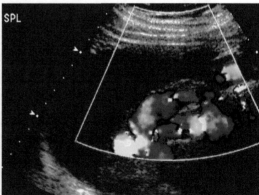

Fig. 17. (*A*) Sagittal view through left lobe showing gastroesophageal varices posterior to the liver. (*B*) Longitudinal view of spleen showing varices at the splenic hilum.

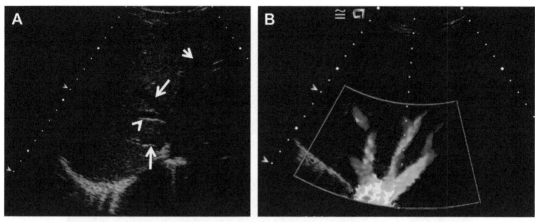

Fig. 18. (*A*) Transverse gray-scale and (*B*) color Doppler images showing the right middle and left hepatic veins (*arrows*) draining posteriorly into the IVC. An accessory vein (*arrowheads*) empties into the IVC at its junction with the middle hepatic vein.

Hepatic vein obstruction

Hepatic vein obstruction (Budd-Chiari syndrome) is most commonly caused by thrombosis in the hepatic veins or vena cava. This is most commonly due to coagulopathy (either idiopathic, pregnancy, or oral contraceptives).[18] Other causes of Budd-Chiari syndrome are obstructing membranes or extrinsic compression from liver masses.

Budd-Chiari clinically presents as hepatomegaly, ascites, and abdominal pain. Features of portal hypertension may be present.

Acute thrombus may be hypoechoic or appear as an echogenic filling defect within the hepatic vein. Doppler shows absence of flow.[4] The vein shrinks as the thrombus fibroses. Chronic thrombus may be hyperechoic or isoechoic to the liver parenchyma, resulting in the vein becoming less visible. In chronic venous obstruction, intrahepatic collateral channels develop to bypass the obstruction as a result. These appear as tortuous nonanatomic vessels with venous waveforms that meander toward the IVC,[4] and thus away from the transducer (Video 4). This is a characteristic finding of hepatic vein obstruction. These pathways can be intrahepatic or extrahepatic.

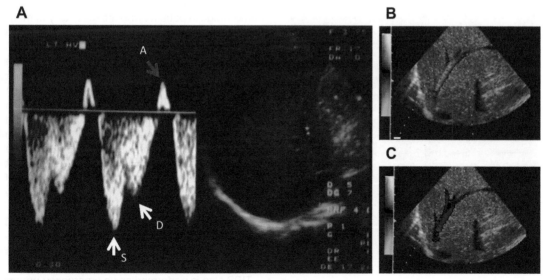

Fig. 19. (*A*) Hepatic vein Doppler waveform. Antegrade flow is away from the transducer and therefore below the baseline. It is composed of the S-wave followed by the D-wave (*white arrows*). During atrial systole, flow is reversed (A-wave [*red arrow*]). Color Doppler obtained during (*B*) ventricular systole and (*C*) atrial systole showing reversal of flow.

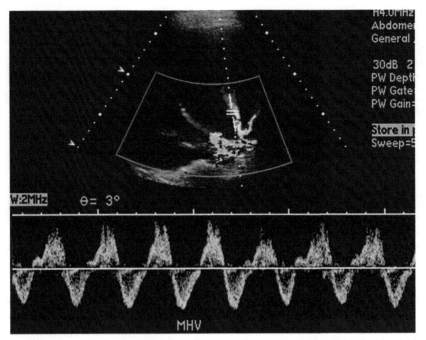

Fig. 20. Congestive cardiac failure. The Doppler spectrum shows exaggerated pulsatility, with the retrograde A-wave equal or greater than the antegrade component.

If there is partial obstruction, cardiac pulsation is attenuated, and the hepatic vein Doppler spectrum may show a monophasic waveform (**Figs. 22** and **23**).

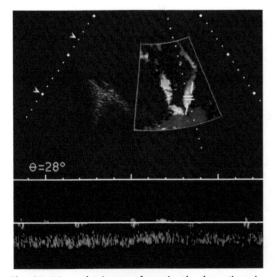

Fig. 21. Monophasic waveform in the hepatic vein. This can be seen in cirrhosis due to loss of liver compliance, as in this case (note irregular liver contour and ascites) or hepatic vein obstruction.

TRANSJUGULAR INTRAHEPATIC PORTOSYSTEMIC SHUNTS

Bleeding from esophageal varices is a serious complication of portal hypertension, with a mortality rate of more than 30%. Creation of a portosystemic shunt to decompress the portal system is an effective therapeutic option to prevent variceal hemorrhage in patients who are refractory to medical treatment.[19] Transjugular shunts or TIPS have replaced surgical shunts over the past 20 years. TIPS is a percutaneous imaging-guided procedure in which a channel is constructed within the liver connecting the portal vein with the middle or right hepatic vein, thus diverting blood from the portal to the systemic circulation. The shunt is formed by placing an expandable metal stent within the hepatic parenchyma. Polytetrafluoroethylene (PTFE)-covered stents,[20] introduced in the past decade, have resulted in marked improvement of long-term shunt patency. An alternative to the conventional TIPS is the direct intrahepatic portosystemic shunt, which in a transabdominal approach is used to create a shunt through the hepatic parenchyma between the portal vein and the inferior vena cava.[21]

TIPS also is performed as an emergency procedure in patients with uncontrollable active bleeding, although it is associated with a mortality of 30% to 50% in this setting. Other indications for

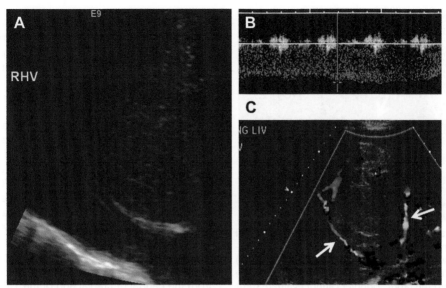

Fig. 22. (*A*) Hepatic vein stenosis secondary to chronic thrombus with echogenic thick wall (*B*) Doppler spectrum shows monophasic waveform. (*C*) Extrinsic compression of right and middle hepatic veins (*arrow*) by a liver metastasis.

TIPS include refractory ascites, Budd-Chiari syndrome, hepatic veno-occlusive disease, hepatic hydrothorax, hepatorenal syndrome, and hepatopulmonary syndrome. Creation of a TIPS successfully reduces the portosystemic pressure gradient in more than 90% of cases.[21]

Contraindications for TIPS are severe congestive cardiac failure, pulmonary hypertension, multiple hepatic cysts, hepatic encephalopathy, portal vein thrombosis, and thrombosis of all the hepatic veins.

Doppler ultrasound is the preferred screening modality for evaluation of TIPS patency. Evaluation of TIPS includes imaging the shunt with gray-scale and color, and obtaining velocities in the stent and flow direction in the portal veins and hepatic veins. A baseline evaluation is performed within 1 week after placement. Surveillance is performed at 3 to 6 monthly intervals if there is clinical concern for shunt patency. Microbubbles of air trapped within the fabric of covered

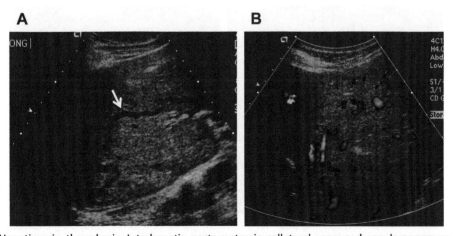

Fig. 23. Hepatic vein thrombosis. Intrahepatic porto-systemic collateral venous channels appear as tortuous nonanatomic vessels (*arrow*) on gray scale (*A*). These collaterals characteristically show flow away from the transducer and toward the IVC, appearing blue on color Doppler (*B*).

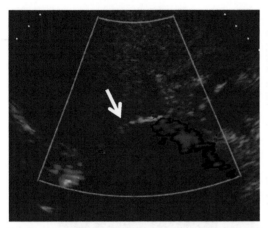

Fig. 24. Recently placed covered TIPS stent. The wall of the stent is visible as an echogenic line with acoustic shadowing (*arrow*) connecting the portal vein (*red*) and hepatic vein (*blue*). It is opaque to ultrasound due to air within the fabric. Doppler cannot evaluate stent patency until the air dissipates.

stents will render them opaque to ultrasound for the first few days after placement (**Fig. 24**). This may take up to a week to resolve. A TIPS stent appears as an echogenic cylindrical structure running through the hepatic parenchyma from the right portal vein to the right or middle hepatic veins, whereas color Doppler will show flow from the portal or caudal end to the hepatic end (**Fig. 25**).

Complications of TIPS

Transcapsular puncture and intraperitoneal hemorrhage are significant procedural complications. After the procedure, 40% to 45% of patients report worsening of portal hypertension as a result of the shunting of portal blood into the systemic circulation.

A deployed TIPS stent has a diameter of 10 to 12 mm. The caudal end of the TIPS should lie within the portal vein and the cranial end in the hepatic vein. The stent can be placed too far into the portal vein or it may migrate into the IVC or even the right atrium (**Fig. 26**). Once epithelialization has occurred around the metal struts, a malpositioned stent may be impossible to remove, making future liver transplantation more difficult.[22]

TIPS thrombosis or occlusion usually occurs in the immediate postprocedure period. It can result from the caudal or cranial end of the TIPS retracting into the liver parenchyma, resulting in closing of the track. TIPS stenosis occurs as a result of pseudointimal hyperplasia, which develops due to contact between traversed biliary radicles and the lumen. This insidious complication develops within weeks of stent placement and leads to significant stenosis in 18% to 78% of bare metal stents.[21] With PTFE-covered stents, the incidence of encephalopathy and stenosis are lower: approximately 8% to 20%. PTFE-covered stents are now the standard of care device for TIPS.

If identified early enough, a thrombosed or stenosed stent can be revised.

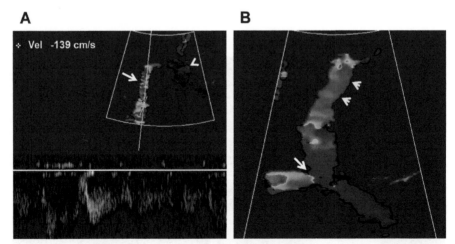

Fig. 25. (*A*) Patent TIPS (*arrow*) running posteriorly from the portal vein (*arrowhead*). Angle-corrected velocity within the TIPS is 139 cm/s, which is normal. (*B*) Reversal of flow in intrahepatic portal vein (*yellow arrowheads*) in a patent TIPS (*white arrow* marks the caudal end of the TIPS). The main portal vein has antegrade flow and appears in red.

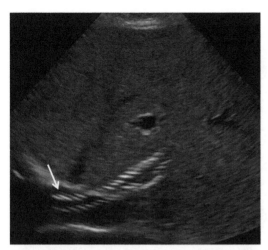

Fig. 26. Malpositioned TIPS. The cephalic end of the TIPS (*arrow*) has extended beyond the liver and lies in the IVC. almost reaching the right atrium.

No flow is seen in a thrombosed TIPS (**Fig. 27**). If flow is present, angle-corrected velocities are obtained in the proximal mid and distal TIPS stent, in that portion of the stent that lies entirely within hepatic parenchyma. In a functioning TIPS, velocities within the stent should be between 90 and 190 cm/s.[5] The Doppler waveform is monophasic or may demonstrate cardiac pulsatility. The creation of a new portosystemic shunt leads to alterations in portal hemodynamics that should be documented on the baseline scan. The portosystemic pressure gradient causes portal blood to be pulled into the stent from both directions, leading to an increase in velocity in the main portal vein in an antegrade direction, whereas hepatofugal

flow may develop in the portal vein branches inside the liver (see **Fig. 25**).

Stenosis tends to occur in the mid stent or hepatic vein end of the stent, or within the hepatic vein. Low stent velocities of less than 90 cm/s are suspicious for stenosis. An elevated velocity of more than 190 cm/s at a focal point within the stent may represent stenosis,[5] especially if low velocities are also found proximally (**Fig. 28**). Conversely, diffusely high velocities throughout the stent are not a sign of stenosis. Changes in velocity of more than 50 cm/s over time also should be considered suspicious for stenosis.[23] The presence of new collateral vessels or ascites are indirect indicators of TIPS failure. Other signs of stenosis include a fall in antegrade main portal vein velocity and a reversion of the hepatofugal flow in the intrahepatic portal vein branches to hepatopetal. Patients are referred for angiography when the Doppler ultrasound is suspicious for obstruction (**Box 2**).

Arterio-venous fistulae and *false aneurysms* result from penetrating arterial injury due to trauma, or as a complication of liver biopsy of other intervention. Doppler ultrasound is an effective method of detecting these complications. A false aneurysm is a collection of extravasated blood and thrombus that is contained by the surrounding hepatic parenchyma. It communicates with the artery through a narrow neck that marks the site of injury. On gray-scale ultrasound it appears as a well-defined cystic mass. Color Doppler demonstrates that the cystic portion is composed of swirling blood that has a characteristic appearance described as the Yin-Yang sign caused by the rotation of blood within the cavity of the false aneurysm (**Fig. 29**A, Video 5). Rapid, pulsatile, to-and-fro flow is seen at the neck, with blood

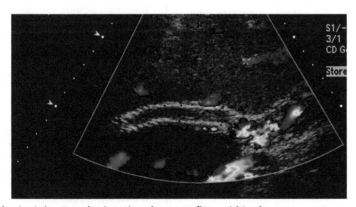

Fig. 27. TIPS thrombosis. Color Doppler imaging shows no flow within the stent.

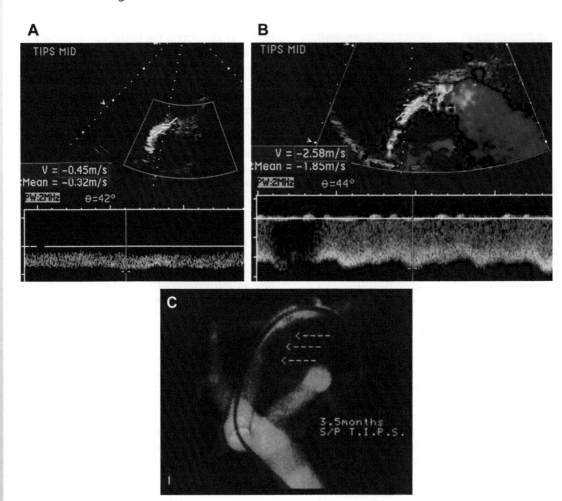

Fig. 28. TIPS stenosis in 2 patients. (*A*) Slow velocity of 45 cm/s at proximal end of the TIPS. (*B*) Different patient with focally elevated velocity of 258 cm/s in mid TIPS. (*C*) Angiogram showing stent stenosis due to pseudointimal hyperplasia (*arrows*). Abnormally low or high velocities are signs of TIPS stenosis. Velocities are reduced proximal (caudad) to the stenosed area, and elevated velocities are seen at the stenosis.

entering the false aneurysm in systole and exiting during diastole. An arteriovenous fistula results when penetrating injury creates a communication between a hepatic artery branch and a portal or hepatic vein branch. Color Doppler shows the fistula as an area of high-velocity turbulent flow in the hepatic parenchyma (see **Fig. 29**B). The receiving vein is dilated and may show arterial waveforms.

WHAT THE REFERRING PHYSICIAN NEEDS TO KNOW

Doppler ultrasound is the first-line modality for imaging a wide range of liver disease. It is quick, accurate, can be performed portably, and has no adverse effects. Doppler ultrasound is the preferred screening modality for evaluation of TIPS patency and portal hypertension. A baseline

---

Box 2
Doppler findings in TIPS

- Covered TIPS are normally opaque to ultrasound for a few days after insertion and patency cannot be assessed during this period.

- Low intrashunt velocities of less than 90 cm/s are a sign of TIPS stenosis

- Focally elevated intrashunt velocities of greater than 190 cm/s (with lower velocities proximal and distal) are a sign of TIPS stenosis

- Hepatofugal flow in the intrahepatic portal veins and increased velocity in the main portal vein post-TIPS are normal and indicate a functioning stent. Conversely, if the direction of flow in the intrahepatic portal veins changes from fugal to petal, it may indicate a developing stenosis.

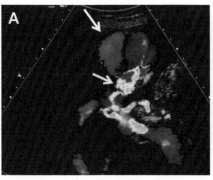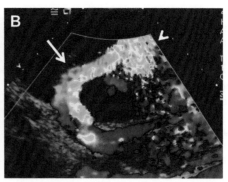

Fig. 29. (A) False aneurysm secondary to liver biopsy. Contained leak from a branch of hepatic artery with swirling blood creating a Yin-Yang sign (*white arrow*). Yellow arrow marks the neck. (*B*) Arteriovenous fistula. The fistula appears as an intense area of color with turbulent flow, which appears as a mixture of colors (*arrowhead*). Draining vein (*blue*) and feeding artery (multicolored, running parallel to vein) are visible (*long arrow*).

evaluation is performed within 1 week after placement. Surveillance is performed at 3 to 6 monthly intervals if there is clinical concern for shunt patency.

SUMMARY

Doppler ultrasound is a noninvasive and accurate modality for evaluation of the liver and liver vasculature. Its real-time capability allows rapid diagnosis in a wide range of hepatic pathology.

SUPPLEMENTARY DATA

Videos related to this article can be found online at http://dx.doi.org/10.1016/j.cult.2014.07.001.

REFERENCES

1. Tessler FN, Gehring BJ, Gomes AS, et al. Diagnosis of PVT: the value of color Doppler imaging. AJR Am J Roentgenol 1991;157:293–6.
2. Pozniak M, Allan P. Clinical Doppler ultrasound. 3rd edition. London: Churchill Livingstone; 2013.
3. Epiel C, Abshagen K, Vollmar B. Regulation of hepatic blood flow: the hepatic arterial buffer response revisited. World J Gastroenterol 2010; 16(48):6046–57.
4. McNaughton DA, Abu-Yousef MM. Doppler US of the liver made simple. Radiographics 2011;31(3): 161–88.
5. Pellerito J, Polak JF. Introduction to vascular sonography. 6th edition. Elsevier; 2013. Chapter 30.
6. Berzigotti A, Piscaglia F, EFSUMB Education and Professional Standards Committee. Ultrasound in portal hypertension–part 2–and EFSUMB recommendations for the performance and reporting of ultrasound examinations in portal hypertension. Ultraschall Med 2012;33(1):8–32 [in English, German].
7. Weinreb J, Kumari S, Phillips G, et al. Portal vein measurements by real-time sonography. AJR Am J Roentgenol 1982;139(3):497–9.
8. Schneider AW, Kalk JF, Klein CP. Hepatic arterial pulsatility index in cirrhosis: correlation with portal pressure. J Hepatol 1999;30(5):876–81.
9. Betrosian AP, Agarwal B, Douzinas EE. Acute renal dysfunction in liver disease. World J Gastroenterol 2007;13(42):5552–9.
10. Platt JF, Ellis JH, Rubin JM, et al. Renal duplex Doppler ultrasonography: a noninvasive predictor of kidney dysfunction and hepatorenal failure in liver disease. Hepatology 1994;20(2):362–9.
11. Ryan KJ, Ray CG. Sherris medical microbiology. 4th edition. New York: McGraw Hill; 2003.
12. Andrade ZA. Schistosomiasis and liver fibrosis. Parasite Immunol 2009;31:656–63.
13. Schuppan D, Afdhal N. Liver cirrhosis. Lancet 2008; 371(9615):838–51.
14. Maheshwari A, Thuluvath PJ. Management of acute hepatitis C. Clin Liver Dis 2010;14(1):169–76.
15. Wilkins T, Malcolm JK, Raina D, et al. Hepatitis C: diagnosis and treatment. Am Fam Physician 2010; 81(11):1351–7.
16. Nelson DK, Lanzino G, Moran CJ, et al. Global epidemiology of hepatitis B and C in people who inject drugs: results of systematic reviews. Lancet 2011;378(9791):571–83.
17. Hirschfield GM, Gershwin ME. The immunobiology and pathophysiology of primary biliary cirrhosis. Ann Rev Pathol 2013;8:303–30.
18. Cura M, Haskal Z, Lopera J. Diagnostic and interventional radiology for Budd-Chiari. Radiographics 2009;29(3).

19. Loffroy R, Estivalet L, Cherblanc V, et al. Transjugular intrahepatic portosystemic shunt for the management of acute variceal hemorrhage. World J Gastroenterol 2013;19(37):6131–43. http://dx.doi.org/10.3748/wjg.v19.i37.6131.

20. Hausegger KA, Karnel F, Georgieva B, et al. Transjugular intrahepatic portosystemic shunt creation with the Viatorr expanded polytetrafluoroethylene-covered stent-graft. J Vasc Interv Radiol 2004;15:239–48.

21. Fidelman N, Kwan S, LeBerge J, et al. The transjugular intrahepatic portosystemic shunt: an update. Am J Roentgenol 2012;199:746–55. http://dx.doi.org/10.2214/AJR.12.9101.

22. da Silva RF, Arroyo PC Jr, Duca WJ, et al. Migration of transjugular intrahepatic portosystemic shunt to the right atrium: complications in the intraoperative period of liver transplantation. Transplant Proc 2008;40(10):3778–80. http://dx.doi.org/10.1016/j.transproceed.2008.06.061.

23. Middleton WD, Teefey SA, Darcy MD. Doppler evaluation of transjugular intrahepatic portosystemic shunts. Ultrasound Q 2003;19(2):56–70.

Contrast Evaluation of Liver Masses

Mark Abel, MBBS[a],*, Wey Chyi Teoh, MBBS[b], Edward Leen, MD[c]

KEYWORDS

- CEUS • Ultrasound • Contrast • Liver • Review • Microbubble

KEY POINTS

- Contrast-enhanced ultrasound (CEUS) is highly useful in the detection and characterization of focal liver lesions (FLLs) as well as in monitoring of ablation therapy.
- Ultrasound contrast agents (UCAs) are pure intravascular tracers with excellent safety profiles, ideally suited for evaluating perfusion changes.
- Limitations include poor penetration and nonlinear propagation artifacts.

Videos of color Doppler demonstrating feeding artery and spoke wheel configuration of an FNH, CEUS of the same FNH in the arterial phase, and typical appearance of hypervascular liver metastases on CEUS accompany this article at http://www.ultrasound.theclinics.com/

INTRODUCTION

There are an estimated 782,000 diagnoses and 746,000 deaths attributed to primary liver cancer annually.[1] The liver is also the second most common site for metastatic spread, with significantly more patients suffering from liver metastases than primary cancer.[2]

Ultrasound is the most commonly used imaging modality of the liver.[3] It is inexpensive, portable, nonionizing and has an excellent safety record.[4,5] Traditional gray-scale and color Doppler ultrasound imaging have inherent limitations. First, detection of FLLs is complicated by similar echogenicity of the lesion and the surrounding liver parenchyma. Second, accurate characterization of FLLs is problematic with different pathologic lesions having overlapping or nondiscrete gray-scale imaging features. Last, although color and spectral Doppler imaging allows visualization of gross blood

flow characteristics, it cannot determine microvascular status or enhancement qualities.[6]

The advent of UCAs has improved characterization of liver masses by comparing the altered enhancement dynamics of a lesion with the adjacent liver parenchyma.[7] In addition, the ability to perform real-time evaluation of FLLs in all vascular phases has conferred CEUS a temporal resolution superior to most other imaging modalities.[8,9] CEUS is highly useful in differentiating FLLs, with reported accuracies of up to 92% to 95%.[10–14] Its use has reduced the need for further imaging or biopsies.[15]

In 2012, the World Federation for Ultrasound in Medicine and Biology (WFUMB) and European Federation of Societies for Ultrasound in Medicine and Biology (EFSUMB) in conjunction with the Asian Federation of Societies for Ultrasound in Medicine and Biology, American Institute of Ultrasound in Medicine, Australasian Society for

The authors have nothing to disclose.
 a Department of Surgery & Cancer, Hammersmith Hospital, Imperial College London, Du Cane Road, London W12 0HS, UK; b Department of Radiology, Changi General Hospital, 2 Simei Street 3, Singapore, Singapore 529889; c Department of Imaging, Hammersmith Hospital, Imperial College NHS Trust, Du Cane Road, London W12 0HS, UK
* Corresponding author.
E-mail address: mark.abel@nhs.net

Ultrasound in Medicine, and International Contrast Ultrasound Society published a set of guidelines to standardize the use of CEUS in liver imaging.[8]

This review article covers the technical considerations of CEUS, UCA evaluation of common liver masses, and its use in ablation therapy, limitations of technique, pitfalls, and future prospects.

PART 1: TECHNICAL CONSIDERATIONS
Ultrasound Contrast Agents

Physical properties
UCAs contain gas bubbles, referred to as *microbubbles*. Most of the UCAs in current clinical use belong to the second-generation. The typical second-generation microbubble has a stable outer shell comprising a thin (10–200 nm thick) biocompatible material (eg, phospholipids) and an inner core of hydrophobic gas (eg, perfluorocarbon, sulfur hexafluoride, or nitrogen), which has a high molecular weight, reduced solubility, and diffusivity.[16] These properties increase resistance to arterial pressure, preventing microbubbles from dissolving in the bloodstream.

A microbubble is approximately 3 to 5 μm in diameter, slightly smaller than a human red blood cell but much larger than the molecules of CT and magnetic resonance (MR) contrast agents. They are confined within the blood pool because they cannot extravasate through the vascular endothelium into the interstitium. They remain, however, small enough to move into the microcirculation of the pulmonary capillaries for safe excretion.[13] The gaseous component of UCAs is respired out in the lungs after approximately 10 to 15 minutes, whereas the shell is either broken down in the liver or excreted by the kidney.[17]

Most UCAs are gradually cleared from the blood pool after the fifth minute. An exception is Sonazoid (Daiichi-Sankyo, GE Tokyo, Tokyo, Japan), which remains in the human liver for several hours. This is because the Sonazoid microbubbles are phagocytozed by Kupffer cells, long after it is cleared from the blood pool. Sonazoid has thus been compared with superparamagnetic iron oxide agents used for MR hepatic imaging. It is the only commercial available UCA with an effective postvascular phase.[18]

Microbubble interaction with ultrasound
Although microbubbles increase the backscatter of ultrasound beams and produce highly echogenic signals, oscillating microbubbles are required for effective contrast imaging.

The natural resonance frequencies of microbubbles (where they are driven into maximal oscillations) are between 3 and 5 MHz. This is coincidentally similar to frequencies used in abdominal imaging.[13] On exposure to ultrasound waves of low acoustic pressure, a microbubble volumetrically expands and contracts in a controlled manner, undergoing stable cavitation. At high acoustic pressures, the microbubble reaches an unstable size and collapses, undergoing inertial cavitation (**Fig. 1**).

Oscillating microbubbles produce asymmetric, nonlinear signals. Human tissue returns largely linear signals and a minimal amount of nonlinear signals at low acoustic pressure. The harmonics arising from the nonlinear signals of the oscillating microbubbles are processed by specialized contrast ultrasound software to produce an image solely depicting microbubble echoes.[19]

> *Commercially approved UCAs*
> - SonoVue (Bracco SpA, Milan, Italy) consists of a sulfur hexafluoride gas contained within a phospholipid shell. It is currently approved for use in Europe, China, Korea, Hong Kong, Singapore, India, New Zealand, and Brazil.
> - Sonazoid consists of perfluorobutane within a phospholipid shell. It is licensed for use in Japan and South Korea.
> - Definity/Luminity (Lantheus Medical, Billerica, Massachusetts) consists of perflutren within a lipid shell. It is licensed in Canada, Mexico, Israel, New Zealand, India, Australia, Korea, Singapore, and United Arab Emirates.
> - Optison (GE Healthcare, Princeton, New Jersey) consists of human serum albumin with a perflutren core. It is currently being trialled for liver imaging.
> - Levovist (Bayer AG, Schering AG, Berlin, Germany) consists of galactose, palmitic acid, and air. It is a first-generation UCA, which has been approved for liver imaging. It is currently no longer available, although production has recommenced in Japan.
> - To date, no UCAs have been approved by the US Food and Drug Administration (FDA) for evaluation of abdominal abnormalities. Optison and Definity are FDA approved, however, for cardiac imaging and can legally be used off-label in the abdomen.

Enhancement phases
The normal liver has a dual blood supply, with approximately one-third coming from the hepatic artery and two-thirds from the portal vein.[20] Vascular phases of a CEUS liver study are similar to CT and MR imaging, progressing from the arterial to portovenous phase and ending with the late (delayed) phase. The enhancement pattern of an

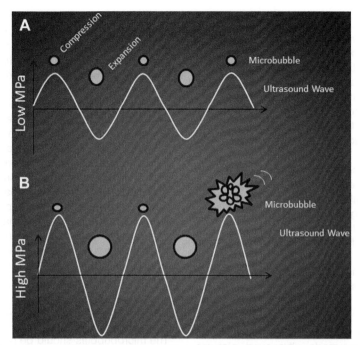

Fig. 1. Microbubble oscillation. (*A*) Stable cavitation at low acoustic pressure. (*B*) Inertial cavitation at high acoustic pressure.

FLL throughout the vascular phases is crucial to its identification.

The arterial phase begins with the arrival of UCA in the hepatic artery. Depending on the circulatory status of the patient, this is typically between 10 and 20 seconds postinjection. The portovenous phase begins when the UCA enters the main portal vein and this occurs at approximately 30 to 45 seconds. The arterial and portovenous phases overlap, because the former lasts up to 45 seconds. The late phase begins after 120 seconds and lasts up to the disappearance of microbubbles from the circulation, at approximately 4 to 6 minutes. An additional postvascular phase is described for Sonazoid, which begins 10 minutes after injection and lasts up to an hour or longer (**Table 1**).

Side effects and contraindications

UCA has a significantly superior safety profile compared with CT or MR contrast agents, with far fewer allergic or anaphylactic reactions reported. It is not nephrotoxic or hepatotoxic.[4,21] The most common adverse effects include dizziness, nausea/vomiting, and pruritus, which are usually minor and transient. Some patients may experience moderate hypotension, although this is likely a vasovagal response.[22] The only contraindication for Sonazoid is allergy to eggs.[12] Other than known hypersensitivity to sulfur hexafluoride (SonoVue) and perflutren (Definity), they are also contraindicated in patients with worsening congestive cardiac failure, acute coronary syndromes, severe pulmonary hypertension, acute respiratory distress syndromes, and suspected cardiac shunts.[23,24] Serious nonfatal adverse reactions to UCAs are rare and occur in approximately 0.01% to 0.03% of patients, the majority of which are anaphylactoid in nature.[25,26] There is no association linking UCA use and higher inpatient mortality risk.[27,28]

While administrating UCA, resuscitation equipment and trained staff must be available to manage adverse events, including acute anaphylaxis. Postinjection, patients should be observed for a minimum of 30 minutes prior to discharge.

UCAs are not licensed for use in pediatric patients, although they have been widely administered off-label in children. Few adverse events have been reported, with no serious events or deaths.[29] There are few data in use of UCAs during pregnancy or while breastfeeding.

Table 1
Displaying vascular phases and timings

Vascular Phase	Start Time	End Time
Arterial phase	10–20 s	30–45 s
Portovenous phase	30–45 s	120 s
Late phase	>120 s	4–6 min
Postvascular/Kupffer phase	10 min	>1 h

Equipment

Low mechanical index imaging

The mechanical index (MI) of an ultrasound system is an approximate translation of the transmitted ultrasound beam's acoustic pressure. To minimize the destruction of microbubbles and prolong their presence within the bloodstream, low MI imaging is required. A low MI also reduces the amount of nonlinear harmonic signals that arise from soft tissue.

Although insufficient acoustic power gives poor signal returns, technological advances have enabled good-quality imaging at low MI. This is achieved by using a short sequence of pulses that are modulated in amplitude, phase, or a combination of both.[30] MI settings of less than or equal to 0.3 are typically recommended for CEUS imaging. Optimal imaging parameters vary between device manufacturers and can be much lower.[8]

Imaging mode

CEUS imaging is viewed using side-by-side or overlying brightness-mode ultrasound pictures. The former uses a dual-screen view that separates the display into adjacent contrast-only mode and a low MI B-mode image. The latter overlays the contrast mode onto B-mode images.

The B-mode image is important for anatomic guidance. In addition, linear reflections from biopsy needles or ablation probes used in interventional procedures cannot be displayed in contrast-only mode, making parallel imaging necessary for instrument guidance.[13]

Analysis and quantification software

Specialist software has been developed to allow quantification of perfusion parameters and to aid objective identification of FLLs through synchronous image analysis during scanning or postprocedure evaluation. Most advanced software products enable the acquisition of good-quality cine loops by incorporating motion compensation and/or respiratory gating. Examples of commercially available products include SonoLiver (TomTec Imaging Systems, Unterschleissheim, Germany), VueBox (Bracco Suisse SA—Software Applications, Geneva Switzerland), and QLAB (Philips, Bothell, Washington).

Using such software, enhancement patterns can be quantified as time intensity curves by selecting regions of interest within a lesion, allowing comparison with nearby liver parenchyma, and interval monitoring to observe perfusion changes. By incorporating parametric imaging, the dynamic enhancement pattern of a lesion can be objectively visualized, increasing the confidence of diagnosis **(Fig. 2)**.

Examination Procedure

UCA administration

The microbubbles should be prepared per manufacturers' guidelines. UCAs can be injected as a bolus or continuous infusion.

Bolus injection The bolus injection method allows rapid distribution of microbubbles into the hepatic vasculature. Contrast injection should be performed via a stop valve and 20-gauge (or larger) cannula inserted into a cubital vein, without further tubing. The UCA is given as a bolus followed by a flush of 0.9% normal saline. Dosing should be calculated according to manufacturers' guidance to ensure even distribution of UCA and to avoid attenuation artifacts from excessive microbubbles. Bolus injections can be repeated as required once previously injected microbubbles are cleared. This can be achieved rapidly by temporarily increasing MI to aid microbubble destruction.[31]

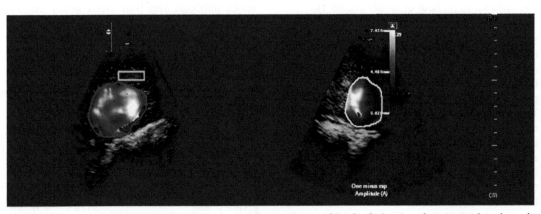

Fig. 2. CEUS parametric imaging. The dynamic vascular pattern within the lesion is color mapped and can be compared with appended color scale.

Infusion injection For infusions, the UCA is first reconstituted before dilution with normal saline in a syringe. The suspension must be continuously agitated to ensure the microbubbles remain formed and evenly distributed. The agent is then injected at a constant rate via a syringe pump. Once a steady stream of microbubbles has been achieved (2–3 minutes), dynamic flow characteristics can be ascertained using flash imaging, a technique where a short burst of increased acoustic pressure obliterates bubbles in the imaging plane. The microbubbles then reaccumulate, allowing observation of enhancement characteristics. Repeat flashes may be required to increase diagnostic confidence.[31,32] The need for additional equipment and complex set-up makes this a less preferred administration method.

Imaging

Prior to contrast injection, imaging using conventional gray-scale and Doppler ultrasound should be carried out to identify the target lesion(s) and optimal imaging positions.

For subsequent contrast mode imaging, the dynamic range, image depth, focal depth, and focal zone size should be adjusted prior to contrast injection. A stop clock is used to display the timings of the enhancement phases. Cine-loop acquisition of the examination allows retrospective frame-by-frame review, because enhancement changes can occur rapidly in the arterial phase.

In the first 2 minutes of the examination (arterial and portovenous phases), image capturing should be carried out without interruption in a single plane. In the late phase, frequent intermittent scanning is performed until microbubble disappearance. Vascular-phase UCA examinations should last at least 5 to 6 minutes. For Sonazoid use, the late-phase imaging is deemed less important and is usually replaced by postvascular phase imaging, which begins after 10 minutes.

Imaging tips

- The imaging plane should preferably be parallel to movement of the diaphragm to maintain lesion visualization throughout the examination.

- Breath holding/gentle breathing in the first 30 seconds is encouraged to ensure visualization of rapid arterial changes.

- The frame rate should be increased to at least 10 Hz for vascular imaging.

- The output power (MI) can gradually be increased to visualize microbubble contrast for deep-seated lesions.

PART 2: UCA EVALUATION OF LIVER MASSES
Characterization of FLL

Accurate characterization of liver lesions can be challenging. A single imaging modality often yields inconclusive or equivocal results, requiring further imaging with alternative modalities. Characterization of an FLL is the most common CEUS application. It can offer a confident diagnosis when pathognomonic enhancement characteristics are observed. In Japan, CEUS is recognized as a first-line investigation for hepatocellular carcinoma (HCC).[33]

Prior to performing a CEUS study, a patient's medical history and risk factors for liver malignancy must be ascertained. Any prior liver imaging should be reviewed and compared.

Enhancement nomenclature

Enhancement indicates perfusion and absence of enhancement denotes avascular status. The enhancement intensity of an FLL is described in comparison to that of adjacent tissue.

- Hyperenhancing indicates relative increased vascularity.

- Hypoenhancing indicates relative decreased vascularity.

- Isoenhancing indicates similar vascular status.

- Nonenhancing indicates complete avascular status.

- Wash-in indicates progressive enhancement.

- Washout indicates progressive reduction in enhancement.

Common benign lesions

Hemangioma Hemangiomas are the most common benign hepatic neoplasm. They are overgrowths of vascular endothelial cells and mesenchymal in origin. Typically, a hemangioma shows peripheral-nodular enhancement in the arterial phase. It fills in completely or partially from the portovenous phase and remains isoenhancing to liver parenchyma in the late phase (**Fig. 3**). Correct diagnosis is achieved in up to 95% when these typical features are seen.[10] Filling in can be rapid in small lesions[34] and real-time imaging allows the identification of flash-filling hemangiomas, which can be missed by CT and MR.[13]

Of caution, small and rapidly enhancing high-flow hemangiomas may be mistaken for well-differentiated HCCs, whereas the nonenhancing thrombosed portions of a hemangioma may be mistaken for washout.[35]

Focal nodular hyperplasia Focal nodular hyperplasias (FNHs) are benign hyperplastic lesions that form in response to underlying arteriovenous malformations. Characteristic features include a spoke wheel vascular pattern, a feeding vessel, and presence of a central scar.[36] Confident diagnosis can occasionally be made with Doppler ultrasound.[37] One of the 3 typical features can be seen in 75% of lesions greater than 3 cm, reducing to 30% in smaller lesions.[38]

After UCA injection, a FNH typically shows rapid spoke wheel enhancement before centrifugal and homogeneous filling in during the arterial phase. An erratic filling in pattern is appreciated in 30% of FNHs.[8] During the portovenous and late phases, the lesion may remain hyperenhancing or become isoenhancing. The central scar, if present, is nonenhancing or hypoenhancing (**Fig. 4**, Videos 1 and 2). Rarely, FNH lesions can show complete washout, the majority after 75 seconds.[39] In such cases, an incorrect diagnosis of malignancy may be made if typical features are absent.

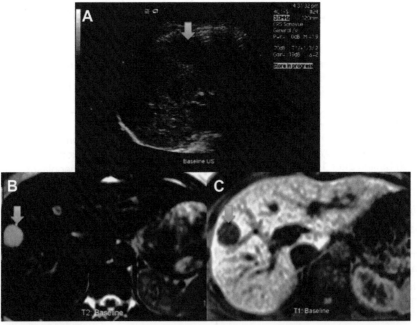

Fig. 3. Indeterminate solid nodule seen in the liver (*blue arrows*): (*A*) B-mode ultrasound shows a well-circumscribed hypoechoic nodule in segment 8; (*B, C*) corresponding MR images of the same lesion, which is T2 hyperintense and T1 hypointense. CEUS and CEMRI evaluation of the indeterminate nodule: (*D–F*) CEUS of shows peripheral nodular enhancement in the arterial phase, with gradual centripetal filling in from the portovenous phase. The late phase shows persistent enhancement; (*G–I*) contrast-enhanced MR images, showing similar changes in the corresponding phases. Findings are typical for liver hemangiomas on CEUS and CEMRI.

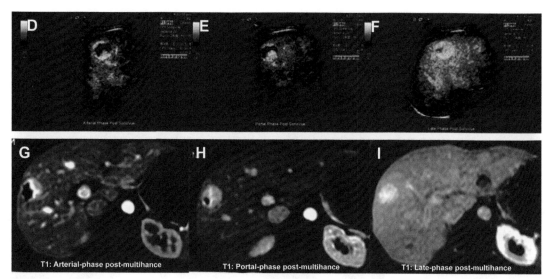

T1: Arterial-phase post-multihance   T1: Portal-phase post-multihance   T1: Late-phase post-multihance

Fig. 3. (*continued*)

Hepatocellular adenoma Hepatocellular adenomas are rare benign lesions related to excessive estrogen. They occur mainly in women of child-bearing age and are strongly associated with oral contraceptive pill use and anabolic/androgenic steroids. Rupture or malignant development is possible, so surgical management is advised for hepatocellular adenomas greater than 3 cm.[40] Arterial-phase imaging demonstrates peripheral hyperenhancement followed by rapid centripetal filling.[41] They become isoenhancing in the portovenous and late phases. Occasionally, they show slight washout, which may lead to an incorrect diagnosis of HCC.[41,42] Although the typical enhancement characteristics of hepatocellular adenomas are not pathognomonic, a patient's demographics and clinical history can aid identification.

Typical enhancement pattern

- Rapid peripheral arterial enhancement and centripetal fill in.

- Isoenhancing in the portovenous and late phases.

Caution

- Hepatocellular adenomas occasionally show soft washout.

Cystic lesions Simple cysts can often be confidentially diagnosed using routine ultrasound, where they appear as thin-walled, well-defined anechoic lesions with distal acoustic enhancement.[43] Debris or hemorrhagic material within a cyst may be difficult, however, to differentiate from a solid nodule.

CEUS is useful for evaluation of complex cysts, because the lack of intracystic solid enhancement or enhancing nodular rim excludes malignant disease (**Fig. 5**).[44]

Infection/Inflammation Hepatic abscesses can show marginal rim and septae arterial enhancement, resulting in a honeycomb appearance.[45] If hyperenhancement is evident, early washout is commonly seen within 30 seconds of contrast injection. Lack of enhancement of the liquefied portions is the most prominent feature.[39] The rare inflammatory pseudotumors have varied enhancement patterns throughout all phases with no significant distinguishing features on CEUS.[46]

Focal fatty changes Focal fatty infiltration (echogenic) and focal fatty sparing (hypoechoic) typically occur around the ligamentum teres, adjacent to the gallbladder fossa and bordering the porta hepatitis. Atypical locations can make diagnosis difficult. It is important to differentiate these from malignant lesions in high-risk patients. CEUS imaging shows focal fatty changes as isoenhancing areas compared with surrounding liver parenchyma throughout all vascular phases (**Fig. 6**).[14]

Common malignant lesions
Cirrhotic liver The cirrhotic liver is predisposed to HCC, with 90% of HCCs occurring in a stepwise progression.[47] Regenerative nodules, which are formed during the attempted repair of a cirrhotic liver, have a dual blood supply similar to normal liver parenchyma. Progression to a dysplastic nodule causes the loss of normal arterial and portovenous blood supplies. On further evolution to

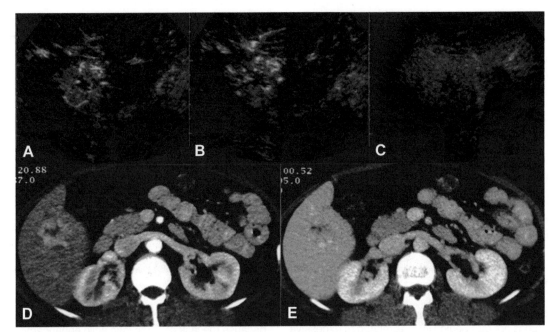

Fig. 4. FNH with central scar. (*A–C*) CEUS shows an arterial enhancing lesion with a central scar. The lesion becomes isoenhancing with the liver in the late phase. The scar remains nonenhancing. (*D, E*) The lesion shows similar characteristics on CECT, with a nonenhancing central scar.

HCC, the lesion gains supply of abnormal unpaired arteries, leading to net arterialization of the tumor. This angioneogenesis increases as the tumor progresses to a poorly differentiated HCC (**Fig. 7**).

Although HCC commonly occurs in a background of liver cirrhosis, it can also occur in normal liver. Certain conditions, such as nonalcoholic fatty liver disease, are known to promote hepatic carcinogenesis in the absence of cirrhosis.[7,48]

Regenerative nodule The typical regenerative nodule is isoenhancing in all phases.[14]

Dysplastic nodule Dysplastic nodules are collections of hepatocytes that contain dysplastic characteristics but do not meet histologic criteria for malignancy. With increasing dysplasia, intranodular portal tracts are lost and are replaced by unpaired arteries.[49] Depending on the degree of dysplasia, a dysplastic nodule can be hypoenhancing, isoenhancing, or hyperenhancing during the arterial phase, becoming isoenhancing or minimally hypoenhancing during the portovenous and late phases. A high-grade dysplastic nodule (HGDN) can have enhancement characteristics that overlap with a well-differentiated HCC.[50] Because HGDNs are considered premalignant, some centers advocate resection or ablation rather than surveillance.[51]

Typical enhancement pattern

- Regenerative nodules are isoenhancing in all phases.
- Low-grade degenerative nodules are iso- or hypoenhancing in the arterial phase. They are isoenhancing in the portovenous and late phases.
- High-grade degenerative nodules can be hyperenhancing in the arterial phase and show slight washout in the late phase.

Caution

- High-grade degenerative nodules can have enhancement characteristics similar to a well-differentiated HCC.

Hepatocellular carcinoma HCC has the most variable enhancement pattern of all malignant lesions. The classic enhancement pattern for HCC is arterial hyperenhancement followed by washout in the late phase (**Figs. 8** and **9**).[13] Practitioners must be aware that HCCs can be isoenhancing or even hypoenhancing during the arterial phase. HCCs typically demonstrate a dysmorphic, basket-like pattern of arterial supply with centripetal fill in. A feeding artery and S-shaped vessels are occasionally evident within or adjacent to the tumor during the arterial phase.[3,7] Heterogeneous enhancement is common in larger tumors.[52]

The washout timing of HCC is variable, although usually slower compared with other malignant tumors. Extended imaging until the disappearance of UCA in the vascular phase (5–6 min) is essential to avoid overlooking HCCs (**Fig. 10**).[53] The more dedifferentiated a tumor, the faster it washes out.[54] Sonazoid shows such lesions as enhancement defects in the postvascular phase.

HCCs occasionally show arterial hyperenhancement but do not wash out. This can be seen in well-differentiated HCCs, which maintain substantial portal tracts and may be mistaken for benign disease.[55] The index of suspicion for an arterial enhancing lesion must, therefore, remain high, particularly in a background of cirrhotic liver disease.

Portal vein thrombosis, which is not uncommon in liver cirrhosis, increases arterial-phase enhancement and decreases portovenous-phase enhancement of the liver parenchyma. This may reduce the disparity between highly arterialized HCCs and adjacent liver, making characterization difficult.[56]

Typical enhancement pattern

- HCCs classically show arterial enhancement and subsequent washout.
- The more dedifferentiated the HCC, the faster the washout.

Caution

- HCCs can be iso- or hypoenhancing in the arterial phase.
- Well-differentiated HCCs may not wash out.
- Poorly differentiated HCCs wash out rapidly.
- Portal vein thrombosis may reduce the disparity between highly arterialized HCCs and adjacent liver.

Cholangiocarcinoma The majority of cholangiocarcinomas are arterially hyperenhancing due to neoangiogenesis. Four different arterial enhancement patterns are reported: peripheral rim enhancement, heterogeneous hyperenhancement, homogeneous hyperenhancement, and heterogeneous hypoenhancement.[57] Tumors with a high concentration of cancerous cells show increased arterial hyperenhancement, whereas those with proportionally more fibrotic tissue enhance less. The peripheral rim enhancement pattern is more commonly seen in livers without concomitant pathology, whereas heterogeneous hyperenhancement is seen more frequently in patients with cirrhosis or chronic hepatitis.[58] Periductal infiltrating intrahepatic cholangiocarcinomas are more likely to

display heterogeneous enhancement due to increased fibrotic tissue. Cholangiocarcinomas wash out by the late phase in CEUS imaging (**Fig. 11**)[39,59] but may show delayed enhancement on contrast-enhanced CT (CECT) or contrast-enhanced MR imaging (CEMRI) studies.

Retraction of the liver surface by the tumor as a consequence of fibrotic proliferation is a helpful radiological clue that should raise suspicion of cholangiocarcinoma. This is readily identified on routine gray-scale imaging. Cholangiocarcinomas also wash out early, not unlike poorly differentiated HCC or metastases.[60]

Typical enhancement pattern

- Cholangiocarcinoma shows arterial enhancement and early washout.

Caution

- Enhancement pattern mimics poorly differentiated HCCs and liver metastases.

Metastases Metastases typically present on CEUS with arterial hyperenhancement, because the tumor contains greater arterial supply than adjacent liver parenchyma. Rapid growth of metastases often results in a ring or halo enhancement, which is attributable to the presence of peripheral arterial vessels and a necrotic core with diminished vascular flow (**Fig. 12**, Video 3). Metastatic lesions wash out early and remain hypoenhancing, starting from the late arterial or early portovenous phase. Some metastases may appear hypoenhancing throughout the vascular phases and this is seen more commonly in colorectal and bronchogenic primary cancers.[3,7]

Metastases may mimic poorly differentiated HCCs or cholangiocarcinomas on CEUS. Clues that help differentiate them include patient history, presence of cirrhosis (increased likelihood of HCC), and multiple lesions (increased likelihood of metastases).

Typical enhancement pattern

- Metastases show arterial enhancement and early washout.
- Metastases show halo enhancement with a hypoenhancing necrotic core.

Caution

- Some metastases can be hypoenhancing in all phases.
- Enhancement pattern mimics that of a poorly differentiated HCC and cholangiocarcinoma.

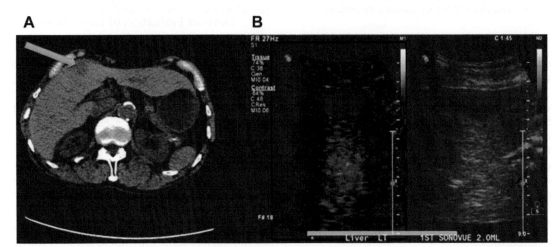

Fig. 5. Incidentally picked up subcapsular low-density focus on CT (*blue arrow*). (*A*) The low-density focus is in segment 4, measuring 50 Hounsfield units. This is suggestive of a solid lesion. It cannot be characterized further on this unenhanced CT study. (*B*) CEUS reveals the lesion to be a cyst with no enhancing intracystic component. The slightly raised echoes within the lesion (seen on parallel B-mode image) are attributed to debris or proteinaceous material.

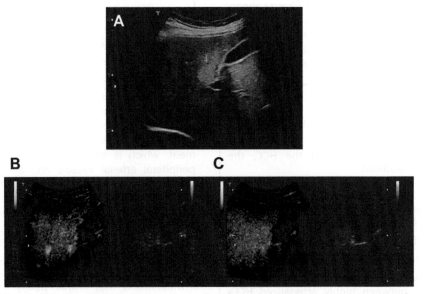

Fig. 6. Focal fatty infiltration. (*A*) B-mode image reveals a vague hyperechoic area anterior to the main portal vein (*orange arrow*). (*B*, *C*) The hyperechoic area remains isoenhancing to the liver in the late arterial and portovenous phases on CEUS.

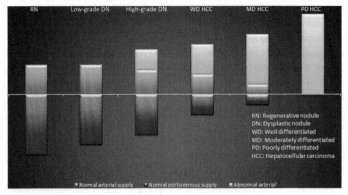

Fig. 7. HCC pathogenesis. Changes in blood supply as a lesion progresses from a regenerative nodule to a poorly differentiated HCC.

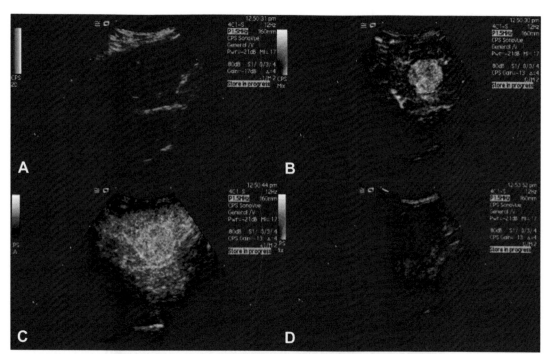

Fig. 8. Typical enhancement pattern of a HCC on CEUS. (*A*) Near isoechoic mass on B-mode ultrasound. (*B*) The mass shows homogeneous hyperenhancement in the arterial phase. (*C*) The mass shows near isoenhancement to the liver in the portovenous phase. (*D*) The mass shows washout and is hypoenhancing to the liver in the late phase.

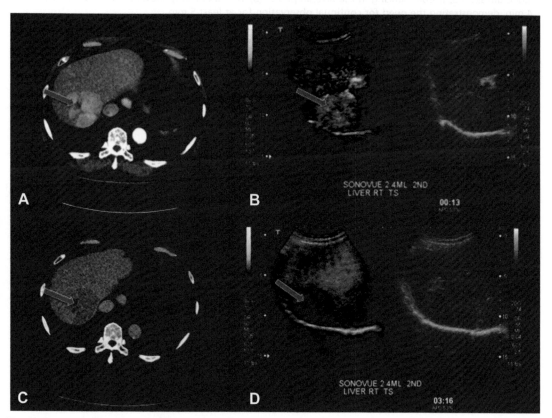

Fig. 9. Corresponding CT and CEUS images of a HCC (*red arrows*). (*A, B*) CT and CEUS images of an arterially enhancing mass in segment 7-8. (*C, D*) CT and CEUS images of the same lesion showing washout in the delayed (late) phase.

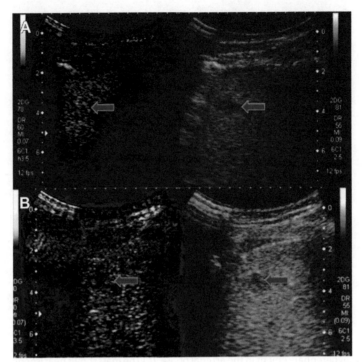

Fig. 10. Enhancement variation of HCC tumor (*red arrows*). (*A*) The tumor, which is slightly hypoechoic on B-mode ultrasound, is isoenhancing in the arterial phase. (*B*) The tumor only shows definite washout from the 3–4 min, demonstrating the need for continual observation for at least 5 min.

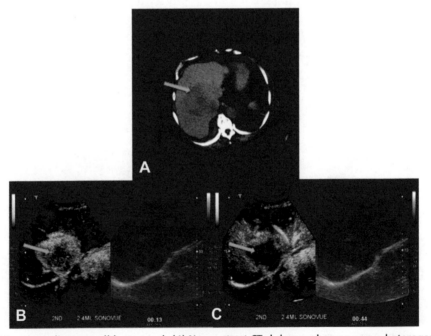

Fig. 11. Indeterminate liver mass (*blue arrows*). (*A*) Noncontrast CT abdomen shows a vague heterogeneous mass in the segment 8. (*B*) CEUS shows an arterial enhancing heterogeneous mass. (*C*) The lesion washes out rapidly by the early portovenous phase. Biopsy of the lesion reveals a cholangiocarcinoma.

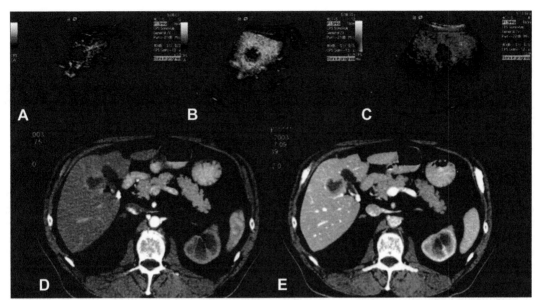

Fig. 12. Rim-enhancing liver metastasis. (*A–C*) CEUS of liver metastasis shows rim enhancement from the arterial phase, with washing out in the portovenous and late phases. The central portion, which consists of necrotic tissue, is nonenhancing. (*D, E*) Corresponding CECT of the same liver metastasis in arterial and portovenous phases.

Lymphoma Primary hepatic lymphoma is rare. The majority of cases occur in immunocompromised patients and men during their 50s.[61] Few data have been published on the enhancement patterns of hepatic lymphoma. Reported enhancement characteristics are typical of malignant lesions, with hyperenhancement during the arterial phase and washout by the late phase.[62,63]

Lesion Detection

CEUS can increase the sensitivity of hepatic lesion detection,[64–67] depicting tumors as small as 3 mm.[68] CEUS detection of small liver metastases can also be superior to dynamic CT in well-performed examinations.[69] As such, the WFUMB-ESFUMB guidelines recommend the use of CEUS as a rule-out test for small metastasis and abscess.[8]

Agents with a postvascular phase (Sonazoid) are particularly useful for this purpose given that malignant lesions are typically devoid of Kupffer cells (**Fig. 13**).[70] Up to half of well-differentiated HCCs do not wash out, however, and avascular lesions (such as cysts) may be mistaken for enhancement defects. Therefore, injection of a further bolus of Sonazoid is advocated to relook at the arterial phase of all detected lesions.[71]

Intraoperative Contrast Ultrasound

Intraoperative ultrasound (IO-US) has been used to assist surgical decision making during liver resections by identifying FLLs. Addition of UCA (IO-CEUS) is shown to be more sensitive than CECT, CEMRI, and IO-US at detecting and characterizing lesions. IO-CEUS can alter the intended surgical procedure in 25% to 30% of cases.[72,73] This translates to a higher rate of curative procedures, fewer remaining positive margins, and improved organ-sparing surgery.[74,75] To perform CE-IOUS, dedicated high-

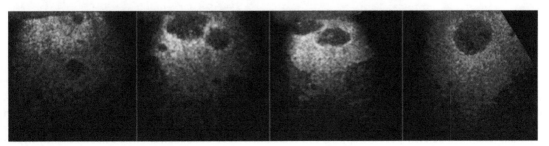

Fig. 13. Detection of liver metastases. Sonazoid contrast with postvascular phase. The liver metastases were clearly seen as enhancement defects.

frequency intraoperative probes are recommended. The duration of contrast enhancement is shorter in IO-CEUS because the microbubbles are destroyed faster due to the closer proximity of the probe to the liver.

CEUS in Ablation Therapy

CEUS improves probe placement by depicting smaller tumors more clearly and increasing contrast resolution between the lesion periphery and surrounding tissue.[76] Studies have shown that addition of UCA to guide interventions has resulted in improved outcomes for ablative procedures compared with unenhanced ultrasound.[77,78] CEUS is especially beneficial where CECT, CEMRI, or routine ultrasound cannot clearly visualize the target lesion.[79]

Periprocedural CEUS is shown comparable with CECT at 24 hours in detecting remaining disease and determining treatment success.[80,81] Remnant disease detected right after ablative treatment can be rectified immediately, avoiding further anesthetic and extended hospital stay. CEUS should be performed approximately 5 minutes postablation to allow for dissipation of gas formed during the procedure (**Fig. 14**).

Postablation monitoring with CEUS is also useful for detecting local recurrence.[82] Operators should be aware of a uniform enhancing hyperemic rim that is frequently seen for up to a month post-treatment. This should not be mistaken for tumor recurrence.

Limitations

CEUS suffers from the same limitations as routine ultrasound; a poor-quality unenhanced scan is unlikely to provide good CEUS images. Subdiaphragmatic lesions can be challenging to detect and characterize. It is also difficult to image deep lesions, particularly in patients who are obese or who have severe fatty liver or cirrhosis.[83] Practitioners should be aware that the ultrasound waves are attenuated by microbubbles, a phenomenon known as self-shadowing. This is important because an excessively high dose of microbubbles limits penetration. In addition, when ultrasound waves propagate through microbubbles, they are altered and contribute to nonlinear

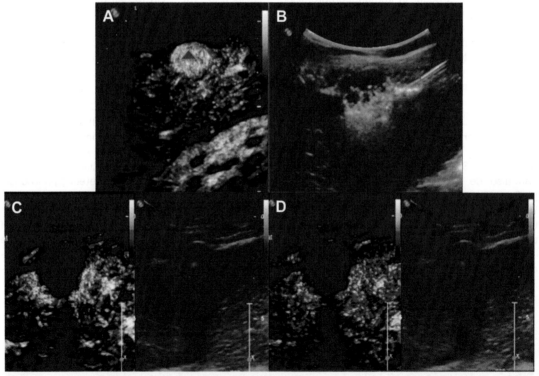

Fig. 14. CEUS in ablation therapy. (A) Preablation CEUS confirms the presences of an arterial enhancing HCC (*orange triangle*). (B) B-mode image of the lesion taken during radiofrequency ablation. Note the presence of an ablation needle (*orange star*). The presence of gas (ring-down artifacts with shadowing) makes it difficult to evaluate this lesion immediately post-therapy. (C, D) Postablation CEUS evaluation shows a smooth, slightly hyperemic rim. This should not be mistaken for remnant tumor. The ablation site is nonenhancing in the portovenous late phase.

echoes (nonlinear propagation), leading to imaging artifacts in the far field.[84]

Although the smallest detectable lesion by CEUS is 3 to 5 mm, diagnostic confidence increases with lesions greater than 1 cm. This is not unexpected, because the smaller the lesion, the harder it is to appreciate its enhancement pattern.

Pitfalls

It is important to be vigilant of the overlapping enhancement patterns of benign and malignant lesions. Bhayana and colleagues[39] reported that 97% of cancerous tumors show washout and this has a positive predictive value of 72%. Although contrast washout is the key finding used for differentiating benign and malignant lesions, approximately 30% of benign lesions exhibit washout, whereas some HCCs do not.

The ability to differentiate the tumor is much more complex, with a specificity of only 64%.[39] The classic arterial hyperenhancement followed by washout is seen not only in HCC but also cholangiocarcinoma, lymphomas, and metastases.

HCC is by far the most common malignant tumor, with a majority showing slow washout.[85] In doubtful cases, additional imaging evaluation with CECT or CEMRI is advised. Biopsy for histologic correlation is advised if the diagnosis remains doubtful.

PART 3: FUTURE PROSPECTS
Tumor Perfusion Quantification

Response Evaluation Criteria in Solid Tumors is the current standard used for assessing treatment response in liver cancer treatment.[86] It is, however, designed to measure reduction in tumor volumes after cytotoxic therapy, limiting its usefulness in assessing the response of cytostatic agents.[87] As purely intravascular agents, microbubbles are perfectly suited for quantifying perfusion changes.[31] Dynamic CEUS is a potential biomarker for assessing treatment response, especially for antiangiogenic agents.[88,89]

3-D and 4-D Imaging with Microbubbles

3-D imaging can better appreciate the entire tumor morphology and volume whereas 4-D imaging

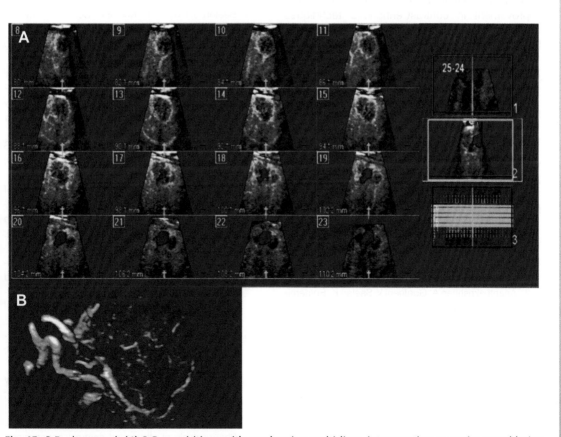

Fig. 15. 3-D ultrasound. (*A*) 3-D acquisitions with overlapping multislices, interrogating an entire postablation site. The recurrent tumor bulk (*solid*) can be better appreciated. (*B*) 3-D rendering of an FNH, showing its central artery and radiating branches.

allows 3-D imaging to be performed real time. The concurrent use of a multislice software package that displays the acquired 3-D images in sequential images may make it easier to detect small lesions (**Fig. 15**). Characterization of an FLL can also be improved with real-time 3-D rendering of a lesion's vasculature.

Targeted Imaging

Microbubbles lined with surface antigens to target specific cell receptors are in development; targets include vascular endothelial growth factor 2 and $\alpha_v\beta_3$ integrin.[90] This may prove valuable in lesion detection and differentiation. It can also improve treatment planning by identifying cell surface mutations, which are susceptible or impervious to particular treatment regimes.

SUMMARY

CEUS is a valuable tool that is cost effective, safe, and nonionizing. Its real-time application and the use of purely intravascular contrast agents are unique features not present in other imaging modalities. Continuous technological advances and improvement in contrast-enhanced techniques will serve to firmly establish the roles of CEUS in hepatic imaging.

ACKNOWLEDGMENTS

The authors acknowledge Christina Kalli for her pictorial contributions to this article.

SUPPLEMENTARY DATA

Videos related to this article can be found online at http://dx.doi.org/10.1016/j.cult.2014.07.003.

REFERENCES

1. IARC, GLOBOCAN. Estimated liver cancer incidence, mortality and prevalence worldwide in 2012. Lyon (France): World Health Organistaion; 2012.
2. Ananthakrishnan A, Gogineni V, Saeian K. Epidemiology of primary and secondary liver cancers. Semin Intervent Radiol 2006;23(1):47–63.
3. Postema M, Gilja OH. Contrast-enhanced and targeted ultrasound. World J Gastroenterol 2011; 17(1):28–41.
4. Ter Haar G. Ultrasonic imaging: safety considerations. Interface Focus 2011;1(4):686–97.
5. Westwood M, Joore M, Grutters J, et al. Contrast-enhanced ultrasound using SonoVue(R) (sulphur hexafluoride microbubbles) compared with contrast-enhanced computed tomography and contrast-enhanced magnetic resonance imaging for the characterisation of focal liver lesions and detection of liver metastases: a systematic review and cost-effectiveness analysis. Health Technol Assess 2013;17(16):1–243.
6. Cosgrove D, Lassau N. Imaging of perfusion using ultrasound. Eur J Nucl Med Mol Imaging 2010; 37(Suppl 1):S65–85.
7. Leen E. The role of contrast-enhanced ultrasound in the characterisation of focal liver lesions. Eur Radiol 2001;11(Suppl 3):E27–34.
8. Claudon M, Dietrich CF, Choi BI, et al. Guidelines and good clinical practice recommendations for Contrast Enhanced Ultrasound (CEUS) in the liver - update 2012: A WFUMB-EFSUMB initiative in cooperation with representatives of AFSUMB, AIUM, ASUM, FLAUS and ICUS. Ultrasound Med Biol 2013;39(2):187–210.
9. Goh V, Gourtsoyianni S, Koh DM. Functional imaging of the liver. Semin Ultrasound CT MR 2013; 34(1):54–65.
10. Strobel D, Seitz K, Blank W, et al. Contrast-enhanced ultrasound for the characterization of focal liver lesions–diagnostic accuracy in clinical practice (DEGUM multicenter trial). Ultraschall Med 2008;29(5):499–505.
11. Beaton C, Cochlin D, Kumar N. Contrast enhanced ultrasound should be the initial radiological investigation to characterise focal liver lesions. Eur J Surg Oncol 2010;36(1):43–6.
12. Hatanaka K, Kudo M, Minami Y, et al. Differential diagnosis of hepatic tumors: value of contrast-enhanced harmonic sonography using the newly developed contrast agent, Sonazoid. Intervirology 2008;51(Suppl 1):61–9.
13. Wilson SR, Burns PN. Microbubble-enhanced US in body imaging: what role? Radiology 2010; 257(1):24–39.
14. Martie A, Bota S, Sporea I, et al. The contribution of contrast enhanced ultrasound for the characterization of benign liver lesions in clinical practice - a monocentric experience. Med Ultrason 2012;14(4): 283–7.
15. Leen E, Ceccotti P, Kalogeropoulou C, et al. Prospective multicenter trial evaluating a novel method of characterizing focal liver lesions using contrast-enhanced sonography. AJR Am J Roentgenol 2006;186(6):1551–9.
16. Stewart VR, Sidhu PS. New directions in ultrasound: microbubble contrast. Br J Radiol 2006; 79(939):188–94.
17. Quaia E. Assessment of tissue perfusion by contrast-enhanced ultrasound. Eur Radiol 2011; 21(3):604–15.
18. Yanagisawa K, Moriyasu F, Miyahara T, et al. Phagocytosis of ultrasound contrast agent microbubbles by Kupffer cells. Ultrasound Med Biol 2007;33(2):318–25.

19. Stride E, Saffari N. Microbubble ultrasound contrast agents: a review. Proc Inst Mech Eng H 2003;217(6):429–47.

20. Lautt WW. Hepatic circulation: physiology and pathophysiology. San Rafael (CA): Morgan & Claypool Life Sciences; 2009.

21. Thomsen HS. Contrast media safety-an update. Eur J Radiol 2011;80(1):77–82.

22. Piscaglia F, Bolondi L. The safety of Sonovue® in abdominal applications: retrospective analysis of 23188 investigations. Ultrasound Med Biol 2006; 32(9):1369–75.

23. Drug safety labeling changes definity (perflutren lipid microsphere) injectable suspension. Maryland: US Food and Drug Administration; 2008.

24. European Medicine Agency. Report: UK, Sonovue, 2013.

25. Herzog CA. Incidence of adverse events associated with use of perflutren contrast agents for echocardiography. JAMA 2008;299(17):2023–5.

26. Wei K, Mulvagh SL, Carson L, et al. The safety of deFinity and Optison for ultrasound image enhancement: a retrospective analysis of 78,383 administered contrast doses. J Am Soc Echocardiogr 2008;21(11):1202–6.

27. Kusnetzky LL, Khalid A, Khumri TM, et al. Acute mortality in hospitalized patients undergoing echocardiography with and without an ultrasound contrast agent: results in 18,671 consecutive studies. J Am Coll Cardiol 2008;51(17):1704–6.

28. Main ML, Ryan AC, Davis TE, et al. Acute mortality in hospitalized patients undergoing echocardiography with and without an ultrasound contrast agent (multicenter registry results in 4,300,966 consecutive patients). Am J Cardiol 2008;102(12): 1742–6.

29. Darge K, Papadopoulou F, Ntoulia A, et al. Safety of contrast-enhanced ultrasound in children for non-cardiac applications: a review by the Society for Pediatric Radiology (SPR) and the International Contrast Ultrasound Society (ICUS). Pediatr Radiol 2013;43(9):1063–73.

30. Eckersley RJ, Chin CT, Burns PN. Optimising phase and amplitude modulation schemes for imaging microbubble contrast agents at low acoustic power. Ultrasound Med Biol 2005;31(2):213–9.

31. Leen E, Averkiou M, Arditi M, et al. Dynamic contrast enhanced ultrasound assessment of the vascular effects of novel therapeutics in early stage trials. Eur Radiol 2012;22(7):1442–50.

32. Arditi M, Frinking PJ, Zhou X, et al. A new formalism for the quantification of tissue perfusion by the destruction-replenishment method in contrast ultrasound imaging. IEEE Trans Ultrason Ferroelectr Freq Control 2006;53(6):1118–29.

33. Bota S, Piscaglia F, Marinelli S, et al. Comparison of international guidelines for noninvasive diagnosis of hepatocellular carcinoma. Liver Cancer 2012;1(3–4):190–200.

34. Maruyama M, Isokawa O, Hoshiyama K, et al. Diagnosis and management of giant hepatic hemangioma: the usefulness of contrast-enhanced ultrasonography. Int J Hepatol 2013;2013:802180.

35. Dietrich CF, Mertens JC, Braden B, et al. Contrast-enhanced ultrasound of histologically proven liver hemangiomas. Hepatology 2007;45(5):1139–45.

36. Kim TK, Jang HJ, Burns PN, et al. Focal nodular hyperplasia and hepatic adenoma: differentiation with low-mechanical-index contrast-enhanced sonography. AJR Am J Roentgenol 2008;190(1): 58–66.

37. Wang W, Chen LD, Lu MD, et al. Contrast-enhanced ultrasound features of histologically proven focal nodular hyperplasia: diagnostic performance compared with contrast-enhanced CT. Eur Radiol 2013;23(9):2546–54.

38. Bartolotta TV, Taibbi A, Matranga D, et al. Hepatic focal nodular hyperplasia: contrast-enhanced ultrasound findings with emphasis on lesion size, depth and liver echogenicity. Eur Radiol 2010; 20(9):2248–56.

39. Bhayana D, Kim TK, Jang HJ, et al. Hypervascular liver masses on contrast-enhanced ultrasound: the importance of washout. AJR Am J Roentgenol 2010; 194(4):977–83.

40. Chaib E, Gama-Rodrigues J, Ribeiro MA Jr, et al. Hepatic adenoma. Timing for surgery. Hepatogastroenterology 2007;54(77):1382–7.

41. Dietrich CF, Schuessler G, Trojan J, et al. Differentiation of focal nodular hyperplasia and hepatocellular adenoma by contrast-enhanced ultrasound. Br J Radiol 2005;78(932):704–7.

42. Jang HJ, Yu H, Kim TK. Contrast-enhanced ultrasound in the detection and characterization of liver tumors. Cancer Imaging 2009;9:96–103.

43. Vachha B, Sun MRM, Siewert B, et al. Cystic lesions of the liver. Am J Roentgenol 2011;196(4): W355–66.

44. Sutherland T, Temple F, Lee WK, et al. Evaluation of focal hepatic lesions with ultrasound contrast agents. J Clin Ultrasound 2011;39(7):399–407.

45. Ding H, Wang WP, Huang BJ, et al. Imaging of focal liver lesions: low-mechanical-index real-time ultrasonography with SonoVue. J Ultrasound Med 2005;24(3):285–97.

46. Kong WT, Wang WP, Cai H, et al. The analysis of enhancement pattern of hepatic inflammatory pseudotumor on contrast-enhanced ultrasound. Abdom Imaging 2014;39(1):168–74.

47. International Consensus Group for Hepatocellular Neoplasia. Pathologic diagnosis of early hepatocellular carcinoma: a report of the international consensus group for hepatocellular neoplasia. Hepatology 2009;49(2):658–64.

48. Tokushige K, Hashimoto E, Kodama K. Hepatocarcinogenesis in non-alcoholic fatty liver disease in Japan. J Gastroenterol Hepatol 2013;28(Suppl 4): 88–92.

49. Giorgio A, Calisti G, di Sarno A, et al. Characterization of dysplastic nodules, early hepatocellular carcinoma and progressed hepatocellular carcinoma in cirrhosis with contrast-enhanced ultrasound. Anticancer Res 2011;31(11): 3977–82.

50. Sugimoto K, Moriyasu F, Shiraishi J, et al. Assessment of arterial hypervascularity of hepatocellular carcinoma: comparison of contrast-enhanced US and gadoxetate disodium-enhanced MR imaging. Eur Radiol 2012;22(6):1205–13.

51. Park YN. Update on precursor and early lesions of hepatocellular carcinomas. Arch Pathol Lab Med 2011;135(6):704–15.

52. Xu HX, Lu MD, Liu LN, et al. Discrimination between neoplastic and non-neoplastic lesions in cirrhotic liver using contrast-enhanced ultrasound. Br J Radiol 2012;85(1018):1376–84.

53. Jang HJ, Kim TK, Burns PN, et al. Enhancement patterns of hepatocellular carcinoma at contrast-enhanced US: comparison with histologic differentiation. Radiology 2007;244(3):898–906.

54. Nicolau C, Catala V, Vilana R, et al. Evaluation of hepatocellular carcinoma using SonoVue, a second generation ultrasound contrast agent: correlation with cellular differentiation. Eur Radiol 2004; 14(6):1092–9.

55. Catalano O, Lobianco R, Cusati B, et al. Hepatocellular carcinoma: spectrum of contrast-enhanced gray-scale harmonic sonography findings. Abdom Imaging 2004;29(3):341–7.

56. Ceccotti P, Leen E, Kalogeropoulou CP, et al. Portal vein thrombosis may alter the correct evaluation of hepatocellular carcinoma with the sonographic contrast pulse sequence technique. J Ultrasound Med 2006;25(12):1619–23.

57. Chen LD, Xu HX, Xie XY, et al. Enhancement patterns of intrahepatic cholangiocarcinoma: comparison between contrast-enhanced ultrasound and contrast-enhanced CT. Br J Radiol 2008; 81(971):881–9.

58. Li R, Zhang X, Ma KS, et al. Dynamic enhancing vascular pattern of intrahepatic peripheral cholangiocarcinoma on contrast-enhanced ultrasound: the influence of chronic hepatitis and cirrhosis. Abdom Imaging 2013;38(1):112–9.

59. Vilana R, Forner A, Bianchi L, et al. Intrahepatic peripheral cholangiocarcinoma in cirrhosis patients may display a vascular pattern similar to hepatocellular carcinoma on contrast-enhanced ultrasound. Hepatology 2010;51(6):2020–9.

60. Xu HX, Lu MD, Liu GJ, et al. Imaging of peripheral cholangiocarcinoma with low-mechanical index contrast-enhanced sonography and SonoVue: initial experience. J Ultrasound Med 2006;25(1):23–33.

61. Avlonitis VS, Linos D. Primary hepatic lymphoma: a review. Eur J Surg 1999;165(8):725–9.

62. Foschi FG, Dall'Aglio AC, Marano G, et al. Role of contrast-enhanced ultrasonography in primary hepatic lymphoma. J Ultrasound Med 2010;29(9): 1353–6.

63. Trenker C, Kunsch S, Michl P, et al. Contrast-enhanced ultrasound (CEUS) in hepatic lymphoma: retrospective evaluation in 38 cases. Ultraschall Med 2014;35(2):142–8.

64. Salvatore V, Bolondi L. Clinical impact of ultrasound-related techniques on the diagnosis of focal liver lesions. Liver Cancer 2012;1(3–4):238–46.

65. Dietrich CF, Kratzer W, Strobe D, et al. Assessment of metastatic liver disease in patients with primary extrahepatic tumors by contrast-enhanced sonography versus CT and MRI. World J Gastroenterol 2006;12(11):1699–705.

66. Larsen LP, Rosenkilde M, Christensen H, et al. The value of contrast enhanced ultrasonography in detection of liver metastases from colorectal cancer: a prospective double-blinded study. Eur J Radiol 2007;62(2):302–7.

67. Cantisani V, Ricci P, Erturk M, et al. Detection of hepatic metastases from colorectal cancer: prospective evaluation of gray scale US versus SonoVue(R) low mechanical index real time-enhanced US as compared with multidetector-CT or Gd-BOPTA-MRI. Ultraschall Med 2010;31(5):500–5.

68. Leoni S, Piscaglia F, Golfieri R, et al. The impact of vascular and nonvascular findings on the noninvasive diagnosis of small hepatocellular carcinoma based on the EASL and AASLD criteria. Am J Gastroenterol 2010;105(3):599–609.

69. Moriyasu F, Itoh K. Efficacy of perflubutane microbubble-enhanced ultrasound in the characterization and detection of focal liver lesions: phase 3 multicenter clinical trial. AJR Am J Roentgenol 2009;193(1):86–95.

70. Numata K, Luo W, Morimoto M, et al. Contrast enhanced ultrasound of hepatocellular carcinoma. World J Radiol 2010;2(2):68–82.

71. Kudo M, Hatanaka K, Maekawa K. Defect reperfusion imaging, a newly developed novel technology using sonazoid in the treatment of hepatocellular carcinoma. J Med Ultrasound 2008;16(3):169–76.

72. Leen E, Ceccotti P, Moug SJ, et al. Potential value of contrast-enhanced intraoperative ultrasonography during partial hepatectomy for metastases: an essential investigation before resection? Ann Surg 2006;243(2):236–40.

73. Martin RC 2nd, Reuter NP, Woodall C. Intra-operative contrast-enhanced ultrasound improves image enhancement in the evaluation of liver tumors. J Surg Oncol 2010;101(5):370–5.

74. Torzilli G. Contrast-enhanced intraoperative ultrasonography in surgery for liver tumors. Eur J Radiol 2004;51(Suppl):S25–9.

75. Nanashima A, Tobinaga S, Abo T, et al. Usefulness of sonazoid-ultrasonography during hepatectomy in patients with liver tumors: a preliminary study. J Surg Oncol 2011;103(2):152–7.

76. Minami Y, Kudo M. Review of dynamic contrast-enhanced ultrasound guidance in ablation therapy for hepatocellular carcinoma. World J Gastroenterol 2011;17(45):4952–9.

77. Solbiati L, Ierace T, Tonolini M, et al. Guidance and monitoring of radiofrequency liver tumor ablation with contrast-enhanced ultrasound. Eur J Radiol 2004;51(Suppl):S19–23.

78. Minami Y, Kudo M, Chung H, et al. Contrast harmonic sonography-guided radiofrequency ablation therapy versus B-mode sonography in hepatocellular carcinoma: prospective randomized controlled trial. AJR Am J Roentgenol 2007;188(2):489–94.

79. Rajesh S, Mukund A, Arora A, et al. Contrast-enhanced US-guided radiofrequency ablation of hepatocellular carcinoma. J Vasc Interv Radiol 2013;24(8):1235–40.

80. Inoue T, Kudo M, Hatanaka K, et al. Usefulness of contrast-enhanced ultrasonography to evaluate the post-treatment responses of radiofrequency ablation for hepatocellular carcinoma: comparison with dynamic CT. Oncology 2013;84(Suppl 1):51–7.

81. Meloni MF, Andreano A, Zimbaro F, et al. Contrast enhanced ultrasound: roles in immediate post-procedural and 24-h evaluation of the effectiveness of thermal ablation of liver tumors. J Ultrasound 2012;15(4):207–14.

82. Salvaggio G, Campisi A, Lo Greco V, et al. Evaluation of posttreatment response of hepatocellular carcinoma: comparison of ultrasonography with second-generation ultrasound contrast agent and multidetector CT. Abdom Imaging 2010;35(4):447–53.

83. Alzaraa A, Gravante G, Chung WY, et al. Contrast-enhanced ultrasound in the preoperative, intraoperative and postoperative assessment of liver lesions. Hepatol Res 2013;43(8):809–19.

84. Tang MX, Eckersley RJ. Nonlinear propagation of ultrasound through microbubble contrast agents and implications for imaging. IEEE Trans Ultrason Ferroelectr Freq Control 2006;53(12):2406–15.

85. Fan ZH, Chen MH, Dai Y, et al. Evaluation of primary malignancies of the liver using contrast-enhanced sonography: correlation with pathology. AJR Am J Roentgenol 2006;186(6):1512–9.

86. Eisenhauer EA, Therasse P, Bogaerts J, et al. New response evaluation criteria in solid tumours: revised RECIST guideline (version 1.1). Eur J Cancer 2009;45(2):228–47.

87. Chun YS, Vauthey JN, Boonsirikamchai P, et al. Association of computed tomography morphologic criteria with pathologic response and survival in patients treated with bevacizumab for colorectal liver metastases. JAMA 2009;302(21):2338–44.

88. Jain RK. Normalization of tumor vasculature: an emerging concept in antiangiogenic therapy. Science 2005;307(5706):58–62.

89. Gauthier M, Leguerney I, Thalmensi J, et al. Estimation of intra-operator variability in perfusion parameter measurements using DCE-US. World J Radiol 2011;3(3):70–81.

90. Kiessling F, Fokong S, Koczera P, et al. Ultrasound microbubbles for molecular diagnosis, therapy, and theranostics. J Nucl Med 2012;53(3):345–8.

Elastography of the Abdomen

Richard G. Barr, MD, PhD, FACR, FSRU[a,b,*]

KEYWORDS

- Elastography • Liver fibrosis • Cirrhosis • Liver • Strain • Stiffness • Ultrasound • Pancreas

KEY POINTS

- There are 2 types of elastography, strain elastography that is qualitative and shear wave elastography that is quantitative.
- Although malignant focal liver lesions are statistically stiffer than benign lesions, there is a large overlap. Therefore, for any individual lesion, elastography is limited in characterizing the lesion as benign or malignant.
- Shear wave elastography is an excellent method for noninvasive evaluation of liver fibrosis.
- Elastography can characterize fluid collections as serous or mucinous.
- Stiffness measurements of the liver and or spleen may be a noninvasive method of assessing hepatic venous pressure.

INTRODUCTION

Ultrasound elastography is a new technique that generates images based on the stiffness of tissue as opposed to anatomy. Many disease states have changes in stiffness that can be detected by elastography. Ultrasound elastography has been used to evaluate multiple organs.[1,2] There are 2 elastography techniques presently available: strain elastography (SE) and shear wave (SWE) imaging.[3,4]

Focal liver masses have a mixed appearance on elastography, with a large overlap in the stiffness of benign and malignant lesion making characterization of focal liver masses problematic with elastography.[5] However, diffuse liver disease, such as fibrosis, can be graded and monitored with SWE. Shear waves do not propagate in simple fluid.[3] Initial studies suggest shear wave imaging may be helpful in characterization of a cystic lesion as serous or mucinous in nature.[1] Evaluation of other abdominal organs has been limited.

Diffuse liver disease is one of the major health problems in the world. Hepatitis is a group of liver disorders characterized by liver inflammation and necrosis of hepatocytes. Hepatitis can be acute or chronic if these changes persist for at least 6 months. Hepatitis C (HCV) and hepatitis B (HBV) viruses are the leading causes of chronic liver disease. It is estimated that 180 and 350 million people worldwide are infected with HCV and HBV, respectively. Annual mortality is estimated at 500,000 to 700,000 and 350,000 as a result of HBV-related and HCV-related liver diseases, respectively.[6–8]

In patients with HCV, failure to spontaneously eradicate infection occurs in 50% to 90% of cases depending on the route of transmission, presence

Funding Sources: R.G. Barr has a research grant from Bracco Diagnostics. R.G. Barr has equipment grants from Siemens Ultrasound, Philips Ultrasound, SuperSonic Imagine, and Esaote Ultrasound. R.G. Barr has received compensation for educational presentations from Philips Ultrasound, Siemens Ultrasound and SuperSonic Imagine.
Conflict of Interest: R.G. Barr is a member of advisory panels for Siemens Ultrasound, Philips Ultrasound, and Toshiba America Medical Systems.
[a] Department of Radiology, Northeastern Ohio Medical University, Rootstown, OH 44272, USA; [b] Southwoods Imaging, 7623 Market Street, Youngstown, OH 44512, USA
* Southwoods Imaging, 7623 Market Street, Youngstown, OH 44512.
E-mail address: rgbarr@zoominternet.net

Ultrasound Clin 9 (2014) 625–640
http://dx.doi.org/10.1016/j.cult.2014.07.002
1556-858X/14/$ – see front matter © 2014 Elsevier Inc. All rights reserved.

of symptomatic hepatitis, and age at which infection occurred.[9] In Western countries, liver disease caused by HCV is the main indication for liver transplantation.

Chronic liver damage results in hepatic fibrosis characterized by an increase in extracellular matrix material produced by fibroblast-like cells in the hepatic parenchyma.[10] Consequently, the liver becomes stiffer than normal and the distortion of normal liver architecture can cause portal hypertension. Fibrosis is the feature mostly related to the progression of chronic hepatitis. It may progress toward liver cirrhosis, leading to hepatic failure, increased risk of hepatocellular carcinoma (HCC), and eventually, death.

The histologic evaluation of liver biopsies is carried out using scoring systems that produce values for various categories of inflammation (grade) and fibrosis (stage). There are several scoring systems all categorizing similar features. In the assessment of HCV chronic hepatitis, the most reproducible scoring system is the Metavir. On the Metavir scoring system, liver fibrosis is evaluated semi-quantitatively and staged on a 5-point scale from 0 to 4 (F0, absent; F1, enlarged fibrotic portal tract; F2, periportal or initial portal-portal septa but intact architecture; F3, architectural distortion but no obvious cirrhosis; and F4, cirrhosis).[11]

Liver disease progression takes place over several decades and is accelerated by the presence of cofactors, such as alcohol consumption, diabetes mellitus, older age of acquisition, human immunodeficiency virus (HIV) coinfection, or coinfection with other viruses.[6] Depending on the presence of cofactors, between 10% and 40% of patients with chronic HCV infection will develop cirrhosis.[12] The prognosis of chronic liver disease is strongly dependent on the extent of liver fibrosis with life-threatening complications that may occur in patients with cirrhosis. Death related to the complications of cirrhosis occurs at an incidence rate of approximately 4% per year, whereas HCC occurs in this population at an estimated incidence rate of 1% to 5% per year.[13] Thus, a precise estimate of the degree of liver fibrosis is essential for surveillance, treatment decisions, and estimation of prognosis.[14–16]

Assessment of liver disease severity is recommended before therapy. As reported in 2012 EASL guidelines for the management of HCV infection,[6] treatment should be initiated promptly in patients with advanced fibrosis (Metavir score F3-F4) and strongly considered in patients with moderate fibrosis (Metavir score F2).

The cirrhotic transformation of the liver is associated with structural and biological changes responsible for an increase in portal pressure.[17]

Although liver biopsy remains the standard for establishing the diagnosis of diffuse liver disease, it is an invasive method associated with patient discomfort and, in rare cases, serious complications,[18–20] and it is limited by significant intra-observer and interobserver variability and sampling errors.[21–23] A noninvasive method of determining liver fibrosis could lead to improved screening for early fibrosis allowing for treatment at a stage that has improved outcomes. Furthermore, this will allow for a noninvasive method to monitor the effect of treatments.

PRINCIPLES OF ELASTOGRAPHY

Elastography is a new technique in ultrasound, which can provide clinically useful information that was previously not available. Elasticity imaging or elastography is an imaging modality based on tissue stiffness rather than anatomy. Palpation has been used to evaluate for a malignancy for over a thousand years.[24] Ultrasound elastography can be considered as the imaging equivalent of palpation being able to quantify the stiffness of a lesion, which was previously judged only subjectively by physical examination.

There are 2 types of elastography: SE and SWE imaging.[3] SE produces an image based on how tissues respond to a displacement force from an external or patient source. This displacement force allows for a qualitative assessment of the lesion. SWE applies a special strong low-frequency acoustic radiation force impulse (ARFI) pulse (push pulse) that results in shear wave propagation that can be measured as a velocity. Because the shear wave speed through tissues depends on the stiffness of the tissue, a quantitative value of the stiffness can be obtained. A more detailed discussion of these techniques can be found elsewhere.[4]

SE

SE determines the relative strain or elasticity of tissue within a field-of-view (FOV).[3] The more an object deforms when a force is applied, the higher the strain and the softer the lesion. To determine the strain of a tissue or lesion, one must evaluate how the lesion deforms when an external force is applied. For example, if an almond was in a bowl of gelatin and the gelatin was pushed down on, the gelatin would deform, indicating it has high strain and is therefore soft. However, the almond would not deform, having low strain, and is therefore hard.

SE is performed on standard ultrasound equipment with specific software that evaluates the frame-to-frame differences in deformation in tissue when a force (stress) is applied. The force can be from patient movement, such as breathing, heartbeat, or external compression with rhythmic motion of the ultrasound transducer as the source of the movement.[3] The technique required to obtain the optimal images varies by system.[3] In SE, the absolute strain modulus value cannot be calculated because the amount of the push (force) cannot be accurately measured. The real-time SE image is displayed with a scale based on the relative strain of the tissues within the FOV.

Results can be displayed in gray-scale or with various color displays; preference is often determined by the user's exposure to elastography and preference in interpretation. In the gray-scale map, soft is coded white, while hard is coded black. It is important to remember that in SE a relative scale is displayed and should not be confused with shear wave imaging where an absolute stiffness value is obtained and color-coded on a per-pixel basis. Several factors affecting the elastogram are important in performing SE, including what tissues are included in the FOV, amount of precompression, and tissue movement. These factors are discussed in detail elsewhere.[3,25,26]

Elastography Using an ARFI Pulse

The use of a low-frequency ultrasound ARFI pulse (push pulse) can be used as a source of tissue displacement. This technique is called ARFI.[27–29] This push pulse generates both axial displacement and shear waves. Shear wave imaging is described in later discussion. When the axial displacement is measured, the technique is similar to SE called Virtual Touch Imaging© (VTI; Siemens Ultrasound, Mountain View, CA, USA).

There are several differences between SE and VTI. One important difference is that radiation force in ARFI imaging is maximized at the point of focus, whereas in SE strain is more uniform laterally in the image based on transducer compression and the amount of stress applied locally and changes with depth. Therefore, a strain ratio for VTI should not be used as a semiquantitative method. A quantitative value of stiffness cannot be obtained using VTI. The ARFI pulse power is limited by guidelines of energy input into a body and thus can be limited by depth penetration. In general, the ARFI push pulse is limited in producing displacement deeper than 8 to 9 cm in abdominal applications.

If an ARFI push pulse is used to generate the tissue displacement, no manual displacement should be used. The probe should be held steady and the patient asked to hold their breath and remain motionless during the acquisition.

SWE

A second technique to determine the elastic properties of a tissue is SWE. In this technique, an initial ARFI pulse (push pulse) is applied to the tissue that induces a shear wave perpendicular to the ultrasound beam. This technique is similar to dropping a stone (the push pulse) into a pond of water. The ripples generated correspond to the shear waves. Conventional B-mode ultrasound sampling techniques are used to calculate the speed of the shear wave generated through the tissues. This technique is diagrammed in **Fig. 1**. The velocity of the shear wave is proportional to stiffness. The hardness of a lesion can be displayed as the speed of the shear wave (Vs) (meters/s [m/s]) through the tissue, or the strain modulus (kiloPascals [kPa]).[4] With SWE, a quantitative measure of the tissue stiffness is obtained either in point of interest or in an FOV with pixel-by-pixel color-coding of the Vs (2-dimensional [2D]-SWE).

Three shear wave systems for abdominal applications are presently available. In the ACUSON

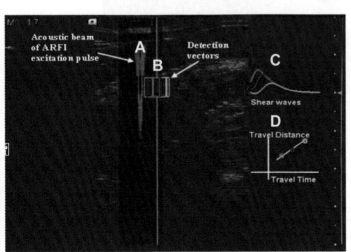

Fig. 1. By applying a high-energy ARFI pulse (*A*), shear waves are generated that propagate perpendicular to the push pulse. Conventional ultrasound is used to monitor the shear waves within the tissue (*B*). The shear waves have higher signal intensity closer to the push pulse and the amplitude of the peak decreases with distance from the push pulse (*C*). By plotting the time to peak and the distance from the push pulse (*D*), the velocity of the shear wave can be calculated. It can be expressed either as the velocity in m/s or with some assumptions of the Young's modulus in kPa.

S3000 ultrasound system (Siemens), a measurement in a small region of interest (ROI) can be obtained (Virtual Touch tissue quantification). A single image is obtained with the measurement of the shear wave speed in the selected ROI displayed. A similar technique is available on the IU22 and the EPIQ (Philips Ultrasound, Bothell, WA, USA) called ElastPQ. In the Aixplorer (SuperSonic Imagine, Aix-en-Provence, France), the effect of the push pulses is amplified by sending a series of pulses successively focused at increasing depths faster than the shear wave's velocity, so that a mach cone front is generated. A high imaging frame rate is achieved by transmitting a plane wave that insonates the entire FOV in a single burst. The result is that the shear wave velocity can be measured and displayed (m/s or kPa) as a quantitative color overlay image at a frame rate of around 1 frame per second.

ELASTOGRAPHY OF THE LIVER
Focal Liver Lesions

Both SE and SWE can be used to evaluate focal liver lesions.[5,30–32] Because SE is qualitative, a lesion can be compared with "normal" liver to determine if the lesion is harder or softer than the background liver. However, this technique is limited in that the background liver may have variable stiffness depending on the degree of steatosis

or fibrosis. In addition, both benign and malignant lesions can be soft or hard compared with normal liver. With SWE, a stiffness measurement is obtained; however, because of the wide variability of a given pathologic abnormality's stiffness, characterization of a lesion as benign or malignant is problematic. For example, in a series by Yu and Wilson,[5] hemangioma had a range of Vs of 0.87 to 4.01 m/s with an average of 0.71 m/s, whereas HCC had a range of 0.77 to 4.34 m/s with an average of 1.01 m/s. Overall, the difference in Vs of malignant 2.57 ± 1.01 m/s and benign lesions 1.73 ± 0.8 was statistically significant ($P<.01$); however, the large overlap between benign and malignant makes the technique unreliable for focal liver mass characterization in any given case. **Fig. 2** is a selected shear wave elastogram of a patient with multiple metastatic lesions from colorectal carcinoma demonstrating the variability of metastatic lesions in the same patient. At this time, the use of elastography is not recommended for characterization of focal liver lesions.

Elastography can be used to improve visualization of a lesion for biopsy (**Fig. 3**) and may be useful in following lesions after treatment.[33]

Diffuse Liver Disease

Liver fibrosis is a significant worldwide problem. As fibrosis progresses, there is increasing loss of

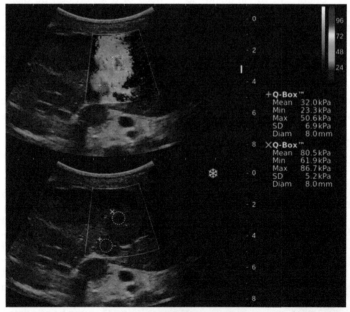

Fig. 2. 2D shear wave elastogram of the liver in a patient with diffuse metastatic disease from colorectal carcinoma demonstrates the marked difference in the stiffness of 2 metastatic lesions (*white circles*), one with mean value of 32 kPa and the other with a value of 81 kPa. The wide range of stiffness seen with both benign and malignant lesions overlaps, significantly limiting the use of shear wave imaging in characterization of focal liver lesions.

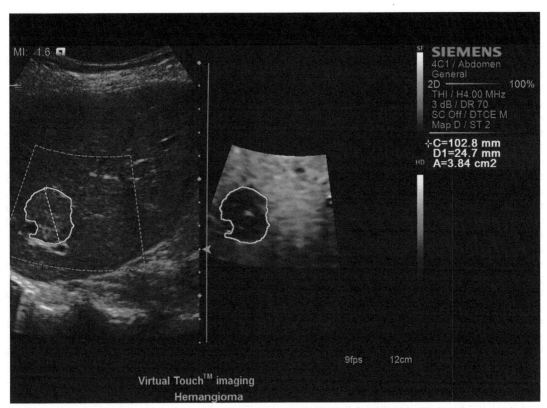

MI: 1.6

SF **SIEMENS**
4C1 / Abdomen
General
2D ———————— 100%
THI / H4.00 MHz
3 dB / DR 70
SC Off / DTCE M
Map D / ST 2

÷C=102.8 mm
D1=24.7 mm
HD A=3.84 cm2

9fps   12cm

Virtual Touch™ imaging
Hemangioma

Fig. 3. VTI of a liver hemangioma. The image on the left is the B-mode image. The hemangioma is poorly visualized on B-mode. The image on the right is the VTI image. The lesion is stiffer than surrounding liver and therefore displaced blacker than the surrounding liver. (*Courtesy of* D. Clevert, MD, Munich, Germany.)

liver function and higher risk of liver cancer. This chronic liver disease is characterized by the deposition of fibrous tissue within the liver. The stage of liver fibrosis is important to determine prognosis, surveillance, and treatment options. Early-stage fibrosis is reversible, whereas the disease that has progressed to cirrhosis is likely irreversible. Presently, the only method of staging the fibrosis has been by liver biopsy.[15] Liver biopsy is considered the gold standard for fibrosis assessment and stage classification and is also able to grade necro-inflammatory activity. In addition to being invasive with potential complications that can be severe in up to 1% of cases,[34,35] a liver biopsy represents roughly only 1/50,000 of the liver volume, and there is interobserver variability at microscopic evaluation.[21] Therefore, noninvasive methods for liver fibrosis assessment have been an intense field of research, including elastographic methods using ultrasound and magnetic resonance imaging.

There has been a proliferation of different methods of liver elastography for the evaluation of liver fibrosis that are not equivalent, which means that cutoff values are system-specific and cannot be readily compared between systems.

There are many confounders that can influence elastography results. These confounders include patient-dependent factors, such as congestive heart failure,[36] exacerbations of acute hepatitis associated with transaminase elevations,[37] and ingestion of food,[38] all of which make the liver stiffer. Artificially elevated stiffness measurements can be seen with extrahepatic cholestasis,[36] with the use of β-blockers,[39] as well as by holding inspiration (Valsalva). Measurements should be taken during a breath-hold in a neutral breathing position. Measurements taken in the left lobe of the liver are often unreliable and less reproducible.[40–42] Stiffness values are higher in the first 1.5 cm to 2.0 cm from the liver capsule and measurements in this location should not be performed. Large vessels should also not be included in the area being measured.[42,43]

Transient Elastography

Transient elastography (TE), introduced in 2003, is the first ultrasound-based elastography technique for the liver and has the largest body of published works. It is performed using the Fibroscan© (Echosens, Paris, France). TE is performed with self-standing dedicated equipment with specific probes through an intercostal approach. The probe contains an electrodynamic transducer that is used to generate a 50-Hz center frequency and 2-mm peak-to-peak amplitude (with M probe) transient displacement. A single-element ultrasound transducer (3.5 MHz with M probe) is mounted on the axis of the vibrator. The transducer is used in conventional pulse-echo acquisition to provide A-mode and M-mode images to the operator in real-time for liver localization. When measurement is triggered, ultrafast pulse-echo sequence is performed with a pulse repetition frequency of 6 kHz during the propagation of the controlled shear wave. The acquisition lasts 80 ms, and strain induced in the liver by the propagation of the shear wave is measured using the standard autocorrelation approach between successive ultrasound lines. The patient lies on his back with the right arm behind the head. It is recommended that 10 valid measurements be performed to have a complete examination, and the median of all valid measurements is used as the final liver stiffness (LS) result. Values are measured in kiloPascals. Measurements of the liver in humans range between 1.5 kPa and 75.0 kPa. The volume of the liver parenchyma examined by TE is at least 100 times greater than a liver biopsy. Various probes are available for patients of various body types. Intra-observer and interobserver reproducibility of TE measurements is excellent (intraclass correlation coefficient [ICC] 0.98 for both) in nonobese subjects.[44] TE values are higher in men than women.

TE cannot be performed in patients with perihepatic ascites. B-mode imaging cannot be performed with FibroScan©. In a study of 13,369 examinations obtaining LS measurements with the standard probe, failure occurred in 3.1% and results were unreliable in 15.8% of cases.[38] Failure rates were associated with body mass index (BMI) greater than 30 kg/m², age greater than 52 years, and type 2 diabetes. In another study, the failure rate with the standard probe correlated with the BMI. The failure rate was 7% for BMI greater than or equal to 30 kg/m², 19% for BMI greater than or equal to 35 kg/m², and 59% for BMI greater than or equal to 40 kg/m². However, the failure rate was significantly decreased in these patients when using the XL probe.[45]

In patients with chronic HCV, LS values greater than 6.8 to 7.6 kPa signify a high probability of significant fibrosis ($F \geq 2$) on biopsy. The cutoff values for predicting cirrhosis ($F = 4$) range between 11.0 and 13.6 kPa.[46,47] Although TE is less accurate in distinguishing between contiguous stages of fibrosis, it can differentiate absence and mild fibrosis from significant fibrosis and cirrhosis. A meta-analysis in recurrent HCV posttransplantation demonstrated 98% sensitivity and 84% specificity of TE for predicting cirrhosis.[48] The use of TE in chronic HCV has been endorsed in the recommendations for the management of viral hepatitis by the European Association for the Study of the Liver.[6]

In chronic HBV patients, a recent meta-analysis[49] found the mean area under receiver operator curves (AUROCs) for the diagnosis of significant fibrosis (F2) and cirrhosis (F4) of 0.859 and 0.929, respectively. In chronic HBV patients, acute inflammation is not uncommon and can affect the LS measurement. It has been suggested that the cutoff values should be modified to account for alanine aminotransferase levels.[50]

Studies performed in patients with nonalcoholic fatty liver disease (NAFLD) and nonalcoholic steato-hepatitis (NASH) have found steatosis does not appear to affect LS measurements,[45,51,52] because it does not change the speed of shear waves but does attenuate them. Wong[53] compared TE to liver biopsy in 246 consecutive NAFLD patients and found a 91% sensitivity and 75% specificity for predicting severe fibrosis ($F \geq 3$), using a cutoff value of 7.9 kPa.

TE has been used to assess many other diffuse liver diseases with similar good results.[54] TE has been evaluated to screen a general community-based population for significant liver fibrosis. In 1190 patients older than 45 evaluated for a medical checkup, 7.5% had LS measurements greater than 8 kPa. The liver biochemistry was normal in these patients; however, a cause of chronic liver disease was found in 43%.[55]

The use of TE for predicting complications of cirrhosis, such as portal hypertension and mortality, has been studied. The AUROCs for predicting clinically significant portal hypertension (hepatic venous pressure gradient ≥ 12 mm Hg) were 0.94 to 0.99 for cutoffs ranging from 13.6 to 21 kPa.[56,57] Measurements of splenic stiffness have also been evaluated and showed better correlation with portal pressure ($r = 0.89$) in patients with cirrhosis than LS.[58] Spleen stiffness values had high AUROC values (0.966) for the identification of patients with portal hypertension with hepatic venous pressure gradients greater than or equal to 10 mm Hg.[58] TE cutoff values from 19.8 to 47.5 kPa were able to predict grade 2 or 3 esophageal varices with AUROCs of 0.72 to 0.78.[59–61] Because of the wide variance in values between studies, TE cannot replace upper gastrointestinal (GI) endoscopy for identifying patients with varices.[2]

In a large prospective study of patients with chronic HCV, TE was more accurate than liver biopsy in predicting prognosis. Patients with TE greater than 9.5 kPa had a significantly reduced 5-year survival.[62]

Two prospective studies have evaluated the risk of HCC developing over a 3-year period in 866 HCV[63] and 1130 HBV patients.[64] The risk of developing HCC paralleled the increase in LS, not only separating patients with or without cirrhosis, but also grouping patients in different risk classes within those with already established cirrhosis.

European Federation of Societies for Ultrasound in Medicine and Biology (EFSUMB) has made the following recommendation for clinical use of TE:

1. TE can be used to assess the severity of liver fibrosis in patients with chronic viral hepatitis, provided that confounding factors are taken into account, and especially to distinguish patients with nil/mild fibrosis from those with significant fibrosis and to identify those with cirrhosis.
2. TE is useful for assessment of liver fibrosis in patients with NAFLD, in patients with alcoholic liver diseases, and in patients coinfected with HIV and HCV. Other types of chronic liver disease might also be investigated, but the evidence is more limited.
3. TE is useful for assessment of liver fibrosis in patients with posttransplant recurrence of chronic HCV.
4. TE has some value for predicting the occurrence of complications of liver cirrhosis, portal hypertension, HCC, and liver-associated mortality. It cannot replace upper GI endoscopy for identifying patients with varices.

Shear Wave Speed Measurement

With increasing fibrosis, the liver becomes stiffer, which can be monitored using SWE.[42,65] With this technique, an ROI is placed in a region of the liver taking care not to include large vasculature. An intercostal approach in segment 8 of the liver has been shown to provide more accurate results. Serial measurements are taken while the patient suspends respiration. The average of these measurements is used to estimate degree of liver fibrosis.

Fig. 4 shows the results of a 27-year-old patient with chronic HCV. The stiffness average of 4.77 kPa is consistent with the patient's liver biopsy result of mild fibrosis. **Fig. 5** is an image from a patient with marked cirrhosis demonstrating a markedly elevated stiffness of 66 kPa.

How this new technology can be used in clinical practice is under extensive investigation.[42] The use of this technique may be able to decrease the number of liver biopsies performed for the evaluation of chronic liver disease. Potential uses

of this technique include liver cirrhosis suspected but not obvious on B-mode ultrasound, evaluation of patients with chronic HCV, follow-up of patients to detect a progression of liver disease, and initiation of treatment.

SWE can be performed in a small ROI, point SWE (pSWE), or with a color-coded map of the shear wave speed (in either m/s or kPa) over a larger ROI.

As with TE, patients should fast for at least 4 hours. SWE measurements are performed intercostally in the right lobe of the liver with conventional curved array transducers. The right arm is extended over the patient's head. The probe is aligned in the intercostal space, limiting rib shadowing. The ROI is placed in the liver at least 1.5 to 2 cm below the liver capsule so as not to include large vessels. The recommended depth is between 3 and 7 cm.[2] The patient is asked to suspend respiration without taking a breath in (Valsalva). In pSWE, the scan is triggered and the measured shear wave speed is displayed. One 2D-SWE system allows for real-time imaging of the color-coded mapping of shear wave speed. Scanning for 3 to 4 seconds in the same location is needed for stabilization of the shear wave measurements. If the signal is weak or unstable, the penetration mode can be used.

As with TE, elevated aminotransferase levels are associated with higher LS values with SWE.[66,67] SWE allows measurements at different sites and a comparison of the right and left lobes shows a trend toward higher values in the left[40,41,68]; however, results obtained in the right lobe of the liver were more accurate compared with liver biopsy.[68]

All vendors recommend taking serial measurements and using a mean value for making clinical decisions. The number of measurements recommended varies in the literature from 5 to 10. Values that are obviously inaccurate are discarded. The inaccurate values can be due to transducer movement or patient movement during the data acquisition. Most systems have a quality assessment for an adequate shear wave measurement with no value given in pSWE or no color-coding in 2D-SWE. Quality indicators have been recommended including an interquartile range less than 30% and a success rate of greater than 60%.[69]

Interobserver variability with pSWE has been shown to be good with ICC = 0.87.[41,43] Interoperator reproducibility has also been reported to be good using 2D-SWE.[70]

Cutoff values of 1.21 to 1.34 m/s have been shown to predict significant fibrosis ($F \geq 2$) with an AUROC of 0.85 to 0.89.[71,72] For diagnosis of cirrhosis, SWE cutoff values range from 1.55

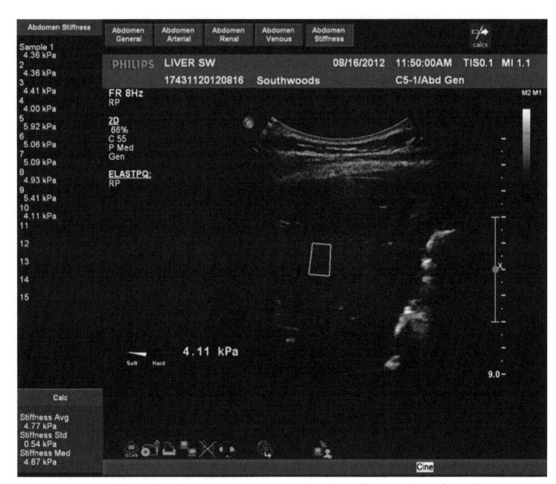

Fig. 4. SWE of a 28-year-old patient with chronic HCV infection. The stiffness average of 4.77 kPa is consistent with the patient's liver biopsy result of mild fibrosis. White rectangle shows FOV where the measurement was obtained. Note that 10 measurements were made. The system calculates the average stiffness, median stiffness, and the standard deviation.

to 2.0 m/s with AUROC of 0.89 to 0.93.[71–73] In a recent meta-analysis of 518 patients with chronic liver disease,[74] the AUROC was 0.87 for predicting significant fibrosis ($F \geq 2$), 0.91 for severe fibrosis ($F \geq 3$), and 0.93 for cirrhosis. The values for 2D-SWE are similar to pSWE with AUROCs of 0.95 to 0.98 for $F \geq 2$, 0.96 for $F \geq 3$, and 0.97 to 0.98 for $F = 4$.[75,76]

The accuracy of SWE for the assessment of liver fibrosis is similar to TE.[71,77] SWE allows for measurements in patients with ascites, whereas TE does not. Preliminary findings using SWE show promising results in patients with NAFLD and NASH[78,79] and posttransplantation.[80]

Recommendations are that pSWE and 2D-SWE can be used to assess the severity of liver fibrosis in patients with chronic viral hepatitis, especially with HCV. Cutoff values between different shear wave methodologies and for different brands of scanners vary using the same methodology.[2]

SE

Most major manufacturers have SE available at least in their high-end systems. SE does not provide a stiffness value. Therefore, several semi-quantitative methods for interpretation have been proposed including the German elasticity score,[81] the Japanese elasticity score,[82] and the liver fibrosis index (LF Index).[83] All are based on visual assessments of the spatial patterns of strain imaging within a ROI. The LF Index uses 9 features to calculate a "stiffness value," including mean and standard deviation of the relative strain value, complexity and ratio of the blue area in the ROI, skewness, kurtosis, entropy, inverse-difference moment, and angular second moment.[42] Several studies using SE have been published.[81,84–89] However, the evidence with this approach is still limited to allow recommendation for its clinical use.[2] **Fig. 6** shows examples of strain imaging of diffuse liver disease.

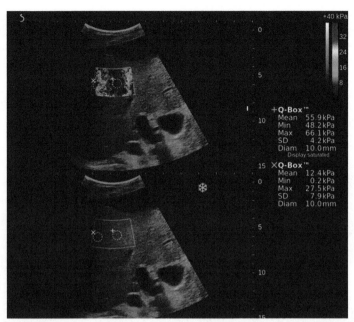

Fig. 5. The shear wave elastogram of a 64-year-old man with advanced alcohol-induced cirrhosis confirms a markedly stiff liver with a value of 55.9 kPa. White circles are the FOV where the measurement of stiffness was taken. The measurement taken in the lateral portion of the FOV should not be used because the accuracy is decreased at the lateral portions of the ROI.

ELASTOGRAPHY OF THE PANCREAS

Pancreatic masses have been evaluated using elastography as both an endoscopic and a transabdominal approach. The pancreas is of uniform intermediate stiffness but, with advancing age, it may become heterogeneous.

With the endoscopic approach, a classification based on a color-scale SE has been used (red as soft, and blue as hard). The normal pancreas is soft and homogeneous, coded green.[90–95] Benign inflammatory pancreatic pathologic abnormality can appear with a honeycomb appearance of predominately blue,[90,92,93] a heterogeneous mixed color pattern with predominately green pattern,[90,92,93] or a homogeneously green pattern.[90,93] Adenocarcinoma has a homogeneous blue pattern (stiff) or appears as a heterogeneous predominantly blue lesion.[90–94] However, this pattern is also observed in half of the chronic pancreatitis patients, so that the specificity of the method in the diagnosis of adenocarcinoma has been reported to be about 60%.[90] Pancreatic neuroendocrine tumors have been reported to have a predominantly blue honeycomb pattern, a homogeneous blue pattern, a green central area surrounded by blue tissue, or a homogeneous green pattern.[93]

Preliminary studies suggest that a homogeneous green pattern can be used to exclude malignancy.[91] However, the clinical usefulness of this technique in distinguishing benign from malignant pathologic abnormalities is limited. Inflammatory lesions of the pancreas can be hard or soft depending on the stage of the inflammation. Neoplasms can have necrotic areas that appear soft in contrast to the viable tumor, which is hard. Itokawa[92] found the strain ratio (strain of lesion compared with strain of normal pancreas) was 23.7 ± 12.7 for mass-forming pancreatitis and 39.1 ± 20.5 for pancreatic cancer.[92]

In differentiating benign and malignant focal pancreatic masses, qualitative[90,91] and semiquantitative strain techniques[92,96–99] have been reported, both showing high overall accuracy. Two meta-analyses published have indicated that endoscopic ultrasound (EUS) elastography has a high sensitivity but lower specificity in differentiation of focal pancreatic masses.[100,101] Computer-aided diagnosis techniques have been suggested to improve the accuracy for the differential diagnosis of focal pancreatic masses.[96,97]

There is less literature on the use of SWE in the evaluation of cystic pancreatic masses. The use of SWE using the point quantification method may be able to distinguish serous from mucinous malignancies. Serous fluid has low viscosity and does not propagate shear waves. A value of XXX or 0 is obtained depending on vendor, indicating shear waves were not identified in the fluid. However,

A

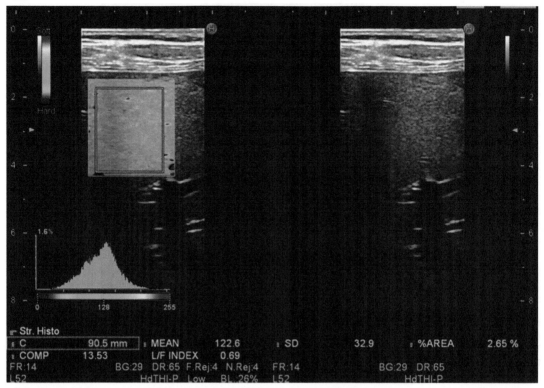

B

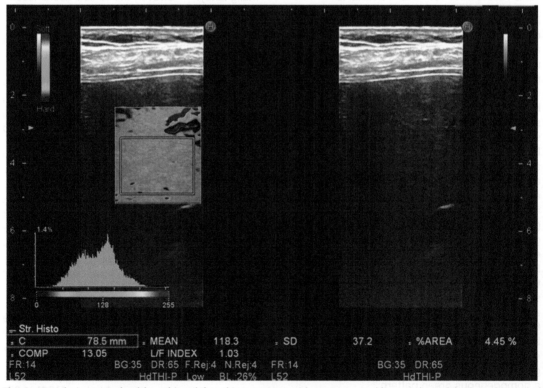

Fig. 6. SE technique in a healthy subject (*A*) and in a patient with compensated liver cirrhosis (*B*). The color-coded elastography ROI is overlaid on conventional B-mode image. Red indicates that tissue is soft, and blue indicates that it is hard. Strain histogram and LF are displayed. (*Courtesy of* G. Ferraioli, MD, Pavia, Italy.)

mucinous cystic lesions have high viscosity that does propagate shear waves. With cystic lesions that contain mucin, a shear wave velocity (expressed in m/s or kPa) will be obtained. Preliminary results using this technique appear promising.[102,103] In the study of D'Onofrio and colleagues, 14 mucinous cystadenomas, 4 pseudocysts, 3 intraductal papillary-mucinous neoplasms, and 2 serous cystadenomas were studied. The values obtained ranged from XXXX/0 to 4.85 m/s in mucinous cystadenomas, from XXXX/0 to 3.11 m/s in pseudocysts, and from XXXX/0 to 4.57 m/s in intraductal papillary-mucinous neoplasms. In serous cystadenomas, all values measured were XXXX/0 m/s. Diagnostic accuracy in benign and nonbenign differentiation of pancreatic cystic lesions was 78%.

Fig. 7 demonstrates the use of point shear wave quantification (A) and the use strain imaging (B) in a patient with acute chronic pancreatitis. A recent study has demonstrated that acute pancreatitis can be diagnosed using SWE with a high sensitivity and specificity. Using a cutoff value of 1.63 m/s, a sensitivity of 100% and a specificity of 98% were obtained. SWE performed better than B-mode ultrasound and CT in the diagnosis of acute pancreatitis.[104]

EFSUMB guidelines and recommendation on the clinical use of ultrasound elastography recommendations are (1) EUS elastography is useful as a complementary tool for the characterization of focal pancreatic lesions; (2) when there is strong clinical suspicion of pancreatic cancer, but the biopsy is inconclusive or negative, a hard focal lesion on elastography and/or suggestive endoscopic contrast-enhanced ultrasound (hypovascular lesion) should guide clinical management by indicating repeat EUS-fine-needle aspiration or direct referral to surgery; (3) EUS elastography cannot be currently recommended for differentiating advanced chronic pancreatitis from pancreatic carcinoma due to their similar tissue stiffness in a large proportion of cases.[2]

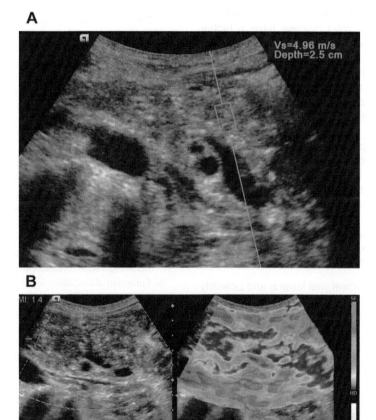

A

Vs=4.96 m/s
Depth=2.5 cm

B

MI: 1.4

Fig. 7. In this patient who presented with abdominal pain, B-mode imaging shows an enlarged pancreas with irregular contour and echotexture, multiple calculi, with mild peripancreatic edema. There is increased shear wave velocity of 4.96 m/s (*A*), suggesting acute pancreatitis. The corresponding SE image (*B*) shows increased stiffness (color scale with red as hard) throughout the entire pancreatic body and tail also suggestive of acute inflammation. (*Courtesy of* A. Mateen, MD, Hyderabad, India.)

ELASTOGRAPHY OF THE GI TRACT

Elastography may show the layered structure of the GI wall but these do not always correspond to the B-mode layers. A technique called strain rate imaging (SRI) has been proposed to assess contractility of the GI walls.[105] SE can be used to assess the stiffness of focal lesions of the GI tract.[106] SE of the GI tract is performed with linear transducers and is available on many scanners. SRI is only available with specific dedicated software currently available only with one scanner.

Shadowing from bowel gas and peristalsis is a major challenge to elastography of the GI tract, degrading image quality and reducing accuracy of semiquantitative elastography measurements. More studies are needed to establish the role of elastography in the evaluation of GI pathologic abnormality and motility.

Preliminary work suggests that elastography may be helpful in assessing whether a stenosis in Crohn disease is caused by inflammation or fibrosis.[107–109] Fibrotic stenosis appears stiff, whereas inflammatory stenosis appears soft. Patients with active Crohn disease have a higher strain ratio between the inflamed and normal regions than patients in remission.[108]

Assessment of the relative strain of the muscle layers of the gastric wall is feasible and allows mapping of the strain distribution.[105] Preliminary work suggests SRI can distinguish contractile activity of the longitudinal from the circular muscle layers that cannot be appreciated on B-mode.[110,111] SRI has been used both in vitro and in vivo to monitor response to drug intervention.[110–112] Ahmed and colleagues[113] were able to identify subgroups of dyspepsia from strain measurements of the gastric wall by SRI.

The EFSUMB guidelines and recommendations on the clinical use of ultrasound elastography state elastography is indicated for the following:

1. Characterizing bowel wall lesions and possibly discerning the active phase of inflammation from fibrotic stenosis using SE.
2. The evaluation of gastric contractility and GI wall strain using SRI.[2]

SUMMARY

Ultrasound elastography can provide additional information over conventional ultrasound in lesion detection or characterization of abdominal masses. However, there is some overlap of the stiffness values of benign and malignant abdominal lesions compared with breast[3,114,115] and prostate,[116] limiting this technique. Additional studies are required to determine the utility of ultrasound elastography in abdominal mass evaluation. Preliminary studies suggest that elastography may be helpful in differentiating fibrotic from inflammatory strictures in Crohn disease.

Evaluation of LS using ultrasound elastography has been extensively studied and shown to be an accurate noninvasive method for staging liver fibrosis. Several techniques including TE and SWE have both been shown to be able to stage liver fibrosis and may be able to access for portal hypertension. Recommendations for the use of TE and SWE for patients with chronic liver disease have been published[2] and it is expected that, with increasing use of ultrasound elastography, the amount of liver biopsies performed for diagnosis and staging of liver fibrosis will significantly decrease. The use of elastography will improve the ability to monitor effectiveness of treatments for chronic liver disease.

REFERENCES

1. Barr RG. US elastography: applications in tumors. In: Luna A, Vilanova JC, Rossi SE, et al, editors. Functional imaging in oncology. New York: Springer Heidelberg; 2014. p. 459–86.
2. Cosgrove D, Piscaglia F, Bamber J, et al. EFSUMB guidelines and recommendations on the clinical use of ultrasound elastography. Part 2: clinical applications. Ultraschall Med 2013;34(3):238–53.
3. Barr RG. Sonographic breast elastography: a primer. J Ultrasound Med 2012;31(5):773–83.
4. Bamber J, Cosgrove D, Dietrich CF, et al. EFSUMB guidelines and recommendations on the clinical use of ultrasound elastography. Part 1: basic principles and technology. Ultraschall Med 2013; 34(2):169–84.
5. Yu H, Wilson SR. Differentiation of benign from malignant liver masses with Acoustic Radiation Force Impulse technique. Ultrasound Q 2011;27(4):217–23.
6. European Association for the Study of the Liver. EASL Clinical Practice Guidelines: management of hepatitis C virus infection. J Hepatol 2011; 55(2):245–64.
7. European Association for the Study of the Liver. EASL clinical practice guidelines: management of chronic hepatitis B virus infection. J Hepatol 2012;57(1):167–85.
8. World Health Organization. Viral hepatitis. Report from the Secretariat. Sixty-third World Health Assembly. 2010.
9. Santantonio T, Wiegand J, Gerlach JT. Acute hepatitis C: current status and remaining challenges. J Hepatol 2008;49(4):625–33.
10. Gressner OA, Weiskirchen R, Gressner AM. Biomarkers of hepatic fibrosis, fibrogenesis and

genetic pre-disposition pending between fiction and reality. J Cell Mol Med 2007;11(5):1031–51.

11. Bedossa P, Poynard T. An algorithm for the grading of activity in chronic hepatitis C. The METAVIR Cooperative Study Group. Hepatology 1996; 24(2):289–93.

12. Afdhal NH. The natural history of hepatitis C. Semin Liver Dis 2004;24(Suppl 2):3–8.

13. Fattovich G, Stroffolini T, Zagni I, et al. Hepatocellular carcinoma in cirrhosis: incidence and risk factors. Gastroenterology 2004;127(5 Suppl 1):S35–50.

14. Lok AS, McMahon BJ. Chronic hepatitis B. Hepatology 2007;45(2):507–39.

15. Seeff LB, Hoofnagle JH. National Institutes of Health Consensus Development Conference: management of hepatitis C: 2002. Hepatology 2002; 36(5 Suppl 1):S1–2.

16. Fleig WE, Krummener P, Lesske J. Criteria for the definition of acute and chronic hepatitis C. Z Gastroenterol 2004;42(8):707–13 [in German].

17. Pinzani M, Gentilini P. Biology of hepatic stellate cells and their possible relevance in the pathogenesis of portal hypertension in cirrhosis. Semin Liver Dis 1999;19(4):397–410.

18. Bravo AA, Sheth SG, Chopra S. Liver biopsy. N Engl J Med 2001;344(7):495–500.

19. Cadranel JF, Rufat P, Degos F. Practices of liver biopsy in France: results of a prospective nationwide survey. For the Group of Epidemiology of the French Association for the Study of the Liver (AFEF). Hepatology 2000;32(3):477–81.

20. Castera L, Negre I, Samii K, et al. Pain experienced during percutaneous liver biopsy. Hepatology 1999; 30(6):1529–30.

21. Regev A, Berho M, Jeffers LJ, et al. Sampling error and intraobserver variation in liver biopsy in patients with chronic HCV infection. Am J Gastroenterol 2002;97(10):2614–8.

22. Bedossa P, Dargere D, Paradis V. Sampling variability of liver fibrosis in chronic hepatitis C. Hepatology 2003;38(6):1449–57.

23. Maharaj B, Maharaj RJ, Leary WP, et al. Sampling variability and its influence on the diagnostic yield of percutaneous needle biopsy of the liver. Lancet 1986;1(8480):523–5.

24. Emerson K. Diseases of the breast. In: Thorn GW, Wintrobe MM, Adams RD, et al, editors. Principals of internal medicine. 7th edition. New York: McGraw-Hill; 1974. p. 582–7.

25. Barr RG, Lackey AE. The utility of the "bull's-eye" artifact on breast elasticity imaging in reducing breast lesion biopsy rate. Ultrasound Q 2011; 27(3):151–5.

26. Barr RG, Zhang Z. Effects of precompression on elasticity imaging of the breast: development of a clinically useful semiquantitative method of precompression assessment. J Ultrasound Med 2012;31(6):895–902.

27. Nightingale K, Soo MS, Nightingale R, et al. Acoustic radiation force impulse imaging: in vivo demonstration of clinical feasibility. Ultrasound Med Biol 2002;28(2):227–35.

28. Fahey BJ, Nightingale KR, Nelson RC, et al. Acoustic radiation force impulse imaging of the abdomen: demonstration of feasibility and utility. Ultrasound Med Biol 2005;31(9):1185–98.

29. Rouze NC, Wang. MH, Palmeri ML, et al. Robust estimation of time-of-flight shear wave speed using a radon sum transformation. IEEE Trans Ultrason Ferroelectr Freq Control 2010;57:2662–70.

30. Guibal A, Boularan C, Bruce M, et al. Evaluation of shearwave elastography for the characterisation of focal liver lesions on ultrasound. Eur Radiol 2013; 23(4):1138–49.

31. Onur MR, Poyraz AK, Ucak EE, et al. Semiquantitative strain elastography of liver masses. J Ultrasound Med 2012;31(7):1061–7.

32. Ying L, Lin X, Xie ZL, et al. Clinical utility of acoustic radiation force impulse imaging for identification of malignant liver lesions: a meta-analysis. Eur Radiol 2012;22(12):2798–805.

33. Kolokythas O, Gauthier T, Fernandez AT, et al. Ultrasound-based elastography: a novel approach to assess radio frequency ablation of liver masses performed with expandable ablation probes: a feasibility study. J Ultrasound Med 2008;27(6):935–46.

34. Seeff LB, Everson GT, Morgan TR, et al. Complication rate of percutaneous liver biopsies among persons with advanced chronic liver disease in the HALT-C trial. Clin Gastroenterol Hepatol 2010; 8(10):877–83.

35. Stotland BR, Lichtenstein GR. Liver biopsy complications and routine ultrasound. Am J Gastroenterol 1996;91(7):1295–6.

36. Millonig G, Friedrich S, Adolf S, et al. Liver stiffness is directly influenced by central venous pressure. J Hepatol 2010;52(2):206–10.

37. Sagir A, Erhardt A, Schmitt M, et al. Transient elastography is unreliable for detection of cirrhosis in patients with acute liver damage. Hepatology 2008;47(2):592–5.

38. Castera L, Foucher J, Bernard PH, et al. Pitfalls of liver stiffness measurement: a 5-year prospective study of 13,369 examinations. Hepatology 2010; 51(3):828–35.

39. Reiberger T, Ferlitsch A, Payer BA, et al. Non-selective beta-blockers improve the correlation of liver stiffness and portal pressure in advanced cirrhosis. J Gastroenterol 2012;47(5):561–8.

40. Karlas T, Pfrepper C, Wiegand J, et al. Acoustic radiation force impulse imaging (ARFI) for non-invasive detection of liver fibrosis: examination standards and evaluation of interlobe differences

in healthy subjects and chronic liver disease. Scand J Gastroenterol 2011;46(12):1458–67.

41. Piscaglia F, Salvatore V, Di Donato R, et al. Accuracy of VirtualTouch Acoustic Radiation Force Impulse (ARFI) imaging for the diagnosis of cirrhosis during liver ultrasonography. Ultraschall Med 2011;32(2):167–75.

42. Ferraioli G, Lissandrin R, Zicchetti M, et al. Diffuse liver diseases. In: Calliada F, Canepari M, Ferraioli G, et al, editors. Sono-Elastography main clinical applications. Pavia (Italy): Edizioni Medico Scientifiche; 2012. p. 13–30.

43. D'Onofrio M, Gallotti A, Mucelli RP. Tissue quantification with acoustic radiation force impulse imaging: measurement repeatability and normal values in the healthy liver. AJR Am J Roentgenol 2010; 195(1):132–6.

44. Fraquelli M, Rigamonti C, Casazza G, et al. Reproducibility of transient elastography in the evaluation of liver fibrosis in patients with chronic liver disease. Gut 2007;56(7):968–73.

45. Myers RP, Pomier-Layrargues G, Kirsch R, et al. Feasibility and diagnostic performance of the FibroScan XL probe for liver stiffness measurement in overweight and obese patients. Hepatology 2012;55(1):199–208.

46. Talwalkar JA, Kurtz DM, Schoenleber SJ, et al. Ultrasound-based transient elastography for the detection of hepatic fibrosis: systematic review and meta-analysis. Clin Gastroenterol Hepatol 2007;5(10):1214–20.

47. Friedrich-Rust M, Ong MF, Martens S, et al. Performance of transient elastography for the staging of liver fibrosis: a meta-analysis. Gastroenterology 2008;134(4):960–74.

48. Adebajo CO, Talwalkar JA, Poterucha JJ, et al. Ultrasound-based transient elastography for the detection of hepatic fibrosis in patients with recurrent hepatitis C virus after liver transplantation: a systematic review and meta-analysis. Liver Transpl 2012;18(3):323–31.

49. Chon YE, Choi EH, Song KJ, et al. Performance of transient elastography for the staging of liver fibrosis in patients with chronic hepatitis B: a meta-analysis. PLoS One 2012;7(9):e44930.

50. Chan HL, Wong GL, Choi PC, et al. Alanine aminotransferase-based algorithms of liver stiffness measurement by transient elastography (Fibroscan) for liver fibrosis in chronic hepatitis B. J Viral Hepat 2009;16(1):36–44.

51. de Ledinghen V, Wong VW, Vergniol J, et al. Diagnosis of liver fibrosis and cirrhosis using liver stiffness measurement: comparison between M and XL probe of FibroScan(R). J Hepatol 2012;56(4): 833–9.

52. Friedrich-Rust M, Wong VW, Vergniol J, et al. Transient elastography with a new probe for obese patients for non-invasive staging of non-alcoholic steatohepatitis. Eur Radiol 2010;20(10):2390–6.

53. Wong VW, Vergniol J, Wong GL, et al. Diagnosis of fibrosis and cirrhosis using liver stiffness measurement in nonalcoholic fatty liver disease. Hepatology 2010;51(2):454–62.

54. Wong GL, Wong VW, Choi PC, et al. Assessment of fibrosis by transient elastography compared with liver biopsy and morphometry in chronic liver diseases. Clin Gastroenterol Hepatol 2008;6(9): 1027–35.

55. Roulot D, Costes JL, Buyck JF, et al. Transient elastography as a screening tool for liver fibrosis and cirrhosis in a community-based population aged over 45 years. Gut 2011;60(7):977–84.

56. Bureau C, Metivier S, Peron JM, et al. Transient elastography accurately predicts presence of significant portal hypertension in patients with chronic liver disease. Aliment Pharmacol Ther 2008;27(12): 1261–8.

57. Vizzutti F, Arena U, Romanelli RG, et al. Liver stiffness measurement predicts severe portal hypertension in patients with HCV-related cirrhosis. Hepatology 2007;45(5):1290–7.

58. Colecchia A, Montrone L, Scaioli E, et al. Measurement of spleen stiffness to evaluate portal hypertension and the presence of esophageal varices in patients with HCV-related cirrhosis. Gastroenterology 2012;143(3):646–54.

59. Sporea I, Ratiu I, Sirli R, et al. Value of transient elastography for the prediction of variceal bleeding. World J Gastroenterol 2011;17(17): 2206–10.

60. Castera L, Le Bail B, Roudot-Thoraval F, et al. Early detection in routine clinical practice of cirrhosis and oesophageal varices in chronic hepatitis C: comparison of transient elastography (FibroScan) with standard laboratory tests and non-invasive scores. J Hepatol 2009;50(1):59–68.

61. Pritchett S, Cardenas A, Manning D, et al. The optimal cut-off for predicting large oesophageal varices using transient elastography is disease specific. J Viral Hepat 2011;18(4):e75–80.

62. Vergniol J, Foucher J, Terrebonne E, et al. Noninvasive tests for fibrosis and liver stiffness predict 5-year outcomes of patients with chronic hepatitis C. Gastroenterology 2011;140(7):1970–9, 1979. e1–3.

63. Masuzaki R, Tateishi R, Yoshida H, et al. Prospective risk assessment for hepatocellular carcinoma development in patients with chronic hepatitis C by transient elastography. Hepatology 2009;49(6): 1954–61.

64. Jung KS, Kim SU, Ahn SH, et al. Risk assessment of hepatitis B virus-related hepatocellular carcinoma development using liver stiffness measurement (FibroScan). Hepatology 2011;53(3):885–94.

65. Yu H, Wilson SR. New noninvasive ultrasound techniques: can they predict liver cirrhosis? Ultrasound Q 2012;28(1):5–11.

66. Yoon KT, Lim SM, Park JY, et al. Liver stiffness measurement using acoustic radiation force impulse (ARFI) elastography and effect of necroinflammation. Dig Dis Sci 2012;57(6):1682–91.

67. Bota S, Sporea I, Peck-Radosavljevic M, et al. The influence of aminotransferase levels on liver stiffness assessed by Acoustic Radiation Force Impulse Elastography: a retrospective multicentre study. Dig Liver Dis 2013;45(9):762–8.

68. Toshima T, Shirabe K, Takeishi K, et al. New method for assessing liver fibrosis based on acoustic radiation force impulse: a special reference to the difference between right and left liver. J Gastroenterol 2011;46(5):705–11.

69. Bota S, Sporea I, Sirli R, et al. Factors that influence the correlation of acoustic radiation force impulse (ARFI), elastography with liver fibrosis. Med Ultrason 2011;13(2):135–40.

70. Ferraioli G, Tinelli C, Zicchetti M, et al. Reproducibility of real-time shear wave elastography in the evaluation of liver elasticity. Eur J Radiol 2012; 81(11):3102–6.

71. Friedrich-Rust M, Wunder K, Kriener S, et al. Liver fibrosis in viral hepatitis: noninvasive assessment with acoustic radiation force impulse imaging versus transient elastography. Radiology 2009; 252(2):595–604.

72. Sporea I, Sirli R, Bota S, et al. Is ARFI elastography reliable for predicting fibrosis severity in chronic HCV hepatitis? World J Radiol 2011;3(7): 188–93.

73. Sporea I, Bota S, Peck-Radosavljevic M, et al. Acoustic Radiation Force Impulse elastography for fibrosis evaluation in patients with chronic hepatitis C: an international multicenter study. Eur J Radiol 2012;81(12):4112–8.

74. Friedrich-Rust M, Nierhoff J, Lupsor M, et al. Performance of Acoustic Radiation Force Impulse imaging for the staging of liver fibrosis: a pooled meta-analysis. J Viral Hepat 2012;19(2):e212–9.

75. Bavu E, Gennisson JL, Couade M, et al. Noninvasive in vivo liver fibrosis evaluation using supersonic shear imaging: a clinical study on 113 hepatitis C virus patients. Ultrasound Med Biol 2011;37(9):1361–73.

76. Ferraioli G, Tinelli C, Dal Bello B, et al. Accuracy of real-time shear wave elastography for assessing liver fibrosis in chronic hepatitis C: a pilot study. Hepatology 2012;56(6):2125–33.

77. Rizzo L, Calvaruso V, Cacopardo B, et al. Comparison of transient elastography and acoustic radiation force impulse for non-invasive staging of liver fibrosis in patients with chronic hepatitis C. Am J Gastroenterol 2011;106(12):2112–20.

78. Yoneda M, Suzuki K, Kato S, et al. Nonalcoholic fatty liver disease: US-based acoustic radiation force impulse elastography. Radiology 2010; 256(2):640–7.

79. Friedrich-Rust M, Romen D, Vermehren J, et al. Acoustic radiation force impulse-imaging and transient elastography for non-invasive assessment of liver fibrosis and steatosis in NAFLD. Eur J Radiol 2012;81(3):e325–31.

80. Crespo G, Fernandez-Varo G, Marino Z, et al. ARFI, FibroScan, ELF, and their combinations in the assessment of liver fibrosis: a prospective study. J Hepatol 2012;57(2):281–7.

81. Friedrich-Rust M, Ong MF, Herrmann E, et al. Real-time elastography for noninvasive assessment of liver fibrosis in chronic viral hepatitis. AJR Am J Roentgenol 2007;188(3):758–64.

82. Tatsumi C, Kudo M, Ueshima K, et al. Noninvasive evaluation of hepatic fibrosis using serum fibrotic markers, transient elastography (FibroScan) and real-time tissue elastography. Intervirology 2008; 51(Suppl 1):27–33.

83. Fujimoto K, Kato M, Kudo M, et al. Novel image analysis method using ultrasound elastography for noninvasive evaluation of hepatic fibrosis in patients with chronic hepatitis C. Oncology 2013; 84(Suppl 1):3–12.

84. Morikawa H, Fukuda K, Kobayashi S, et al. Real-time tissue elastography as a tool for the noninvasive assessment of liver stiffness in patients with chronic hepatitis C. J Gastroenterol 2011;46(3): 350–8.

85. Ferraioli G, Tinelli C, Malfitano A, et al. Performance of real-time strain elastography, transient elastography, and aspartate-to-platelet ratio index in the assessment of fibrosis in chronic hepatitis C. AJR Am J Roentgenol 2012;199(1):19–25.

86. Koizumi Y, Hirooka M, Kisaka Y, et al. Liver fibrosis in patients with chronic hepatitis C: noninvasive diagnosis by means of real-time tissue elastography–establishment of the method for measurement. Radiology 2011;258(2):610–7.

87. Tatsumi C, Kudo M, Ueshima K, et al. Non-invasive evaluation of hepatic fibrosis for type C chronic hepatitis. Intervirology 2010;53(1):76–81.

88. Gulizia R, Ferraioli G, Filice C. Open questions in the assessment of liver fibrosis using real-time elastography. AJR Am J Roentgenol 2008;190(6): W370–1 [author reply: W372–3].

89. Ferraioli G, Gulizia R, Filice C. Real-time elastography in the assessment of liver fibrosis. AJR Am J Roentgenol 2007;189(3):W170.

90. Janssen J, Schlorer E, Greiner L. EUS elastography of the pancreas: feasibility and pattern description of the normal pancreas, chronic pancreatitis, and focal pancreatic lesions. Gastrointest Endosc 2007;65(7):971–8.

91. Hirche TO, Ignee A, Barreiros AP, et al. Indications and limitations of endoscopic ultrasound elastography for evaluation of focal pancreatic lesions. Endoscopy 2008;40(11):910–7.

92. Itokawa F, Itoi T, Sofuni A, et al. EUS elastography combined with the strain ratio of tissue elasticity for diagnosis of solid pancreatic masses. J Gastroenterol 2011;46(6):843–53.

93. Giovannini M, Thomas B, Erwan B, et al. Endoscopic ultrasound elastography for evaluation of lymph nodes and pancreatic masses: a multicenter study. World J Gastroenterol 2009;15(13):1587–93.

94. Iglesias-Garcia J, Larino-Noia J, Abdulkader I, et al. EUS elastography for the characterization of solid pancreatic masses. Gastrointest Endosc 2009;70(6):1101–8.

95. Lee TH, Cha SW, Cho YD. EUS elastography: advances in diagnostic EUS of the pancreas. Korean J Radiol 2012;13(Suppl 1):S12–6.

96. Saftoiu A, Vilmann P, Gorunescu F, et al. Efficacy of an artificial neural network-based approach to endoscopic ultrasound elastography in diagnosis of focal pancreatic masses. Clin Gastroenterol Hepatol 2012;10(1):84–90.e1.

97. Saftoiu A, Vilmann P, Gorunescu F, et al. Neural network analysis of dynamic sequences of EUS elastography used for the differential diagnosis of chronic pancreatitis and pancreatic cancer. Gastrointest Endosc 2008;68(6):1086–94.

98. Saftoiu A, Vilmann P, Gorunescu F, et al. Accuracy of endoscopic ultrasound elastography used for differential diagnosis of focal pancreatic masses: a multicenter study. Endoscopy 2011;43(7):596–603.

99. Iglesias-Garcia J, Larino-Noia J, Abdulkader I, et al. Quantitative endoscopic ultrasound elastography: an accurate method for the differentiation of solid pancreatic masses. Gastroenterology 2010;139(4):1172–80.

100. Pei Q, Zou X, Zhang X, et al. Diagnostic value of EUS elastography in differentiation of benign and malignant solid pancreatic masses: a meta-analysis. Pancreatology 2012;12(5):402–8.

101. Mei M, Ni J, Liu D, et al. EUS elastography for diagnosis of solid pancreatic masses: a meta-analysis. Gastrointest Endosc 2013;77(4):578–89.

102. D'Onofrio M, Gallotti A, Mucelli RP. Pancreatic mucinous cystadenoma at ultrasound acoustic radiation force impulse (ARFI) imaging. Pancreas 2010;39(5):684–5.

103. D'Onofrio M, Gallotti A, Salvia R, et al. Acoustic radiation force impulse (ARFI) ultrasound imaging of pancreatic cystic lesions. Eur J Radiol 2011;80(2):241–4.

104. Goya C, Hamidi C, Hattapoglu S, et al. Use of acoustic radiation force impulse (ARFI) elastography to diagnose acute pancreatiitis at hospital admission: a comparison with ultrasound and computed tomography. J Ultrasound Med 2014;33:1453–60.

105. Gilja OH, Heimdal A, Hausken T, et al. Strain during gastric contractions can be measured using Doppler ultrasonography. Ultrasound Med Biol 2002;28(11–12):1457–65.

106. Waage JE, Havre RF, Odegaard S, et al. Endorectal elastography in the evaluation of rectal tumours. Colorectal Dis 2011;13(10):1130–7.

107. Stidham RW, Xu J, Johnson LA, et al. Ultrasound elasticity imaging for detecting intestinal fibrosis and inflammation in rats and humans with Crohn's disease. Gastroenterology 2011;141(3):819–26.e1.

108. Rustemovic N, Cukovic-Cavka S, Brinar M, et al. A pilot study of transrectal endoscopic ultrasound elastography in inflammatory bowel disease. BMC Gastroenterol 2011;11:113.

109. Ishikawa D, Ando T, Watanabe O, et al. Images of colonic real-time tissue sonoelastography correlate with those of colonoscopy and may predict response to therapy in patients with ulcerative colitis. BMC Gastroenterol 2011;11:29.

110. Matre K, Ahmed AB, Gregersen H, et al. In vitro evaluation of ultrasound Doppler strain rate imaging: modification for measurement in a slowly moving tissue phantom. Ultrasound Med Biol 2003;29(12):1725–34.

111. Ahmed AB, Gilja OH, Gregersen H, et al. In vitro strain measurement in the porcine antrum using ultrasound doppler strain rate imaging. Ultrasound Med Biol 2006;32(4):513–22.

112. Ahmed AB, Gilja OH, Hausken T, et al. Strain measurement during antral contractions by ultrasound strain rate imaging: influence of erythromycin. Neurogastroenterol Motil 2009;21(2):170–9.

113. Ahmed AB, Matre K, Hausken T, et al. Rome III subgroups of functional dyspepsia exhibit different characteristics of antral contractions measured by strain rate imaging - a pilot study. Ultraschall Med 2012;33(7):E233–40.

114. Barr RG. Real-time ultrasound elasticity of the breast: initial clinical results. Ultrasound Q 2010;26(2):61–6.

115. Barr RG, Destounis S, Lackey LB, et al. Evaluation of breast lesions using sonographic elasticity imaging: a multicenter trial. J Ultrasound Med 2012;31(2):281–7.

116. Barr RG, Memo R, Schaub CR. Shear wave ultrasound elastography of the prostate: initial results. Ultrasound Q 2012;28(1):13–20.

Update on the Role of Sonography in Liver Transplantation

 CrossMark

Susan J. Ackerman, MD*, Abid Irshad, MBBS, MD, Madelene Lewis, MD

KEYWORDS

- Liver transplant • End-stage liver disease • Cirrhosis • Organ rejection
- Postoperative complications

KEY POINTS

- The role of ultrasonography in pretransplantation evaluation is primarily to identify any contraindication to transplant.
- Ultrasonography is usually the initial imaging modality performed in the evaluation of the posttransplantation liver.
- Postoperative mechanical complications usually occur at the anastomotic site.
- The most common postoperative vascular complication is hepatic artery stenosis, at approximately 10%.
- Postoperative complications such as infection usually result from biliary leaks, hepatic artery thrombosis, acute graft failure, or preexisting infections.

INTRODUCTION

Liver transplantation (LT) involves the surgical placement of a portion of a liver or a whole liver into a patient in order to restore hepatic function. There are 2 types of donor organs for LT. Cadaveric donor organs are taken from patients who are declared brain dead. The main requirements for a cadaveric transplant are that the donor liver be an appropriate size and of a compatible blood type. In a living donor transplant, a liver segment is taken from a healthy person and donated to a patient needing the transplant. This procedure is possible because the liver has the ability to regenerate, thus the donated segment and the remaining portion of the donor liver grow to a normal size. Most transplants involve a whole liver; however, segmental liver transplantation has occurred with increasing frequency in the past several years.

Most liver transplants are orthotopic, which means the damaged native liver is removed and replaced by the donor liver in the recipient's native hepatic bed. The first LT was performed by Starzl and colleagues at the University of Colorado in 1967. According to the data base of the Organ Procurement and Transplantation Network (OPTN), the total number of LTs performed in the United States from January 1988 to October 2013 is 125,059. Of these, 120,071 were cadaveric and 4988 were living donor liver transplants.[1] LT is the major treatment of patients with end-stage chronic liver disease or acute liver failure. Common indications for LT are listed in **Box 1**.[2] The leading cause for LT is cirrhosis caused by hepatitis C.[3] One-year survival rate for patients receiving

The authors have nothing to disclose.
Portions of this article were previously published in: Ackerman SJ, Irshad A. The role of sonography in liver transplantation. Ultrasound Clin 2007;2(3):377–90.
Department of Radiology, Medical University of South Carolina, 169 Ashley Avenue, Charleston, SC 29425, USA
* Corresponding author.
E-mail address: ackerman@musc.edu

ultrasound.theclinics.com

Box 1
Common indications for LT
• Alcoholic cirrhosis
• Cirrhosis associated with hepatitis B and C
• Autoimmune hepatitis
• Acute liver failure
• Primary sclerosing cholangitis
• Primary biliary cirrhosis
• Malignancy
Data from Bhargava P, Vaidya S, Dick A, et al. Imaging of orthotopic liver transplantation: review. AJR Am J Roentgenol 2011;196:15–25.

Box 2
Contraindications for LT
• Active infection
• Active extrahepatic malignancy
• Severe cardiopulmonary disease
• Thrombosis of the portal and superior mesenteric venous system
• Diffuse hepatic tumor invasion
• Noncompliance
• Active substance or alcohol abuse
Data from Bhargava P, Vaidya S, Dick A, et al. Imaging of orthotopic liver transplantation: review. AJR Am J Roentgenol 2011;196:15–25.

a liver transplant is approximately 87%. Five-year survival rates are 74%.[2]

USE OF ULTRASONOGRAPHY FOR PREOPERATIVE ASSESSMENT

The evaluation of a potential candidate for LT is first to determine the severity of the liver disease by clinical evaluation. After the diagnosis of end-stage liver disease (EDLD) is established, any contraindications to the procedure must be excluded. The final step in preoperative assessment is to evaluate the severity of the patient's disease. Scoring systems that grade the severity of liver disease include the Child-Turcotte-Pugh (CTP) scoring system and the Model for End-Stage Liver Disease (MELD) scoring system. Multiple imaging studies are obtained, including chest radiography, duplex ultrasonography (US), abdominal computed tomography (CT), and occasionally magnetic resonance (MR) angiography or selective angiogram. An important component of transplant assessment is determining the presence of contraindications to surgery. One of the initial imaging modalities used is US. Advantages of US include low cost, ready availability, and that it involves no ionizing radiation. US is useful to exclude any contraindications to transplantation. Cirrhosis is the most common reason for LT and, because cirrhosis is frequently associated with the development of hepatocellular carcinomas (HCC), the initial imaging is gray-scale evaluation of the liver parenchyma. Contraindications for LT are listed in **Box 2**.[2] Relative contraindications include advanced stage HCCs, greater than stage 11. However, given the new techniques in chemoembolization and radiofrequency ablation procedures, the indications may change in the near future.

In evaluation of the hepatic vasculature, it is important to assess portal vein patency. Portal venous thrombosis is a common complication of chronic liver disease, with an occurrence of 5% to 10%.[4,5] A normal portal vein waveform is a continuous, undulating hepatopetal tracing with some variation in flow velocity. In portal hypertension, there is an increase in pressure that accounts for the complications. Doppler analysis of the portal venous flow pattern and the identification of collateral vessels can help to confirm portal hypertension. US is sensitive and specific in the detection of portal vein thrombosis.[3] If the portal vein shows thrombosis or if there is cavernous transformation, the superior mesenteric vein must be patent for transplantation to be feasible. Conventional aortography or MR angiography can be done to evaluate patency if the US findings are equivocal. For standard orthotopic LT (OLTX), the patency of the recipient inferior vena cava (IVC) is important. The hepatic veins should also be assessed, particularly in patients with Budd-Chiari syndrome. In cirrhotic liver, the hepatic vein Doppler waveform shows a loss of plasticity. The hepatic artery is important in the donor liver but not in the recipient. Cirrhosis causes blunting of the hepatic artery systolic component with an increase in the resistive index (RI).[3] The hepatic artery RI decreases in the setting of portal vein thrombosis.

The imaging work-up of a living donor includes evaluation US of the liver. In addition to the evaluation of the solid organs, the hepatic vasculature patency is important to document thrombosis and the hepatic vasculature patency.

US IN THE IMMEDIATE POSTOPERATIVE PERIOD

US is usually the initial imaging modality in evaluation of the posttransplantation liver. It is used routinely for early detection of complications that are clinically occult and when there is evidence of graft dysfunction. It is important to understand the type of surgical procedure that has been performed because there are many variations of liver transplants ranging from a segment or lobe to a whole liver.

The following structures require anastomosis between the recipient and the graft: the portal vein, the hepatic artery, the suprahepatic IVC, the infrahepatic IVC, and the common bile duct. The type of anastomoses may depend on the anatomy of the vessels and the patient's underlying disease process. The immediate posttransplantation US examination includes evaluation of the biliary system, hepatic parenchyma, perihepatic spaces and color Doppler US (CDUS) of the hepatic vasculature. Intraoperative Doppler US of the graft vessels may be performed if there is technical difficulty or the liver is not perfusing adequately. The timing and frequency of postoperative US is variable but there is evidence to suggest that routine CDUS of all hepatic vessels within 24 hours following transplantation is beneficial.[2] Postoperative complications can be mechanical or nonmechanical. Mechanical complications involve the anastomotic sites such as the hepatic artery, main portal vein, IVC, and common bile duct. Nonmechanical complications include rejection, allograft dysfunction, infection, recurrent hepatic malignancy, and posttransplantation lymphoproliferative disease (PTLD). US plays an important role in the detection of mechanical complications.

COMPLICATIONS OF LIVER TRANSPLANTATION
Vascular Complications

Hepatic artery complications
Normal hepatic artery has an antegrade flow throughout the cardiac cycle and has an RI between 0.5 and 0.8. The systolic upstroke is sharp with acceleration time usually less than 0.08 second. For the initial few days, the RI may remain increased and slowly return to normal. An RI of less than 0.6 should raise suspicion for a vascular complication.[6] The hepatic artery complications include thrombosis, stenosis, and pseudoaneurysm.

Hepatic artery thrombosis Hepatic artery thrombosis is the most common complication, with an incidence of 4% to 12% in adults and 9% to 42% in children.[7–9] It is also one of the most serious complications, with a high mortality. Retransplantation may often be required. Predisposing factors for hepatic artery thrombosis include mismatch of the vessel size, cold trauma to the liver, infection, rejection, and poor technique.[7–13]

Complete thrombosis of the hepatic artery leads to nonvisualization of any flow within the main hepatic artery as well as its intrahepatic branches (**Fig. 1**). Doppler US has shown 92% accuracy in the diagnosis of hepatic artery thrombosis.[12] Hepatic edema, severe systemic hypotension, large splenic steal, or severe stenosis may cause a false-positive for hepatic artery thrombosis. Angiography remains the gold standard but use of microbubble US contrast agent also increases the sensitivity of US.[13,14] A progression of a normal waveform into a dampened waveform or an absent diastolic flow should raise a suspicion for an impending thrombosis.

Hepatic artery stenosis Hepatic artery stenosis is also a common complication, with an incidence of 5% to 11% of transplant recipients.[7,8,15,16] This complication occurs within the first few months after transplantation and usually occurs around the area of anastomosis. It can be caused by anastomotic ischemia, clamp injury, and rejection. The Doppler findings include increased velocity greater than 200 cm/s in the narrowed segment. Distal to the stenosis a tardus-parvus distal arterial waveform (systolic acceleration time >0.08 seconds) pattern and low velocities can be seen (**Fig. 2**). Decreased RI of less than 0.5[17,18] can also be seen distal to the stenosis. Upstream from the

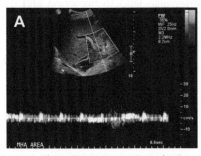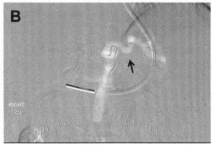

Fig. 1. Hepatic artery thrombosis. Power Doppler image in the area of the main hepatic artery (*A*) shows minimal pulsation without significant flow in the hepatic artery. A CO_2 angiogram of the aorta (*B*) shows preferential flow to the splenic artery (*arrow*) with no flow seen in the main hepatic artery.

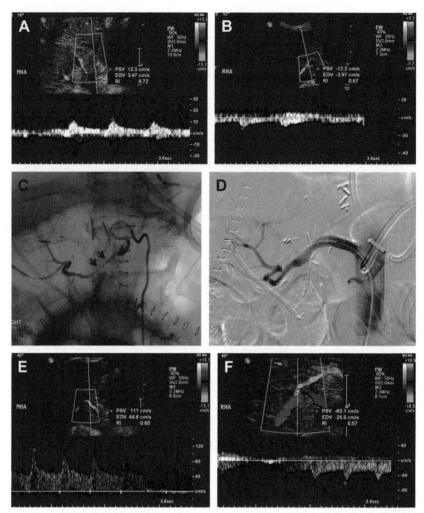

Fig. 2. Hepatic artery stenosis. Doppler US of the main hepatic (*A*) and right hepatic (*B*) arteries shows low peak systolic velocities (12 cm/s) and a tardus-parvus waveform in the main and right hepatic arteries. A hepatic angiogram was performed (*C, D*) that showed stenosis of the main hepatic artery (*arrows, C*) for which a stent was placed subsequently (*D*). Repeat Doppler US after stenting (*E, F*) showed a return to normal velocities and waveforms within the main and right hepatic arteries.

stenosis, a high-resistance pattern with low velocity may be seen. Low-grade narrowing may be missed on Doppler US and angiography may still be considered in the setting of a high clinical suspicion.[7,16,19] Treatment includes balloon angioplasty and vascular reconstruction.

Hepatic artery pseudoaneurysm Pseudoaneurysm (PA) occurs as an uncommon complication with an incidence of about 1% after OLTX.[20] Intrahepatic PA can occur from the trauma from a liver biopsy. Extrahepatic pseudoaneurysms usually occur at the donor-recipient arterial anastomosis and may be caused by infection or technical failure. On gray-scale US, these are seen as a cystic fluid collection near the porta hepatis. Doppler US may show a cystic structure related to the hepatic

artery and either swirling flow (yin-yang type) or turbulent flow. The PA of the hepatic artery can rupture and present with shock. These conditions may also lead to hemobilia and gastrointestinal bleeding if these form fistulous connection with the biliary system. The treatment is usually surgical excision, embolization, or covered stent placement. Extrahepatic PA is usually treated surgically because of the high mortality.

Portal Vein Complications

Portal vein occlusions occur in about 2% of liver transplants.[8,9] Mild narrowing of the portal vein at the anastomosis and mild turbulence of flow are normal findings in the postoperative period.[7] A partial thrombosis or stenosis of the portal vein may also occur. The predisposing factors include hypercoagulable states, misalignment, decreased inflow, increased outflow resistance, previous portal thrombosis, and technical difficulties. Complete thrombosis may show echogenic signals within the portal vein on gray-scale imaging and absence of flow on color and power Doppler imaging. An acute thrombus may occasionally be anechoic on gray-scale imaging. Increased arterial flow in the hepatic artery may be seen as a compensatory secondary finding. Portal vein stenosis may be seen as an area of narrowing on the gray-scale and color imaging. A 3-fold to 4-fold increased velocity in a focal segment of the portal vein should raise suspicion for significant narrowing (**Fig. 3**). A peak anastomotic velocity of greater than 125 cm/s is 73% sensitive and 95% specific for the diagnosis of portal vein stenosis. A 3-fold increase in velocity also has a 73% sensitivity for focal stenosis.[21] A poststenotic vein may show turbulence of flow and dilatation. A portal cavernous transformation may occur from a chronic thrombus. A significant stenosis may lead to graft dysfunction and portal hypertension. In addition, an interval enlargement of spleen may also be seen as a secondary sign of portal hypertension. The treatment of stenosis includes angioplasty, stent placement, or surgical revision.

IVC Complications

IVC complications are rare after transplantation and occur in less than 1% of cases.[22] IVC thrombosis or stenosis may occur at the site of surgical anastomosis. Causes include size discrepancy, external compression by fluid collections, or technical problems during the surgery. Delayed stenosis can occur from fibrosis or chronic thrombosis.

A piggyback cavocaval anastomosis is performed when a portion of the donor IVC is obtained along with the graft and is anastomosed to the recipient IVC at the recipient hepatic venous opening (**Fig. 4**). A piggyback anastomosis may lead to cavocaval dehiscence or Budd-Chiari syndrome because of inadequate venous drainage.[7] Patients may develop hepatomegaly, ascites, pleural effusions, or lower extremity edema. Gray-scale US may show echogenic thrombus or narrowing. The color flow may show turbulence in the area of stenosis with greater than 3-fold to 4-fold velocity compared with the prestenotic segment (**Fig. 5**). Reversal of flow may also be noted if collateral circulation has developed. Loss of normal phasicity in the hepatic veins may also be noted as a secondary sign.[23] Balloon angioplasty and stenting are the usual treatment options.

Hepatic Veins

Hepatic veins are not directly involved in surgical anastomosis and complications of hepatic veins are rare (<1%).[24] As in IVC, thrombosis and stenosis may involve the hepatic veins as well. Budd-Chiari syndrome may recur in patients who receive a transplant for this disease. The Doppler US may show loss of phasicity, which is a nonspecific sign and may be seen with other conditions leading to a decreased hepatic compliance. A persistent monophasic waveform is a sensitive sign for hepatic vein stenosis. In contrast, presence of a triphasic or biphasic waveform also helps by excluding hepatic vein stenosis.

Liver Infarction

Heterogeneous areas in the liver may be seen in the posttransplantation period and can be secondary to rejection, ischemia, hepatitis, cholangitis, or injury. These areas may spontaneously resolve within a few weeks.[15] Infarcts appear

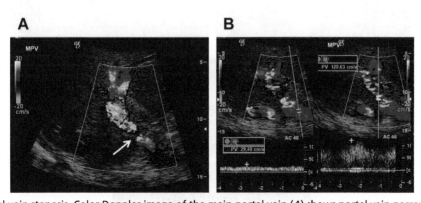

Fig. 3. Portal vein stenosis. Color Doppler image of the main portal vein (*A*) shows portal vein narrowing (*arrow*) with turbulent flow distal to the narrowing. Spectral waveform dual images through the portal vein (*B*) show a velocity of 29 cm/s in an area proximal to the stenosis, whereas the velocity is significantly increased (more than 4-fold) through the area of stenosis, which shows a velocity of 120 cm/s.

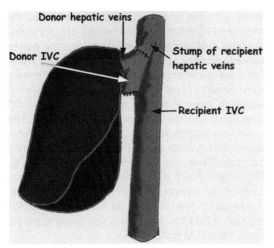

Fig. 4. Piggyback anastomosis shows an anastomosis between the donor IVC and a common stump of the recipient's 3 hepatic veins, with preservation of the recipient IVC. (*From* Quiroga S, Sebastia MC, Margarit C, et al. Complications of orthotopic liver transplantation: Spectrum of findings with helical CT. Radiographics 2001;21:1085–102; with permission.)

hypoechoic on US and may have round or geographic shape. Central necrosis and gas formation may also be seen on US or CT scan (**Fig. 6**). On US, the bright echogenic foci within the parenchyma should raise suspicion for gas. It should be differentiated from pneumobilia, which

is only seen along the portal triads. Infarcts progressively show better delineation of the margins. Large infarcts are usually associated with abnormal Doppler US findings of thrombosis or stenosis in the hepatic artery. CT scan usually shows hypoattenuating peripheral areas.

Splenic Artery Steal Syndrome

Splenic artery steal syndrome is an important but less frequently recognized cause of graft ischemia, with an incidence of about 3% to 8% of OTLX.[25–27] In patients with large spleens and increased pre-transplantation splenic flow, the high flow rates may continue after the transplantation, leading to diversion of significant blood flow away from the transplant. It has also been proposed that an increased portal flow in these patients may be the cause of ischemia. Duplex US usually shows a decreased diastolic flow with a high RI (>0.8–1) in the main as well as intrahepatic arteries (**Fig. 7**). High RI in the posttransplantation period is a common finding and can have a variety of causes such as being a transient postoperative finding, rejection, edema, or systemic hypotension. However, these conditions usually normalize within the first week. A persistent high RI in the arterial system without any other evidence of graft complication should raise suspicion for splenic steal. Increased portal velocity is usually seen in these patients. The diagnosis is confirmed by

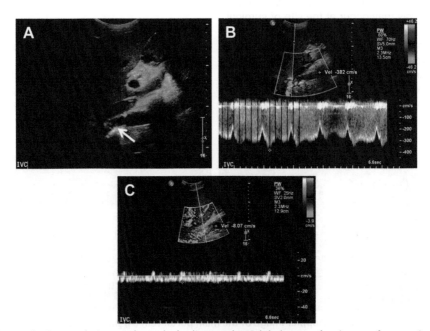

Fig. 5. IVC stenosis. Gray-scale image through the liver and IVC (*A*) shows a focal area of narrowing in the IVC (*arrow*). Doppler US of the IVC shows normal direction of flow with a high velocity (382 cm/s) through the narrowed part (*B*) compared with a significantly lower velocity (8 cm/s) in the IVC proximal to the stenosis (*C*).

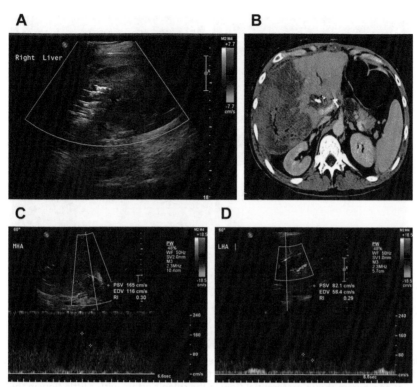

Fig. 6. Liver infarction. Color Doppler US of the right lobe of the liver (*A*) shows no vascular flow in the right lobe. There are echogenic areas suggesting gas in the liver (*arrows*). CT scan of the liver (*B*) confirms a large area of infarction and presence of gas within the liver. Doppler US of the main hepatic artery (*C*) and left hepatic artery (*D*) shows high diastolic flow and low resistive indices of 0.26 to 0.30 either caused by proximal stenosis or compensatory increased diastolic flow secondary to large infarction.

angiography and treatment usually consists of splenic embolization.

Biliary Complications

Biliary complications are common, seen in 6% to 34% of cases of OLTX, and are the second most common cause (after rejection) leading to severe liver dysfunction.[17,28] The major complications include bile leakage, bile duct changes such as strictures, and biliary obstruction. Eighty percent of biliary complications occur within the first 3 to 6 months after transplantation, although bile duct strictures can be seen after many years.[19] Predisposing factors include cold ischemia, difficult anastomosis, and vascular insufficiency. Other complications include stones, fistula, sphincter of Oddi dysfunction, and recurrent biliary disease.

Biliary Obstruction

Biliary strictures can be anastomotic or nonanastomotic. The most common biliary complication is biliary obstruction and is caused by stenosis at the area of anastomosis. US usually shows dilated bile ducts to the level of anastomosis (**Fig. 8**). The

bile ducts are supplied by the small branches of the hepatic arteries. Hence, any complication with the hepatic artery may lead to biliary ischemia, necrosis, and nonanastomotic strictures. Nonanastomotic strictures may also be seen in primary sclerosing cholangitis and infection.[7] The prognosis is worse with nonanastomotic strictures. Compared with endoscopic retrograde cholangiopancreatography (ERCP) and percutaneous transhepatic cholangiography (PTC), which are more invasive, US and MR cholangiopancreatography are usually used as initial noninvasive methods that show dilated biliary ducts. Intrahepatic ductal dilatation has a higher predictive value of the diagnosis of biliary obstruction than the common bile duct diameter.[29] Recurrence of primary sclerosing cholangitis occurs in approximately 20% of cases, usually within 1 year of transplantation.[30] US show dilated, irregular bile ducts with a normal hepatic artery Doppler waveform.

Bile Leak

Biliary leaks or bilomas usually occur within the first month, are secondary to anastomotic

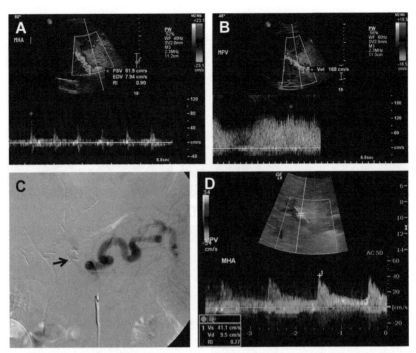

Fig. 7. Splenic steal syndrome. Before and after splenic embolization. (*A*) Doppler US of the hepatic artery shows low diastolic flow with high RI. (*B*) Doppler US through the portal vein shows high-velocity flow in the main portal vein. (*C*) Celiac angiogram shows preferential flow in the splenic artery with a little flow in the hepatic artery (*arrow*). Splenic artery embolization was subsequently performed. (*D*) Doppler US after the splenic artery embolization shows normal waveforms in the hepatic artery.

complications, and are less common in end-to-end biliary anastomosis. If a T tube was inserted, leaks may be seen at the site of T-tube entry. Bile may extravasate in the perihepatic space or may freely distribute within the peritoneal cavity. Patients may present with abdominal pain, distension, or even septic shock. US can usually detect fluid collections but it may be difficult to differentiate from hematoma or ascites. US-guided aspiration may be performed to determine the nature of the fluid. A bile leak can also be confirmed by nuclear medicine hepatobiliary scan or by ERCP. Small bile leaks may spontaneously repair but large leaks may require some kind of intervention. Stent placement through PTC or ERCP is the usual treatment and helps in spontaneous healing of the defect.

Postoperative Fluid Collections

Hematomas are among the most common collections in the immediate posttransplantation period. On US, these are avascular fluid collections that have a complex appearance. They are seen in the first few days after transplantation and usually resolve spontaneously in few weeks. Hematomas rarely need drainage. Hematomas are common in the perihepatic region, especially in the subhepatic space. Ascites and bile leak are other common fluid collections. Compared with hematomas, these appear anechoic. Bile leak (biloma) can be seen as a focal fluid collection around the liver usually in the subhepatic space or as free intraperitoneal fluid on US. Hepatobiliary nuclear scan can confirm the bile leak and differentiate it from other fluid collections. Bile leak can also be confirmed on PTC or ERCP. In the early postoperative period, an increasing fluid collection should raise the suspicion of bile leak. Increase in the ascites can also occur from the IVC or portal vein abnormalities.[4] On CT scan, hematoma usually shows higher attenuation values compared with other collections. MR imaging is more specific in differentiating hematomas because of the signals from the blood products. Right-sided pleural effusion is also a common finding after transplantation.

INFECTIONS

Given the immunocompromised state of these patients, infections may occur in the early posttransplantation period. Infections can occur from surgical complications, acute graft failure, or pre-existing latent infections.[31,32] Fluid collections may become superinfected in these immunocompromised patients. Early postoperative infections

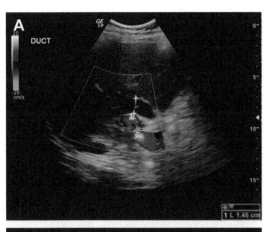

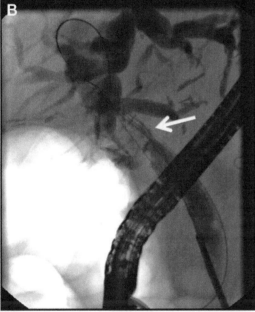

Fig. 8. Biliary stenosis. Color Doppler US of the porta hepatis (*A*) shows dilated common bile duct. Endoscopic retrograde cholangiopancreatography image (*B*) shows markedly dilated intrahepatic ducts and a narrowed segment around the biliary anastomotic area (*arrow*).

are usually intra-abdominal and include intrahepatic and extrahepatic abscesses, cholangitis, peritonitis, and wound infection. Hepatic abscesses occur in about 2% to 4% of adult transplant recipients[31,32] and hepatic thrombosis is a common predisposing cause. Abscesses may also occur in cholangitis and biliary obstruction. US may show single or multiple hypoechoic lesions within the liver that are avascular. Gas may form in these and may show as echogenic foci with dirty shadowing. Purulent abscess may appear on US as particulate ascites.[2] Decreased cell-mediated immunity in these patients also makes them vulnerable to viral infections such as varicella, cytomegalovirus, and recurrent hepatitis B and C. These patients also have a higher risk of fungal and parasitic infections.

MALIGNANCY IN LIVER TRANSPLANTATION

Recurrent and de novo malignancies are the second leading cause of death in patients who have liver transplants following age-related cardiovascular disease.[33] The most common neoplasms in patients who have liver transplants are skin cancer, Kaposi sarcoma, and non-Hodgkin lymphoma.[13,15,34] The common risk factors for malignancy in liver transplant recipients include long-term immunosuppression, history of alcohol use before transplantation, greater rate of chronic viral infections (hepatitis, Epstein-Barr, herpes, and cytomegalovirus) and acute rejection episodes.[2,13,33] The standardized incidence ratios for patients who have liver transplants versus the general population are 2 to 3 for all cancers, up to 20 for lymphoproliferative malignancies, more than 30 for skin cancer, and more than 100 for Kaposi sarcoma.[31] Malignancies in patients after LT can be classified as de novo nonlymphoid malignancies, PTLD, and recurrent malignancy.

DE NOVO NONLYMPHOID MALIGNANCIES

The incidence of de novo malignancies in patients who have liver transplants ranges from 3.1% to 14.4%.[31] It has been shown that suppression of the immune system via immunosuppressive drugs leads to an increased risk of de novo malignancies.[35] LT for alcohol-related liver disease is associated with a greater incidence of de novo cancers than in patients with transplantation for liver disease from other causes.[33]

The most common de novo malignancies after LT are skin cancers including squamous cell carcinoma (SCC), basal cell carcinoma (BCC), and Kaposi sarcoma.[32] BCC and SCC occur in similar numbers; however, the risk with respect to the general population is higher for SCC compared with BCC.[31] The peak time to occurrence is 5 to 10 years after transplantation.[36] Some liver transplant recipients are at increased risk for developing cancer despite immunosuppression and LT. This finding can be seen in patients with primary sclerosing cholangitis and ulcerative colitis, which have an increased risk of developing colorectal cancer. However, the colorectal cancer risk is similar to that of patients with ulcerative colitis without transplants.[31,33] The rates of uterine, ovarian, breast, and prostate cancer are not increased compared with general population rates.[31]

De novo solid organ malignancies are associated with a high mortality, which may be related to tumor aggressiveness in the setting of immunosuppression.[31] Skin cancers have shown better survival rates compared with other de novo malignancies. Long-term immunosuppression should be minimized when possible. Prevention and surveillance according to guidelines for the general population should be followed in all patients with liver transplants to increase the likelihood of early detection.

PTLD

PTLD is a major complication of organ transplantation. It encompasses a spectrum of abnormal conditions of lymphocyte proliferation, which clinically may present as a mild mononucleosislike illness to outright lymphoma. The frequency in adults ranges from 2% to 8.4%.[37] The incidence is higher in pediatric patients. PTLD can involve the liver, lymph nodes, spleen, small bowel, stomach, kidneys, adrenal glands, and mesentery.

Liver involvement may be extrahepatic or intrahepatic, with extrahepatic involvement being more common (**Fig. 9**). Extrahepatic involvement frequently presents with an encasing, ill-defined soft tissue mass at the liver hilum. Intrahepatic involvement is most often a diffuse infiltrative process or, less commonly, multiple hepatic masses.[2]

Epstein-Barr virus has been highly associated with PTLD.[31,37,38] Hepatitis C may also be a risk factor in the development of PTLD.[31] Treatment of PTLD varies based on histology, stage, location, clinical status, graft status, and time from transplantation. Treatment options include reducing immunosuppression, targeting B cells with monoclonal antibodies, or chemotherapy.[38] The mortality for PTLD is up to 40%.[31] Early diagnosis is important to start prompt treatment and prevent evolution to more aggressive disease.

RECURRENT HCC

Recurrent HCC after LT occurs in approximately 20% of patients despite selection criteria and preoperative staging protocols.[35] Tumor size, number of nodules, and the presence of vascular invasion are the most predictive features for recurrence.[35,39] Recurrence usually occurs within 2 years of transplantation and is associated with decreased survival rates. The most common sites of recurrence are the lung, liver, and lymph nodes (**Figs. 10** and **11**).[2,34] Recurrent disease is thought to result from undetected preoperative extrahepatic metastasis or from the release of tumor cells during surgical manipulation. There are few treatment options for recurrence after LT.

REJECTION IN TRANSPLANTATION

The incidence of graft rejection seen in the early years after surgery has been reduced significantly by advances in immunosuppression and surgical techniques.[2] However, rejection remains the most common cause of primary graft dysfunction. The imaging appearance is nonspecific, often with the only abnormality being a heterogeneous appearance of the liver parenchyma. There are no specific Doppler findings diagnostic of rejection. The diagnosis of rejection continues to be established with core biopsy. The role of imaging is

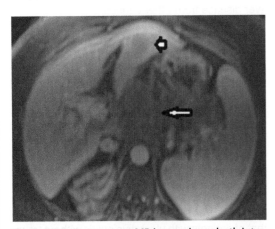

Fig. 9. PTLD. Postcontrast MR image shows both intrahepatic and extrahepatic disease with a mass in the left lobe (*arrowhead*) and a lymph node conglomerate (*arrow*) in the gastrohepatic ligament.

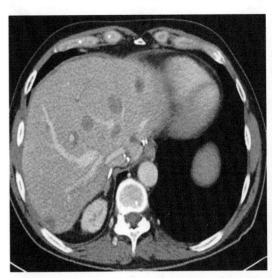

Fig. 10. Recurrent HCC after transplantation. Contrast-enhanced CT image shows recurrent HCC presenting as multiple hepatic masses.

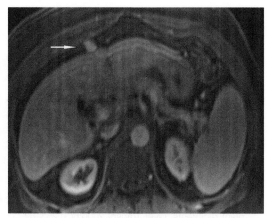

Fig. 11. Recurrent HCC after transplantation. Postcontrast MR image shows recurrent HCC presenting as an enhancing mass (*arrow*) anterior to the liver.

to exclude other complications that have signs and symptoms similar to rejection.[2,35]

ACUTE REJECTION

Patient with acute rejection often experience jaundice and have abnormal liver function tests. It may be associated with fever, pain, and eosinophilia. Acute rejection usually occurs in the early days, weeks, and months after transplantation. However, acute does not refer to time but pathologic findings and reversibility of the diagnosis. The incidence of acute rejection ranges from 12% to 19%.[40] Multiple episodes of acute rejection may occur. Treatment typically consists of high-dose steroids.

CHRONIC REJECTION

Chronic rejection remains a major cause of late graft failure and is irreversible. The incidence of chronic rejection is 2.5% to 17%.[40] It is pathologically characterized pathologically by obliterative vasculopathy, foam cell changes, and bile duct loss. The imaging features are nonspecific and diagnosis is established via liver biopsy.

SUMMARY

The use of US in the preoperative and postoperative liver transplant evaluation is well established. The use of US in the pretransplantation phase is to identify any contraindications to liver transplantation. In the immediate posttransplantation phase, US is used to identify any vascular or biliary complications that may require intervention in order to save the graft. Multimodality imaging such as MR imaging, CT, nuclear medicine, and angiography is also used to definitively diagnose and possibly treat some of these complications.

REFERENCES

1. US Department of Health and Human Services. Annual Report of the US Organ Procurement and Transplantation Network and the Scientific Registry of Transplant Recipients. Transplant Data 2013. Rockville (MD): Health Resources and Services Administration, Healthcare Systems Bureau, Division of Transplantation.
2. Bhargava P, Vaidya S, Dick A, et al. Imaging of orthotopic liver transplantation: review. AJR Am J Roentgenol 2011;196:15–25.
3. Keefee EB. Selection of patients for liver transplantation. In: Maddrey WC, Schiff ER, Sorrell MR, editors. Transplantation of the liver. 3rd edition. Philadelphia: Lippincott Williams & Wilkins; 2001. p. 5–34.
4. Shaw A, Siddhu PS. Ultrasound assessment of the liver transplant candidate. In: Siddhu PS, Baxter GM, editors. Ultrasound of abdominal transplantation. 1st edition. Stuttgart (Germany): Thieme; 2002. p. P76–87.
5. Uzochukwu LN, Bluth EI, Smetherman DH, et al. Early postoperative hepatic sonography as a predictor of vascular and biliary complications in adult orthotopic liver transplant patients. AJR Am J Roentgenol 2005;185:1558–70.
6. Wozney P, Zajko AB, Bron KM, et al. Vascular complications after liver transplantation: a 5-year experience. AJR Am J Roentgenol 1986;147:657–63.
7. Langnas AN, Marujo W, Stratta RJ, et al. Vascular complications after orthotopic liver transplantation. Am J Surg 1991;161:76–82.
8. Nghiem HV. Imaging of hepatic transplantation. Radiol Clin North Am 1998;36:429–43.
9. Berrocal T, Parrón M, Alvarez-Luque A, et al. Pediatric liver transplantation: a pictorial essay of early and late complications. Radiographics 2006;26:1187–209.
10. Flint EW, Sumkin JH, Zajko AB, et al. Duplex sonography of hepatic artery thrombosis after liver transplantation. AJR Am J Roentgenol 1988;151:481–3.
11. Hom BK, Shrestha R, Palmer SL, et al. Prospective evaluation of vascular complications after liver transplantation: comparison of conventional and microbubble contrast-enhanced US. Radiology 2006; 241:267–74.
12. Sidhu PS, Shaw AS, Ellis SM, et al. Microbubble ultrasound contrast in the assessment of hepatic artery patency following liver transplantation: role in reducing frequency of hepatic artery arteriography. Eur Radiol 2004;14:21–30.
13. Quiroga S, Sebastia MC, Margarit C, et al. Complications of orthotopic liver transplantation: spectrum of findings with helical CT. Radiographics 2001;21: 1085–102.
14. Garcia-Críado A, Gilabert A, Bargallo X, et al. Radiology in liver transplantation. Semin Ultrasound CT MR 2002;23:114–29.

15. Nghiem HV, Tran K, Winter TC III, et al. Imaging of complications in liver transplantation. Radiographics 1996;16:825–40.

16. Vit A, De Candia A, Como G, et al. Doppler evaluation of arterial complications of adult orthotopic liver transplantation. J Clin Ultrasound 2003;31:339–45.

17. Crossin JD, Muradali D, Wilson SR. US of liver transplants: normal and abnormal. Radiographics 2003; 23:1093–114.

18. Marshall MM, Muiesan P, Kane PA, et al. Hepatic pseudoaneurysms following liver transplantation: incidence, presenting figures and management. Clin Radiol 2001;56:579–87.

19. Chong WK, Beland JC, Weeks SM. Sonographic evaluation of venous obstruction in liver transplants. AJR Am J Roentgenol 2007;188:W515–21, 1618.

20. Glockner JF, Forauer AR. Vascular or ischemic complications after liver transplantation. AJR Am J Roentgenol 1999;173:1055–9.

21. Lerut J, Rtzakis A, Bron KM, et al. Complications of venous reconstruction in human orthotopic liver transplantation. Ann Surg 1987;205:404–14.

22. Meire H. Transplant liver assessment. In: Meire H, Cosgrove DO, Dewbury K, et al, editors. Abdominal and general ultrasound. 2nd edition. London: Churchill Livingstone; 2000. p. 280–94.

23. Sevmis S, Boyvat F, Aytekin C, et al. Arterial steal syndrome after orthotopic liver transplantation. Transplant Proc 2006;38:3651–5.

24. Uflacker R, Selby JB, Chavin K, et al. Transcatheter splenic artery occlusion for treatment of splenic artery steal syndrome after orthotopic liver transplantation. Cardiovasc Intervent Radiol 2002;25:300–6.

25. Quintini C, Hirose K, Hashimoto K, et al. "Splenic artery steal syndrome" is a misnomer: the cause is portal hyper-perfusion, not arterial siphon. Liver Transpl 2008;14:374–9.

26. Fulcher AS, Turner MA. Orthotopic liver transplantation: evaluation with MR cholangiography. Radiology 1999;211:715–22.

27. Gow PJ, Chapman RW. Liver transplantation for primary sclerosing cholangitis. Liver 2000;20:97–103.

28. Graziadei IW, Wiesner RH, Batts KP, et al. Recurrence of primary sclerosing cholangitis following liver transplantation. Hepatology 1999;29(4):1050–6.

29. Winston D, Emmanoulides C, Busuttil R. Infections in liver transplant recipients. Clin Infect Dis 1995;21: 1077–91.

30. Tachopoulou OA, Vogt DP, Henderson JM, et al. Hepatic abscess after liver transplantation. Transplantation 2003;75:79–83.

31. McCaughan GW, Vajdic CM. De novo malignant disease after liver transplantation? Risk and surveillance strategies. Liver Transpl 2013;19(11): S62–7.

32. Otley CC, Pittelkow MR. Skin cancer in liver transplant recipients. Liver Transpl 2000;6(3):253–62.

33. Fung JJ, Jain A, Kwak EJ, et al. De novo malignancies after liver transplantation: a major cause of late death. Liver Transpl 2001;7(11):S109–18.

34. Caiado AH, Blasbalg R, Marcelino AS, et al. Complications of liver transplantation: multimodality imaging approach. Radiographics 2007;27:1401–17.

35. Zimmerman MA, Ghobrial RM, Tong MJ, et al. Recurrence of hepatocellular carcinoma following liver transplantation. Arch Surg 2008;143(2):182–8.

36. Belloni-Fortina A, Piaserico S, Bordignon M, et al. Skin cancer and other cutaneous disorders in liver transplant recipients. Acta Derm Venereol 2012;92: 411–5.

37. Wu L, Rappaport DC, Hanbidge A, et al. Lymphoproliferative disorders after liver transplantation: imaging features. Abdom Imaging 2001;26:200–6.

38. Kamdar KY, Rooney CM, Heslop HE. Post-transplant lymphoproliferative disease following liver transplantation. Curr Opin Organ Transplant 2011; 16(3):274–80.

39. Schlitt HJ, Neipp M, Weimann A, et al. Recurrence patterns of hepatocellular carcinoma and fibrolamellar carcinoma after liver transplantation. J Clin Oncol 1999;17(1):324–31.

40. Gonzalez JT, Bellido CB, Riera J, et al. Study of liver transplant rejection in alcoholism-induced cirrhosis. Transplant Proc 2013;45:3650–2.

Renal Ultrasound

Joel P. Thompson, MD, MPH*, Shweta Bhatt, MD

KEYWORDS

- Ultrasound • Renal cyst • Renal pseudotumor • Renal pathology • Renal tumor
- Renovascular hypertension • Renovascular pathology

KEY POINTS

- Familiarization with the appearance of common renal congenital variants and renal pseudotumors is key in differentiating these mimics from renal neoplasms.
- Hydronephrosis may be obstructive or nonobstructive in etiology. Urolithiasis is the most common obstructive cause, demonstrated as foci of well-defined echogenicity with sharp posterior shadowing and posterior twinkle artifact on Doppler.
- Renal cystic disease may be caused by both inherited and noninherited causes. The differential diagnosis may be narrowed based on the presence of nephromegaly, discrete cysts versus numerous microcysts, and the identification of multiorgan involvement.
- Renal neoplasms may be detected on renal ultrasound, which is particularly good at demonstrating renal vein involvement. Although CT and MR imaging are often used to characterize lesions, contrast-enhanced ultrasound is emerging as an alternative imaging modality.
- Spectral Doppler ultrasound is useful in the setting of suspected renovascular hypertension, with direct signs including visualization of the stenosis, increased peak systolic velocity greater than 200 cm/s, and increased renal-to-aorta peak systolic velocity greater than 3.5. Indirect signs include tardus parvus waveform distal to the stenosis.

INTRODUCTION

Ultrasonography may be used for the detection, characterization, and follow-up of a wide variety of acute and chronic renal pathology. The sonographic evaluation of adults may detect congenital abnormalities or be used to further characterize abnormalities on other imaging modalities. Ultrasound is often the initial imaging modality in the emergency department for evaluation for suspected obstructive nephropathy. Although CT or MR imaging is often the gold standard, renal masses and pseudotumors may be further characterized and followed using ultrasound. Color and spectral Doppler imaging is useful for the detection of a variety of vascular and nonvascular pathologies.

The objective of this article is to provide an overview of renal pathology with emphasis on the role of ultrasound in their diagnosis and follow-up evaluation.

RENAL ANATOMY

The kidneys are paired retroperitoneal structures on either side of the vertebral column at the level of T12-L3 vertebrae. Each kidney is approximately 10 to 12 cm in length, 4 to 5 cm in width, and 2.5 to 3 cm in thickness.[1] At the medial aspect of each kidney is the concave-shaped renal hilum, which contains the renal artery, renal vein, renal pelvis, and renal sinus fat.

Renal pyramids and their overlying cortex form a lobulated contour. Between each pyramid is an extension of renal cortex, termed *column of Bertin*. The renal cortex contains glomeruli and the renal pyramids comprise collecting tubules. At the tip of each medullary pyramid is a renal papilla, from

Department of Imaging Sciences, University of Rochester School of Medicine and Dentistry, 601 Elmwood Avenue, Box 648, Rochester, NY 14642, USA
* Corresponding author.
E-mail address: Joel_Thompson@urmc.rochester.edu

Ultrasound Clin 9 (2014) 653–681
http://dx.doi.org/10.1016/j.cult.2014.07.011
1556-858X/14/$ – see front matter

which urine empties into a minor calyx. Two to 3 minor calyces empty into a major calyx; 2 to 3 major calyces then empty into the renal pelvis, which is continuous with the ureter.

SONOGRAPHIC TECHNIQUE

Sonographic evaluation of the kidneys is best performed with a low frequency transducer, usually 2 to 5 MHz, depending on a patient's body habitus.[2] Lower frequencies provide deeper tissue penetration; higher frequencies provide improved image resolution. Visualization of the right kidney is often best performed using the liver as an acoustic window via an anterior oblique approach. The left kidney is located more superiorly than the right kidney, and its upper pole can be visualized using the spleen as an acoustic window via an intercostal approach. A subcostal approach may also be used to evaluate the upper poles during a maximum inspiration breath-hold. The lower poles of both kidneys may be targeted using a posterior approach. Decubitus, prone, or upright positioning may, however, enable optimal imaging, particularly of the left kidney, due to adjacent stomach and air-filled bowel.[2]

Both long-axis and transverse views of the kidneys should be obtained, along with evaluation of the renal hilum. The right kidney should be hypoechoic to the liver, whereas the left kidney should be isoechoic or hypoechoic to the spleen (**Fig. 1**). A long-axis measurement of renal length should be recorded for each kidney; a length discrepancy of 2 cm or greater is considered significant and should be further evaluated for a possible cause for the discrepant sizes.

CONGENITAL NORMAL VARIANTS

The adult kidneys are formed from the metanephros, which develops at week 5 of gestation and begins to function at approximately week 9.[3] The metanephros contains the ureteric bud, which forms the calices and ureters, and the metanephrogenic blastema, which forms the renal parenchyma. The kidneys are formed within the pelvis at approximately week 5 of gestation, then ascend and rotate medially approximately 90° until the hila are directed medially. The kidneys attain their normal adult location by the ninth week of gestation.[1]

Renal pseudotumors, or tumor mimics, are often developmental variants resulting from abnormal renal growth. A common pseudotumor is *persistent fetal lobulation* (**Fig. 2**), which is seen when normal fetal lobulations fail to diminish at the end of the fetal period. The indentation between prominent lobules overlies columns of Bertin, which differentiates fetal lobulations from scarring (which overlies renal pyramids).

Prominent columns of Bertin are intrusions of hypertrophied cortical tissue found between medullary pyramids. Prominent columns of Bertin are most often located at the junction between the upper and middle thirds of the kidney and more frequently in the left kidney (left-to-right ratio 2:1).[4] The ultrasound appearance is of a soft tissue mass isoechoic to renal cortex that extends into the hyperechoic renal sinus, usually oriented perpendicular to the renal cortex (**Fig. 3**). The overlying renal contour is usually normal. Occasionally, prominent columns of Bertin may appear more echogenic than overlying cortex due to anisotropic effect.[3,5]

A *dromedary hump* is a focal bulge along the superolateral margin of the left kidney, formed due to impression by the adjacent spleen (**Fig. 4**). Because a dromedary hump comprises cortical tissue, it may be differentiated from a

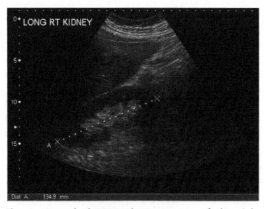

Fig. 1. Normal ultrasound appearance of the right kidney. The liver is used as an acoustic window and is isoechoic to the kidney.

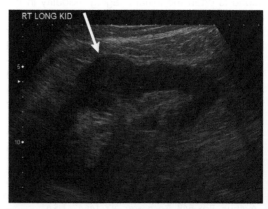

Fig. 2. Persistent fetal lobulation. Longitudinal ultrasound image of the right kidney demonstrates a lobular pseudotumor (*arrow*) comprised of renal cortex, with lateral margins overlying columns of Bertin.

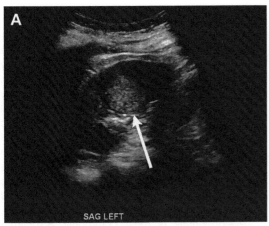 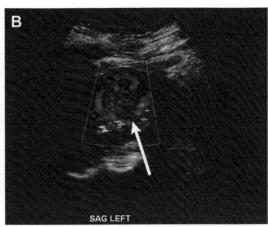

Fig. 3. Column of Bertin. (*A*) On longitudinal ultrasound view of the left kidney, there is a round masslike region (*arrow*) between medullary pyramids that is isoechoic to renal cortex and extends into the renal sinus fat. (*B*) Doppler ultrasound image demonstrates normal renal vascularity peripheral to the column of Bertin (*arrow*).

mass due to its isoechoic appearance to adjacent renal cortex. Obtuse angle with the adjacent contiguous renal capsule margin also favors a benign congenital variant rather than a mass.

A *junctional parenchymal defect* is an extension of renal sinus fat through the renal cortex, formed by partial fusion of 2 embryonic parenchymal masses, termed *renunculi* (**Fig. 5**).[6] These may be differentiated from a scar or renal mass (such as angiomyolipoma) based on their characteristic location: the medial half of the kidney along the anterior upper pole or posterior lower pole.

Congenital renal anomalies may also result from abnormal renal ascent from the pelvis, including horseshoe kidney, crossed renal ectopia, and ectopic location. *Horseshoe kidney* is the most common renal fusion anomaly, caused by abnormal fusion of the metanephrogenic blastema at the lower pole of each kidney. The kidneys are then fused by an isthmus of fibrous tissue or functional cortex at their lower poles (**Fig. 6**); the isthmus does not allow ascent of the kidneys above the inferior mesenteric artery; thus, the kidneys are located lower than in the normal adult.

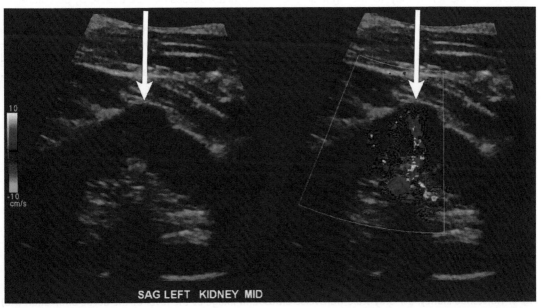

Fig. 4. Dromedary hump. Longitudinal gray-scale (*left*) and color Doppler (*right*) ultrasound view of the kidney demonstrates a dromedary hump along the lateral aspect of the left kidney with normal renal vascularity (*arrows*), which is a focal bulge of normal cortical tissue due to impression by the adjacent spleen. Diagnosis is made by its characteristic location.

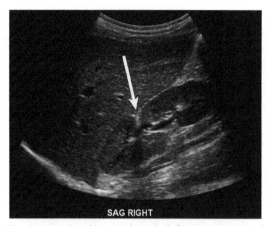

Fig. 5. Junctional parenchymal defect. Longitudinal ultrasound view of the right kidney using the liver as an acoustic window demonstrates a smooth parenchymal defect in the renal cortex with renal sinus fat extending through the defect at the junction of the mid- and upper poles (*arrow*).

Abnormal course of the ureters predisposes these patients to obstruction, calculi, and infection.[7] There are 4 findings suggestive of horseshoe kidney: (1) lower than normal position of the kidneys, (2) medial location of the lower poles close to the spine, (3) long axis more vertical than normal, and (4) visible isthmus.[7,8]

Crossed renal ectopia most often occurs when the upper pole of one kidney fuses to the lower pole of the contralateral kidney during gestation; crossover of the left kidney to the right side is most common, with malrotation of the left kidney.[8] *Ectopic kidneys* without abnormal fusion may also occur, most commonly in the pelvis (**Fig. 7**) but also rarely in the thorax if a diaphragmatic hernia is present.

INFECTION AND INFLAMMATION

Increased renal echogenicity is often seen in the presence of renal parenchymal disease but is a nonspecific finding.[9,10] Increased echogenicity may be identified by comparing the kidneys with adjacent organs (ie, liver and spleen) or by demonstrating increased echogenicity of renal pyramids to the overlying cortex.[11] Echogenic kidneys are broadly classified as medical renal disease and often require a biopsy to confirm the pathology. Systemic medical renal disease usually presents as bilateral increased echogenic kidneys, which may be of normal or increased size (**Fig. 8**).

Pyelonephritis is most commonly associated with an ascending genitourinary tract infection and is a clinical diagnosis; sonographic appearance is usually normal.[9] Renal edema may cause nephromegaly. *Focal or multifocal pyelonephritis* may occur in diabetic or immunocompromised patients and may be seen on ultrasound as either focal increased or decreased echogenicity within the renal cortex, extending from renal medulla to the renal capsule (**Fig. 9**).[12] Focal pyelonephritis may be differentiated from abscess by the absence of a distinct wall.[10] Doppler ultrasound shows decreased perfusion within this area. Pyelonephritis may resolve with conservative management, including antibiotics, or may occasionally lead to formation of *renal abscess* (**Fig. 10**) or *inflammatory pseudotumor* (**Fig. 11**). Renal abscesses may be treated by percutaneous or surgical drainage.

Xanthogranulomatous pyelonephritis is the result of long-standing pyelonephritis, characterized by progressive parenchymal scarring and replacement of tissue with macrophages.

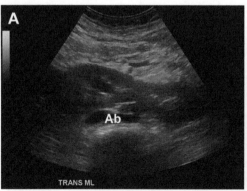
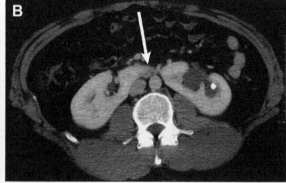

Fig. 6. Horseshoe kidney. (*A*) Gray-scale transverse ultrasound image at the level of the aortic bifurcation (Ab) demonstrates 2 reniform masses connected across the midline by tissue. (*B*) Contrast-enhanced CT image at the level of the distal aorta shows 2 medially located kidneys with enhancing tissue connecting the inferior poles across the midline (*arrow*). Horseshoe kidney is an independent risk factor for renal calculi (seen here in the left upper kidney), hydronephrosis, and transitional cell carcinoma.

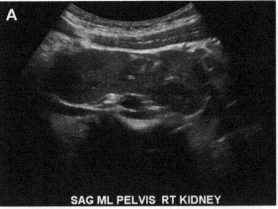
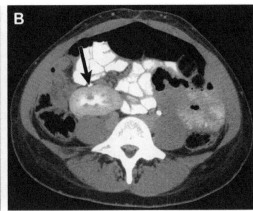

Fig. 7. Ectopic kidney. (*A*) Transverse ultrasound image in the midline pelvis demonstrates a reniform mass, which in the absence of a kidney on ultrasound of the right flank is consistent with an ectopic pelvic right kidney. (*B*) Axial CT image in the lower abdomen during renal excretory phase shows the transversely oriented and inferiorly displaced right kidney (*arrow*).

Sonographically, this appears as an enlarged kidney with replacement of the renal parenchyma by cystic spaces, which often contain debris. Multiple hypoechoic masses may also be present, representing abscesses or granulomas. This is most often found in patients with diabetes or pregnancy with recurrent urinary tract infections; classically, a staghorn calculus is present.

Emphysematous pyelonephritis (EPN) is a surgical emergency that is a result of a severe necrotizing infection of the kidney, which leads to accumulation of gas within the renal tissues (**Fig. 12**). A majority of the cases are unilateral, more often affecting the left kidney, and almost exclusively occur in the setting of diabetes

mellitus. EPN can be further classified according to the extent of involvement in the kidney[13]:

Class I: gas confined to the collecting system
Class II: gas within renal parenchyma
Class III: extension of gas or abscess into perinephric or pararenal space
Class IV: bilateral EPN or EPN in a solitary kidney

Classes I, II, and III EPN without thrombocytopenia or shock are treated by percutaneous nephrostomy placement and intravenous antibiotics. More severe cases are treated surgically with nephrectomy. CT has 100% sensitivity for detection of EPN.

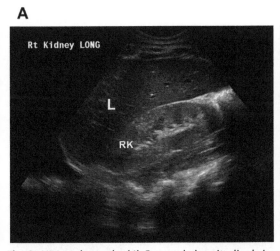
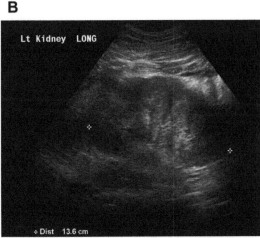

Fig. 8. HIV nephropathy (*A*) Gray-scale longitudinal view of the right kidney demonstrates hyperechoic renal parenchyma compared with the adjacent liver. A right pleural effusion is also visualized. L, liver; RK, right kidney. (*B*) Gray-scale longitudinal image of a mildly enlarged left kidney in the same patient shows hyperechoic medullary pyramids compared with normal renal cortex echogenicity.

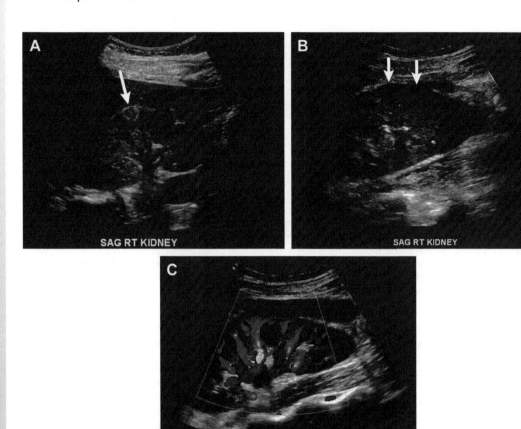

Fig. 9. Pyelonephritis. (*A*) Heterogenous right renal parenchyma in a 23-year-old woman who was 22-weeks pregnant with fever, right flank pain, and *Escherichia coli* urinary tract infection. There is a focal hyperechoic area (*arrow*) in the interpolar region. (*B*) Ultrasound of a different patient shows an enlarged right kidney with peripheral region of decreased echogenicity (*arrows*) in the midkidney without identifiable walls. (*C*) Doppler ultrasound shows increased vascularity to this area, consistent with focal pyelonephritis.

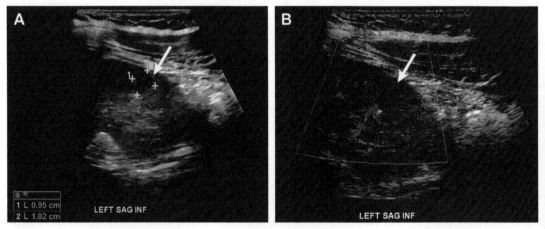

Fig. 10. Renal abscess in a 24-year-old woman with clinical pyelonephritis. (*A*) Longitudinal gray-scale ultrasound image demonstrates a focal hypoechoic lesion (*arrow*) with irregular wall in the left lower kidney. (*B*) Color Doppler image demonstrates that the lesion (*arrow*) has nonvascular walls.

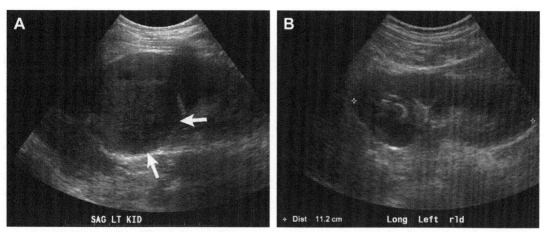

Fig. 11. Inflammatory pseudotumor in a 14-year-old girl with fever and failed treatment of urinary tract infection. (*A*) Longitudinal gray-scale image of the left kidney demonstrates a large 7 × 6 cm solid mass (*arrows*) that is isoechoic to adjacent renal parenchyma. Biopsy of an adjacent perirenal lymph node was performed due to clinical concern for lymphoma or solid tumor, with pathology demonstrating lymphoid hyperplasia. (*B*) After antibiotic therapy, repeat ultrasound 2 months later demonstrates near resolution of the mass.

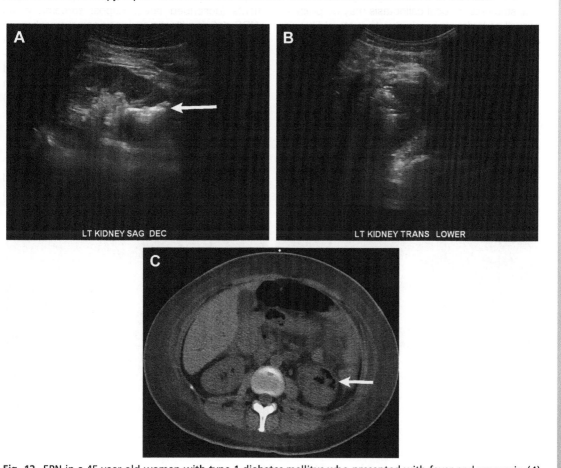

Fig. 12. EPN in a 45-year-old woman with type 1 diabetes mellitus who presented with fever and urosepsis. (*A*) Longitudinal and transverse (*arrow*). (*B*) Gray-scale image demonstrate a heterogenous hyperechoic area in the left lower kidney with posterior reverberation artifact consistent with air. (*C*) Axial nonenhanced CT image through the lower kidneys confirms the presence of air within left renal parenchyma consistent with class II EPN (*arrow*). There is a small amount of perirenal fluid. The patient improved after volume resuscitation and intravenous antibiotics.

Pyonephrosis is a suppurative infection of the renal collecting system, typically as sequela of obstruction. Ultrasound demonstrates hydronephrosis with debris or fluid-fluid levels within the collecting system (**Fig. 13**).

Renal tuberculosis is present in 4% to 8% of patients with pulmonary tuberculosis.[14] The sonographic appearance varies widely and depends on the stage of disease. At initial exposure, *Mycobacterium tuberculosis* organisms are spread hematogenously and trapped in periglomerular capillaries, inciting granuloma formation in the renal cortex.[9] Ultrasound may demonstrate granulomas of variable size and echogenicity.[15] If reactivation occurs, organisms spread via a descending infection from the proximal convoluted tubules down to the bladder. Granulomas may coalesce (forming a tuberculoma) and rupture into the renal calyx or perirenal space, creating an abscess. Papillary necrosis may be present. Calyceal strictures or focal caliectasis may be present as well as hydronephrosis due to ureteral fibrosis and stricture formation. Chronic infection may result in both parenchymal atrophy and dystrophic calcification (termed, *putty kidney*). Evaluation is usually best performed by CT or urography.

HIV-Related Renal Disease

HIV-related renal manifestations are diverse, including HIV-associated nephropathy, opportunistic infections, highly active antiretroviral therapy-related toxicity, and HIV-associated neoplasms.[16] *HIV-associated nephropathy* is the leading cause of renal failure in HIV-positive patients, presenting as decreasing renal function,

proteinuria, and azotemia.[17] Ultrasound evaluation may demonstrate diffusely or geographically hyperechoic kidneys, decreased corticomedullary differentiation, and normal to increased renal size.[16] Diagnosis is established by renal biopsy.

Opportunistic infections include *Pneumocystis jiroveci*, *Candida albicans*, *Aspergillus*, and *Mycobacterium*; ultrasound findings are nonspecific and include increased renal echogenicity, the presence of abscesses, or hydronephrosis due to obstruction (from a fungal ball, for example).

Indinavir sulfate is a protease inhibitor that is used as part of highly active antiretroviral therapy and is associated with radiolucent renal stone formation in up to 20% of patients. Indinavir stones are radiolucent on CT. Ultrasound reveals evidence of ureteral obstruction but confirms diagnosis in a minority of cases.[18]

HIV-associated lymphoma has the same appearance as in nonimmunocompromised patients (described later). Kaposi sarcoma is an AIDS-defining illness and may occur anywhere in the body. Unfortunately, Kaposi sarcoma is often clinically occult before patient death and no specific sonographic appearance has been described to date. HIV-infected individuals also have an increased risk of renal cell carcinoma (RCC) (described later).

HYDRONEPHROSIS

Hydronephrosis is abnormal dilatation of the renal pelvis and calyces, which may be the result of both obstructive and nonobstructive causes (**Table 1**).[19] Hydronephrosis may be categorized as mild,

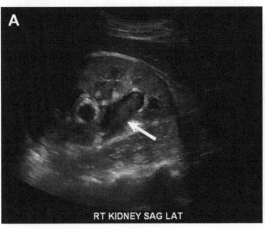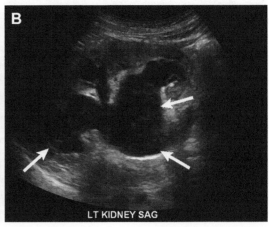

RT KIDNEY SAG LAT   LT KIDNEY SAG

Fig. 13. Pyonephrosis in a 67-year-old man with bilateral hydronephrosis and prostate hypertrophy. (*A*) Longitudinal gray-scale ultrasound image of the right kidney demonstrates moderate hydronephrosis with echogenic debris (*arrow*) within the collecting system, consistent with blood, pus, or debris. (*B*) Longitudinal gray-scale ultrasound image of the left kidney demonstrates severe hydronephrosis with renal parenchymal thinning and echogenic debris (*arrows*) within the collecting system. Urine obtained on nephrostomy tube placement was pustular and grew E Coli.

Table 1
Causes of hydronephrosis

Obstructive causes		
Congenital	UPJ obstruction	
	Ureterocele	
	Posterior urethral valves	
Acquired		
Intrinsic (intraluminal)	Urolithiasis	
	Blood clot	
	Neoplasm (transitional cell carcinoma)	
	Infectious (fungus ball, tuberculosis, *Schistosomiasis*)	
	Inflammatory (postradiation, iatrogenic)	
Extrinsic (extraluminal)	Pregnancy	
	Benign prostatic hypertrophy	
	Neoplastic (genitourinary, colorectal, sarcomas, lymphoma)	
	Infectious (diverticulitis, appendicitis, tubo-ovarian abscess)	
	Inflammatory (pelvic inflammatory disease, postradiation)	
	Retroperitoneal fibrosis	
Functional	Neurogenic bladder	
	Diabetes mellitus	
	Spinal cord injury	
	Anticholinergic drugs	
Nonobstructive causes		
Congenital	Vesicoureteral reflux	
Acquired	Increased urine flow (diuresis, diabetes insipidus)	
	Vesicoureteral reflux (infection, downstream obstruction)	

Adapted from Lin EP, Shweta B, Dogra VS, et al. Sonography of urolithiasis and hydronephrosis. Ultrasound Clin 2007;2:1–16; with permission.

moderate, or severe. Although the definitions of these grades differ among radiologists, mild hydronephrosis generally corresponds to enlargement of the calyces with maintained visualization of papillae. The papillae are not visualized in moderate hydronephrosis. In severe hydronephrosis there is ballooning of the calices and loss of the echogenic renal sinus, with or without thinning of the overlying cortex (**Fig. 14**).[19] Hydroureter may be associated with any category of hydronephrosis. If the bladder is distended when hydronephrosis or hydroureter is identified, postvoid images should be obtained to decrease the likelihood of a false-positive result.

Obstructive Hydronephrosis

Urolithiasis is the most common form of obstructive hydronephrosis, with a lifetime risk of up to 13% in men and 7% in women in the United States and Europe.[20,21] The presence of renal stones are associated with male gender, non-Hispanic white ethnicity, comorbidities such as diabetes and obesity, and increased environmental temperature.[21] Renal colic classically presents as severe, spasmodic flank pain that may radiate to the groin as the stone progresses inferiorly through the ureter. A majority of ureteral calculi become obstructed either at the ureteropelvic junction (UPJ) or the ureterovesicular junction. Although ultrasound has lower sensitivity for identifying ureteral calculi compared with CT (in particular, small calculi <3 mm),[22–25] sonographic evaluation is the modality of choice for patients who should avoid radiation, such as pregnant women and children.

Sonographic findings of nephrolithiasis include well-defined echogenic foci with sharp posterior shadowing. Placing the suspected stone within the focal zone and decreasing the distance between the transducer and the suspected stone improve detection of posterior acoustic shadowing.[26] Most renal calculi demonstrate twinkle artifact, which is rapidly changing red and blue color on Doppler behind the calcification, a result of phase jitter within the machine; spectral tracing in the area of twinkle artifact demonstrates noise (**Fig. 15**). The positive predictive value of twinkle artifact is as high as 94% and increases the sensitivity of sonographic imaging compared with using B-mode alone.[27,28]

Calculi at the ureterovesicular junction should be easily visualized when the bladder is fully

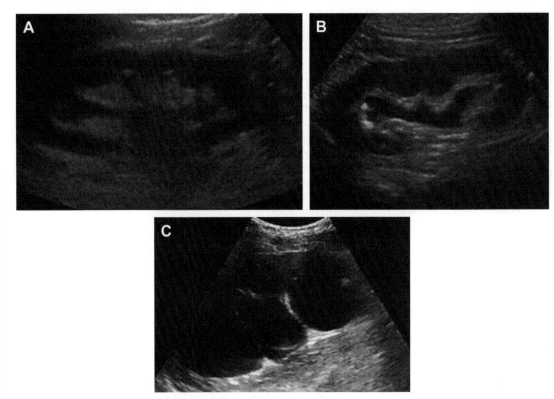

Fig. 14. Grades of hydronephrosis. (*A*) Enlarged caliceal system with intact papillae representing mild hydronephrosis. (*B*) Enlarged calices with flattening of the renal papillae consistent with moderate hydronephrosis. (*C*) Severe hydronephrosis involves marked pelvicaliectasis and thinning of the overlying renal cortex.

distended (**Fig. 16**). Transabdominal evaluation for ureteral jets may be performed, with positive findings including nonvisualization of ureteral jet, decreased frequency of ureteral jets, and decreased peak velocity of the ureteral jet.[29] The clinical utility of ureteral jet evaluation is, however, questionable.[30]

Nephrocalcinosis, or calcification within renal parenchyma, may mimic nephrolithiasis (**Fig. 17**). Medullary nephrocalcinosis may be caused by

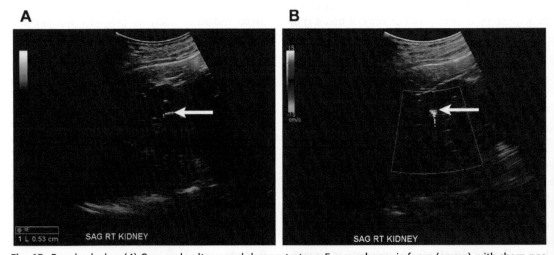

Fig. 15. Renal calculus. (*A*) Gray-scale ultrasound demonstrates a 5 mm echogenic focus (*arrow*) with sharp posterior shadowing. (*B*) Color Doppler ultrasound with focal point at the level of the echogenic focus (*arrow*) shows twinkle artifact.

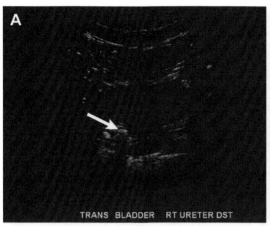
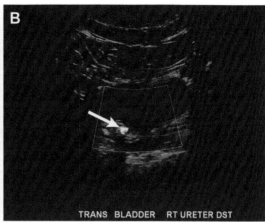

Fig. 16. Calculus at the ureterovesicular junction. (*A*) Transverse ultrasound of the bladder demonstrates a subtle echogenic focus with sharp posterior shadowing just behind the bladder in the region of the right uretovesicular junction (*arrow*). (*B*) Color Doppler ultrasound demonstrates twinkle artifact (*arrow*).

primary hyperparathyroidism, hypervitaminosis D, renal tubular acidosis, and medullary sponge kidney.[31] Cortical nephrocalcinosis may be the result of acute renal cortical necrosis, oxalosis, or chronic glomerulonephritis. Additional causes of false-positive findings may be due to vascular calcifications (typically linear), intrarenal gas (typically demonstrates a dirty shadow), milk of calcium cysts, surgical scar, or calcified neoplasms (**Fig. 18**).

Obstructive hydronephrosis may also be caused by neoplasms (most commonly transitional cell carcinoma), pyonephrosis, fungal balls, blood clots, or ureteral strictures. *Ureteral strictures* may be sequela of infection (described previously), trauma/instrumentation, or prior radiation therapy. These are better diagnosed with CT urography or retrograde ureterography due to limited visualization of the mid- and distal ureters on ultrasound.

Obstructive hydronephrosis may also be the result of extrinsic compression on the genitourinary system. The most common cause of *extrinsic obstructive hydronephrosis* in women is pregnancy. The most common cause in men over age 50 is benign prostatic hypertrophy. Neoplasms (including ovarian and uterine tumors),

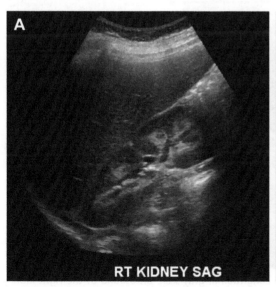
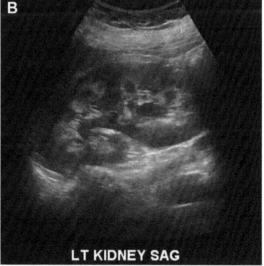

Fig. 17. Nephrocalcinosis in a 19-year-old woman with medullary sponge kidney and history of recent urolithiasis. (*A*) Longitudinal gray-scale ultrasound of the right kidney shows highly echogenic medullary pyramids. (*B*) Similar findings are present in the left kidney. Also noted is mild hydronephrosis, consistent with patient's current pregnancy.

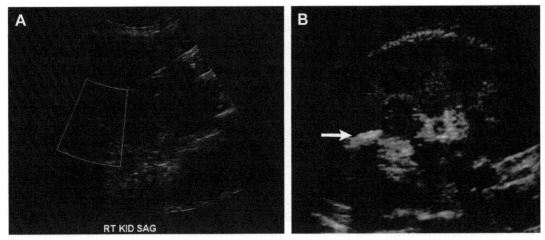

Fig. 18. Mimics of renal calculi. (*A*) Longitudinal gray-scale ultrasound of the right kidney demonstrates a complex right renal cystic lesion with coarse shadowing calcification in a 74-year-old man with history of left nephrectomy for renal cell carcinoma. This did not enhance on follow-up MR imaging (not shown) and was considered a benign complex cyst on follow-up imaging. (*B*) Complex cystic lesion with milk of calcium (*arrow*) in the dependent portion of the cyst with posterior acoustic shadowing.

abdominopelvic fluid collections, or retroperitoneal fibrosis, however, may also cause mass effect on the ureters. These conditions are often best diagnosed with CT.

Obstructive hydronephrosis may also be congenital in etiology. *UPJ obstruction* is the most common cause of hydronephrosis in infancy and early childhood (**Fig. 19**). Causes of UPJ obstruction include functional stenosis (inadequate peristalsis and luminal distention due to abnormally few smooth muscle cells), anatomic obstruction due to smooth muscle hypertrophy or fibrous bands, or abnormal renal pelvic insertion into the ureter.[32] In addition to visualizing

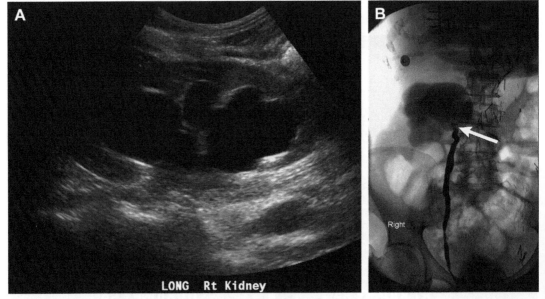

Fig. 19. UPJ obstruction in an 84-year-old woman. (*A*) Longitudinal gray-scale ultrasound of the right kidney demonstrates severe hydronephrosis with renal cortical thinning. (*B*) Anteroposterior fluoroscopic image from retrograde pyelogram demonstrates severe pelvicaliectasis with focal narrowing of the right proximal ureter in the region of the UPJ (*arrow*). Sequela of left nephrectomy and retroperitoneal lymph node dissection for left ureteral transitional cell carcinoma is partially visualized.

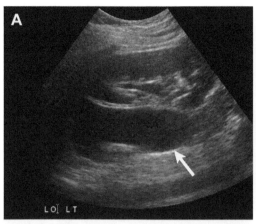
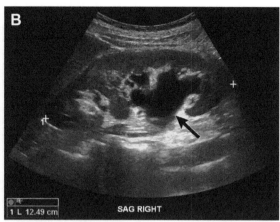

Fig. 20. Duplicated urinary collecting system. (*A*) Longitudinal gray-scale ultrasound of the left kidney demonstrates severe hydronephrosis of the upper moiety (*arrow*). (*B*) Longitudinal gray-scale ultrasound of the right kidney in a different patient demonstrates moderate hydronephrosis of the lower pole (*arrow*) moiety with flattening of the papillae. The upper pole moiety is associated with renal calculi and ureterocele formation, whereas the lower pole moiety is associated with vesicoureteral reflux due to ectopic ureteral insertion.

hydronephrosis on ultrasound, increased echogenicity of medullary pyramids and loss of corticomedullary differentiation are correlated with poor renal function.[33] An additional cause of unilateral or bilateral hydronephrosis in early childhood is a *posterior urethral valve*, which is best depicted by voiding cystourethrogram.

A *duplicated urinary collecting system* is associated with hydronephrosis of the upper pole collecting system due to ureterocele or ectopic insertion into the bladder (typically more inferior and medial compared with the normal lower pole collecting system insertion according to the Weigert-Meyer rule). Ultrasound reveals upper pole hydronephrosis and may reveal a ureterocele, which is a round, anechoic mass protruding into the bladder (**Fig. 20**).[34]

Nonobstructive Hydronephrosis

The most common cause of nonobstructive hydronephrosis is *vesicoureteral reflux*, which is retrograde flow of urine from the urinary bladder into the ureters (**Fig. 21**). Vesicoureteral reflux may be

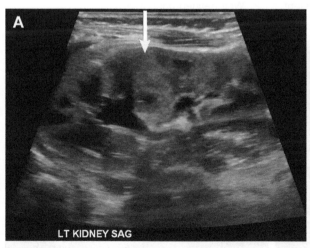
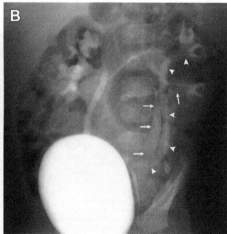

Fig. 21. Vesicoureteral reflux in a 2-month-old with hydronephrosis on prenatal ultrasound. (*A*) Longitudinal image of the left kidney demonstrates mild hydronephrosis. Note the prominent cortical tissue in the medial aspect of the midkidney (*arrow*), which could represent a prominent column of Bertin or cortical tissue with duplicated collecting system. (*B*) Voiding cysturethrogram demonstrates bilateral vesicoureteral reflux. There is partial duplication of the left renal collecting system, with an upper pole ureter (*arrowheads*) and lower pole ureter (*arrows*) emptying into a common distal ureter.

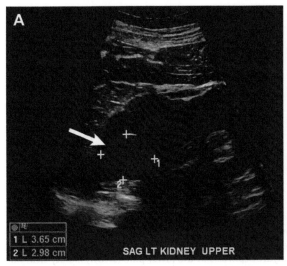
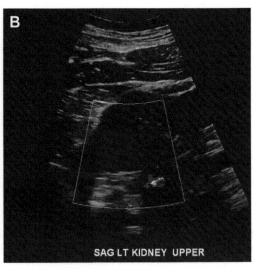

Fig. 22. Simple renal cyst. (*A*) Longitudinal gray-scale ultrasound of the left kidney demonstrates a 3.7 × 3.0 cm anechoic region (*arrow*) with posterior acoustic enhancement, well-defined back wall, and imperceptible side-walls. A second cyst is seen in the lower kidney. (*B*) Corresponding color Doppler ultrasound demonstrates lack of internal vascularity, consistent with a simple cyst.

congenital due to a valvular defect at the vesi-coureteral junction or may be acquired due to downstream obstruction (such as benign prostatic hypertrophy, infection, or trauma). Acquired causes of nonobstructive hydronephrosis can also be the result of *increased urine flow*, such as aggressive intravenous hydration, diuresis, or diabetes insipidus.

RENAL CYSTIC DISEASE

Renal cysts are the most commonly encountered renal lesion.[35,36] Simple renal cysts are present

on approximately 12% of ultrasound examinations; the prevalence increases with age with cysts present in up to 36% of patients in their eighth decade of life.[37] Cysts develop within renal tubules from immature epithelial cells that abnormally secrete tubular fluid and solute rather than absorb it, which explains why renal cysts may enlarge over time.[38]

On ultrasound, a lesion must demonstrate the following characteristics on all views to qualify as a simple renal cyst (**Fig. 22**):

1. Anechoic lumen
2. Well-defined back wall

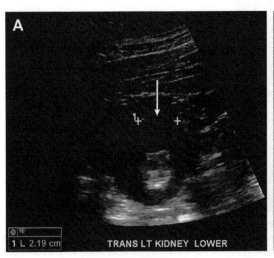
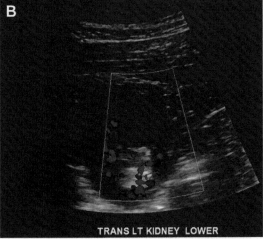

Fig. 23. Complex cyst. (*A, B*) Transverse gray-scale ultrasound of the left kidney shows a cyst with a subtle internal septation (*arrow*) and wall calcification. Corresponding color Doppler ultrasound demonstrates no internal vascularity within the cyst or the septation.

Table 2
Comparison of inherited causes of renal cystic disease

Disease	Sonographic Appearance	Other
Autosomal-dominant polycystic kidney disease (**Fig. 24**)	Classically, nephromegaly with expansile cysts; infants may have enlarged echogenic kidneys with subcapsular cysts	• Most common genetic cause of end-stage renal disease, 1 in 400 to 1 in 1000 live births. • Involves polycystic kidney disease 1 (chromosome 16) or polycystic kidney disease 2 (chromosome 4). • Cysts may arise from any portion of the nephron and enlarge over time. • Most commonly identified between 20 and 40 y of age; may cause pain, hypertension, or calculi. • Increased prevalence of aortic and intracranial aneurysms. • Hepatic cysts usually present in adults.
Autosomal-recessive polycystic kidney disease	Large echogenic kidneys (at birth); moderately enlarged kidneys with pseudomedullary nephrocalcinosis	• One in 20,000 live births; involves polycystic kidney and hepatic disease 1 on chromosome 6. • Dilatation and elongation of collecting ducts creates numerous small (<3 mm) cysts.[40] • More than 60% of patients also have Caroli disease. • Approximately 25% of patients die within the first year of life (dependent on severity of oligohydramnios and pulmonary hypoplasia).
Glomerulocystic disease	Subcapsular cortical cysts; angiomyolipomas may be present (eg, tuberous sclerosis)	• Associated with numerous syndromes, including von Hippel-Lindau and tuberous sclerosis. • Cysts arise from glomeruli. • Renal cysts generally do not lead to renal failure but do increase risk of RCC (75% incidence in patients with von Hippel-Lindau). • Extrarenal manifestations differentiate between syndromes.
Nephronophthisis	Normal-sized kidneys with normal to increased echogenicity; cysts develop at corticomedullary junction	• Autosomal recessive; approximately 1–2 per 100,000 live births. • NPHP1 mutation (chromosome 2) in majority of cases. • Chronic interstitial nephritis, leading to fibrosis and renal failure. Early symptoms include polyuria and polydipsia. • May be associated with a variety of syndromes, including Joubert and Meckel-Gruber.

3. Acoustic enhancement deep to the lesion
4. Imperceptible wall
5. Absent internal vascularity

Lesions that do not fulfill these criteria are considered complex cystic lesions and require further evaluation, usually by contrast-enhanced CT. Contrast-enhanced sonography has, however, recently been shown effective in discriminating between benign or malignant cystic lesions.[39] Mimics of renal cysts include lymphoma, aneurysms and arteriovenous malformatons, and caliceal diverticula.

Cysts may be complicated by hemorrhage or infection and thus demonstrate internal low-level echos and debris; additional imaging or follow-up is recommended to exclude malignancy.

Cysts may contain thin curvilinear calcifications on the periphery, usually due to prior hemorrhage or infection. Thick or amorphous calcifications should, however, prompt further evaluation to exclude malignancy. Likewise, thin internal septations may be seen in otherwise simple cysts (**Fig. 23**), but thickened or irregular septations are suspicious for cystic renal cell carcinoma.

Renal cystic disease may be classified by inherited and noninherited etiologies. Autosomal-dominant polycystic kidney disease is among the most common inherited diseases and is the most common inherited cause of end-stage renal disease.[40] Other causes of inherited disorders associated with renal cysts are listed in **Table 2**.[35] The underlying pathology in many genetic renal cystic diseases is abnormal structure or function

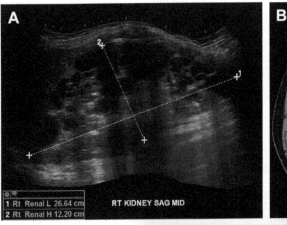
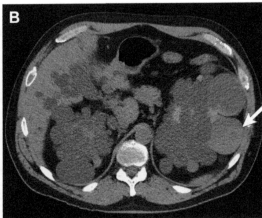
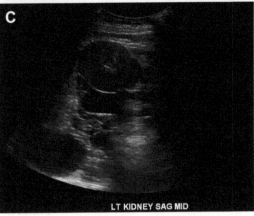

Fig. 24. Autosomal-dominant polycystic kidney disease in a 54-year-old man who presented for evaluation of left flank pain and hematuria. (*A*) Longitudinal panoramic gray-scale ultrasound image of the right kidney demonstrates a massively enlarged right kidney almost totally replaced by cysts. (*B*) Axial nonenhanced CT of the kidneys demonstrates massive enlargement of both kidneys with the majority of volume occupied by numerous cysts. Numerous liver cysts are also present. Note a high attenuation cyst (*arrow*) in the lateral left kidney consistent with recent hemorrhage (the cause of the patient's pain and hematuria). (*C*) Longitudinal Doppler ultrasound images in the same patient 1 month later demonstrate a large cyst with avascular internal debris, likely from prior internal hemorrhage.

Table 3
Comparison of noninherited causes of renal cystic disease

Disease	Sonographic Appearance	Clinical Information
Simple cysts	Normal kidney size and echogenicity; single or multiple simple cysts	• Incidence increases with age, up to 36% of patients in their 8th decade.[37] • Prenatal solitary cysts often resolve before birth.
Acquired cysts	Usually multiple bilateral cysts	• Increased prevalence the longer the patient is on hemodialysis. • Cysts may resolve after renal transplant.
Medullary sponge kidney (see **Fig. 17**)	Normal kidney size; echogenic medullary pyramids	• Cystic dilatation of medullary and papillary collecting ducts. • Increased risk of infection and nephrolithiasis; hypercalciuria. • May be familial.[41] • CT demonstrates cystic ectatic collecting ducts (bunch of grapes or bouquet of flowers) on noncontrast CT and striated paintbrush appearance of medullary pyramids on urogram phase.
Renal cystic neoplasms (**Fig. 25**)	Multiseptated cystic mass that compresses adjacent renal parenchyma	• Cystic nephroma: bimodal distribution occurring in patients <4 and >30 y of age. • Cystic partially differentiated nephroblastoma • Cystic renal cell carcinoma, Wilms tumor, and clear cell sarcoma typically demonstrate solid enhancing nodules on CT.
Renal sinus cysts (nontubular origin) (**Fig. 26**)	Cysts in the renal sinus, single or multiple, noncommunicating	• Urinomas (renal sinus or perirenal) typically due to obstructive uropathy or trauma. • Parapelvic cysts are of lymphatic origin. • Renal sinus cysts and diverticula.
Lithium-induced microcysts (**Fig. 27**)	Normal kidney size; multiple tiny echogenic foci throughout the cortex and medulla	• Due to chronic lithium treatment. • May lead to progressive nephropathy, including nephrogenic diabetes insipidus. • Histology demonstrates glomerulosclerosis, distal tubular dilation with 1–2 mm microcysts, and adjacent fibrosis.[42]

of cilia, which regulate cell proliferation and differentiation.[36] Because cilia are present within multiple organs (including the brain, liver, pancreas, and lungs), ciliopathies commonly have multiorgan associations and are thus recognized as various syndromes. Inherited cystic disease that occurs in utero (such as severe autosomal-recessive kidney disease, renal cystic dysplasia, and multicystic dysplastic kidney) may be associated with poor survival, because poor renal function leads to oligohydramnios, pulmonary hypoplasia, and Potter sequence.

Renal cystic disease may also be noninherited (**Table 3**). Common causes of noninherited renal cystic disease include idiopathic simple cysts, acquired cysts (which are found in the majority of patients on long-term hemodialysis), and lithium-induced microcysts. Medullary sponge kidney has historically been considered a sporadic disorder but has recently been reported that familial clustering may represent autosomal-dominant inheritance with variable penetrance and expressivity.[41]

RENAL NEOPLASMS

Sonography may detect incidental renal masses or be used to further characterize lesions detected by CT or MR imaging.[43] Ultrasound may be used to characterize renal masses, including assessing the size, cystic or solid composition, the presence of vascular invasion, and the presence of internal vascularity.

RCC is the most common primary renal malignant neoplasm. Approximately 4% of RCCs are familial in origin, including tuberous sclerosis and von Hippel-Lindau syndromes.[44] There are 4 main histologic types of RCC that are

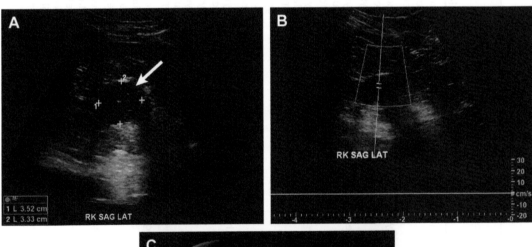

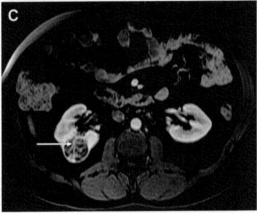

Fig. 25. Cystic RCC in a 44-year-old man presenting with new onset gross hematuria and right flank pain. (*A*) Longitudinal gray-scale ultrasound of the right kidney demonstrates a multiseptated cystic lesion (*arrow*) with increased through transmission. (*B*) Corresponding spectral Doppler ultrasound shows an arterial waveform within a septation. (*C*) T1 fat-suppressed MR image with intravenous contrast during corticomedullary phase demonstrates avid enhancement of the septa (*arrow*), which is consistent with renal cell carcinoma. The patient underwent a partial nephrectomy, with surgical pathology demonstrating clear cell type RCC limited to the kidney.

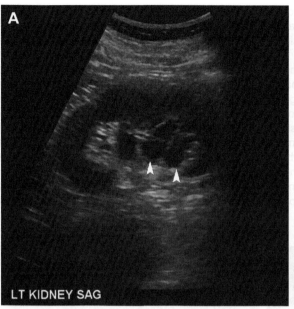
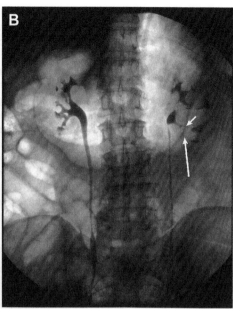

Fig. 26. Renal sinus cyst in a 65-year-old man with bladder and prostate cancer. An ultrasound was ordered due to clinical suspicion for hydronephrosis. (*A*) Longitudinal gray-scale ultrasound of the left kidney reveals multiple small parapelvic/sinus cysts (*arrowheads*). Doppler ultrasound showed no internal vascularity (not shown). (*B*) Retrograde pyelogram performed for staging of bladder cancer confirms that the left parapelvic cysts are not within the collecting system and extrinsically compress the lower calyces (*arrows*).

indistinguishable on imaging: clear cell, papillary, chromophobe, and collecting duct carcinoma. A rare subtype of collecting duct carcinoma, called medullary carcinoma, is associated with young

Fig. 27. Lithium-induced microcysts in a 35-year-old man receiving treatment of multiple psychiatric conditions, including long-term lithium therapy. Longitudinal gray-scale ultrasound performed for nocturia reveals normal size kidneys (approximately 12 cm in length) with multiple tiny echogenic foci throughout the left kidney, corresponding to numerous bilateral microcysts.

persons with sickle cell disease or trait and has a poor prognosis.

Patients may present with hematuria, weight loss, abdominal pain, fever, or fatigue. Although ultrasound is limited in its ability to accurately stage RCC, it is useful for depicting vascular invasion and extension into the renal vein or inferior vena cava (IVC). Important staging criteria include

Stage I: tumor confined within renal capsule
Stage II: tumor extension into perinephric fat or ipsilateral adrenal gland
Stage III: tumor extension into renal vein or IVC, or regional lymph node involvement
Stage IV: tumor extension beyond Gerota fascia or distant metastasis

The appearance of RCC varies from hypoechoic to hyperechoic, with smaller RCCs (<3 cm) more likely to be hyperechoic. Approximately 15% of RCCs may be cystic, perhaps due to internal necrosis.[45] Several sonographic findings may help distinguish between an RCC and an angiomyolipoma. RCCs do not exhibit posterior shadowing (approximately one-third of angiomyolipomas do), whereas hypoechoic rims and intratumoral cysts are only seen in RCCs.[46]

If a lesion is indeterminate on B-mode ultrasound, spectral Doppler may help differentiate RCC from pseudotumor. Spectral Doppler may show a high peak systolic velocity with a low-resistance waveform in RCC, the result of intratumoral arteriovenous shunting and a deficient media layer in tumoral arterial walls (**Fig. 28**).[47,48]

Renal masses detected by ultrasound are most often further characterized using CT or MR imaging. One study demonstrated that MR imaging was more likely to provide a differential diagnosis compared with CT but at a much higher cost.[49] In addition to characterizing the lesion, these modalities provide important staging criteria when choosing an appropriate treatment regimen. Contrast-enhanced ultrasound is an emerging modality for the characterization of renal lesions,

particularly outside the United States. Early data suggest that contrast-enhanced ultrasound is not inferior to or even more accurate than CT in detecting blood flow in hypovascular tumors and characterizing complex renal cysts.[50]

Additional renal neoplasms are outlined in **Table 4**.

The most common benign renal mass is an angiomyolipoma, comprising vessels, smooth muscle, and adipose tissue. Eighty percent of AMLs are sporadic; 20% are associated with tuberous sclerosis and tend to be multiple and bilateral. AMLs larger than 4 cm in diameter or containing pseudoaneurysms greater than 5 mm in diameter

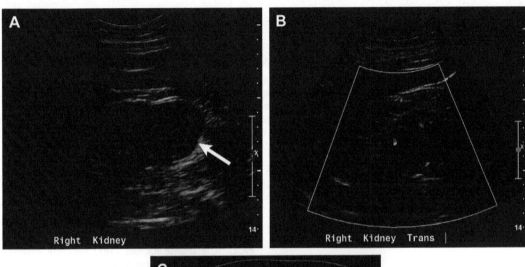

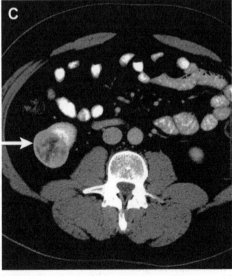

Fig. 28. RCC in a 41-year-old man presenting with abdominal pain. (*A*) Longitudinal gray-scale ultrasound of the right kidney demonstrates a 4.3-cm solid predominantly hyperechoic mass (*arrow*) in the right lower kidney. (*B*) Color Doppler ultrasound demonstrates internal flow. (*C*) Staging contrast-enhanced CT shows an avidly enhancing exophytic lesion (*arrow*) in the right lower kidney. A partial nephrectomy was performed, with surgical pathology showing clear cell type RCC that was confined to the kidney.

Table 4
Malignant renal neoplasms

Type	Overview	Sonographic Appearance
RCC (see **Fig. 28**)	• Most common primary renal malignant neoplasm • 1% Are bilateral, 10% multifocal at presentation	• 50% Hyperechoic, 30% isoechoic (abnormal renal contour), 10% hypoechoic. • Most often solid, but 5% may be cystic. • May have amorphous calcification. • Doppler may show internal vascularity and displaced vessels peripherally.
Transitional cell carcinoma (**Fig. 29**)	• Most common urothelial tumor • 10% Bilateral metachronous or synchronous tumors • Association with Lynch syndrome	• Most too small to be identified on ultrasound. • Bulky intraluminal polypoid mass or thickening and narrowing of lumen. • Pelvicaliectasis may be present. • Vascularity excludes similar-appearing etiologies, such as blood clot and fungus ball.
Lymphoma (**Fig. 30**)	• Most common non-Hodgkin B-cell lymphoma • Most often bilateral renal involvement	• Masses are near-anechoic and can simulate cysts due to homogenous tissue composition (lacks through-transmission). • 5 Potential appearances: 1. Multiple parenchymal lesions (most common) 2. Solitary lesion 3. Diffuse involvement with nephromegaly 4. Perirenal rindlike mass 5. Direct extension from retroperitoneal lymphadenopathy • Lack of posterior enhancement and Doppler may help differentiate from a cyst.
Metastatic disease	• Most common primaries are lung, breast, gastrointestinal tract, and melanoma	• Most commonly multiple bilateral renal masses. • Hypoechoic cortical mass lesion without through transmission.

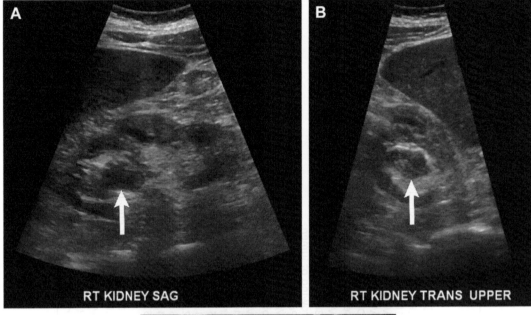

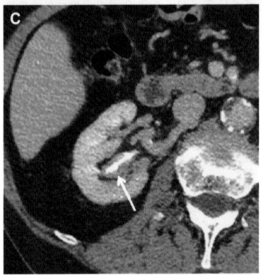

Fig. 29. Papillary urothelial carcinoma in an 82-year-old man with hematuria. (*A*) Longitudinal and transverse gray-scale ultrasound of the right kidney demonstrates a focal dilatation of right upper collecting system with wall thickening and internal debris (*arrow*). (*B*) Transverse gray-scale ultrasound image better demonstrates the internal debris (*arrow*). (*C*) CT urogram during excretory phase demonstrates soft tissue thickening of the calix (*arrow*), consistent with urothelial carcinoma.

are at greater risk of hemorrhage.[51] The classic sonographic appearance of an AML is a well-defined hyperechoic mass, but distinguishing AML from RCC may be difficult. On ultrasound, RCCs do not exhibit posterior shadowing (whereas approximately one-third of AMLs do), whereas hypoechoic rims and intratumoral cysts are only seen in RCCs.[46] On CT, 95% of AMLs larger than 1 cm in size demonstrate macroscopic fat attenuation. Additional benign renal neoplasms are outlined in **Table 5**.

PERIRENAL PATHOLOGY

A diverse range of pathology may affect the perirenal space. Most commonly, inflammatory processes involving the kidney or adjacent organs may result in inflammatory edema collecting adjacent to the kidney. Thickening of perirenal septa may also be observed. Processes, such as abscess or xanthogranulomatous pyelonephritis, may result in an ill-defined complex perinephric fluid collection. Simple fluid in the perirenal space

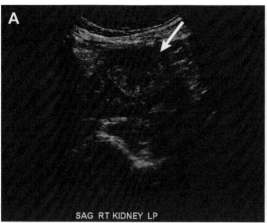 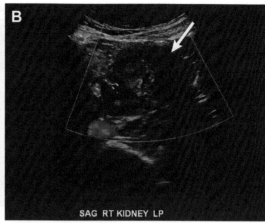

Fig. 30. Marginal zone lymphoma in an 85-year-old man. (*A*) Grayscale ultrasound shows a crescentic mass of heterogenous echogenicity adherent to the right lower kidney (*arrow*). (*B*) Color Doppler ultrasound image demonstrates no internal vascularity (*arrow*).

may represent a urinoma, most commonly the result of ureteral obstruction or trauma.

Renal trauma may present in a variety of ways on ultrasound. Ultrasound has poor sensitivity for detecting low-grade renal parenchymal injury. Sensitivity may be as high as 93%, however, for detecting higher-grade injury, which may be identified as disorganized appearance of the kidney along with expansion and altered echogenicity of

the perirenal space.[52] Perirenal hemorrhage may be hypo-, iso-, or even hyperechoic to renal parenchyma depending on the acuity.

Ultrasound also has limited sensitivity in the identification of *spontaneous perirenal hemorrhage*, particularly in the identification of underlying cause (approximately 50% of which are malignant neoplasms).[53] A normal renal ultrasound does not exclude the presence of perirenal

Table 5
Benign renal neoplasms

	Overview	Sonographic Appearance
Angiomyolipoma (Fig. 31)	• Most common benign renal neoplasm • Contain vessels, muscles, and fat • Increased risk of hemorrhage when >4 cm	• Hyperechoic well-defined mass with echogenicity, like perirenal fat (if >1 cm then CT or MR imaging should demonstrate fat) • Some may demonstrate acoustic shadowing (RCC does not). • Poorly defined posterior wall.
Oncocytoma	• 5% Of renal neoplasms • Arise from renal tubule epithelium	• Nonspecific appearance that overlaps with RCC (differentiated by surgical pathology).
Hemangioma	• May present with macroscopic hematuria	• Nonspecific solid mass, commonly located in renal pyramids or renal pelvis.
Juxtaglomerular cell tumor	• Secretes renin (classically a young woman with severe hypertension) • Rare	• Usually small (<3 cm) hyperechoic cortical mass.
Multilocular cystic nephroma (Fig. 32)	• Consists of large, noncommunicating cystic spaces within a capsule	• Cannot differentiate from cystic RCC.

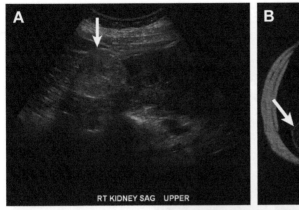

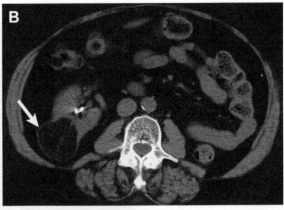

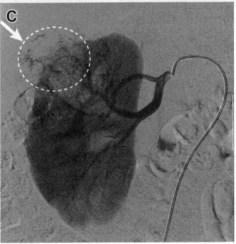

Fig. 31. Angiomyolipoma. (*A*) Longitudinal gray-scale view of the right kidney demonstrates a predominantly hyperechoic well-defined mass (*arrow*) in the upper kidney with some posterior acoustic shadowing. (*B*) Axial nonenhanced CT through the lesion demonstrates an exophytic lesion in the right kidney with macroscopic fat content (*arrow*). (*C*) Angiogram of the right kidney demonstrates a hypovascular mass in the upper kidney (*arrow*), which was prophylactically embolized due to risk of future hemorrhage.

pathology, and further imaging should be performed based on clinical suspicion, particularly in the presence of hematuria.

Infiltrative processes may involve the perirenal space and appear as an hypoechoic rind of tissue surrounding the kidney. Lymphoma, retroperitoneal fibrosis, and Erdheim-Chester disease may have this appearance (**Fig. 33**).[54] Neoplasms may involve the perirenal space, including RCC (by direct extension), lymphoma (a majority of which are diffuse large B cell lymphoma), angiomyolipoma, liposarcoma, and metastases (most commonly lung cancer).

VASCULAR PATHOLOGY

The renal arteries arise from the aorta just inferior to the level of the superior mesenteric artery.[55] The right renal artery passes posterior to the inferior vena cava, and each renal artery is located posterior to the renal vein. There is classically one renal artery to each kidney, although an accessory renal artery may be present in up to 20% of kidneys. Each renal artery divides into segmental and interlobar arteries in the renal hilum. Doppler ultrasound should demonstrate blood flow throughout the renal medulla with a low-resistance spectral waveform.

Renovascular hypertension is the most common cause of secondary hypertension, accounting for 2% to 5% of cases.[56,57] A vast majority of cases (>90%) are caused by atherosclerotic disease and typically involve the origin and proximal one-third of the renal arteries. In the United States, *fibromuscular dysplasia* is the second leading cause of renovascular hypertension, accounting for less than 10% of cases. The most common subtype involves medial fibroplasia, which is characterized

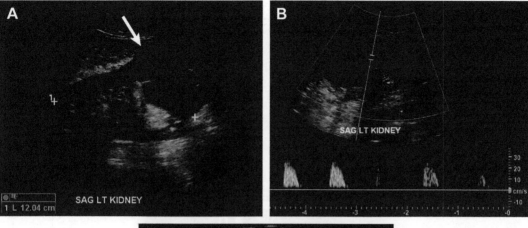

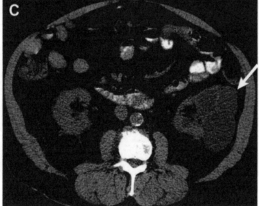

Fig. 32. Multilocular cystic nephroma. (*A*) Longitudinal gray-scale ultrasound image of the left kidney reveals a multiloculated cystic lesion (*arrow*) with increased through transmission in the lower pole. (*B*) Spectral Doppler demonstrates arterial flow within a septa as well as vascularity within a peripheral nodule. (*C*) Axial nonenhanced CT demonstrates a complex exophytic mass (*arrow*) arising from the left lower kidney. Intermediate attenuation within the cystic spaces may represent old hemorrhage or protein content.

by the classic string of beads appearance in the middle one-third of the renal artery.[58] Intimal fibroplasia is much less common and is characterized by focal concentric stenosis or long, smooth narrowing. *Large-vessel vasculitis*, such as giant-cell ateritis or Takayasu arteritis may also cause renovascular hypertension and is much more common in the Far East and the Indian subcontinent; Takayasu arteritis may cause up to 60% of renovascular hypertension in India.[59,60] Rarer causes of renovascular hypertension include middle aortic syndrome in children (associated with Williams syndrome), extrinsic compression on renal arteries (most commonly due to neurofibromatosis), and aortic or renal artery dissection.

Diagnostic ultrasound provides both anatomic and functional assessment of patients with suspected renovascular hypertension and findings may be direct or indirect. Direct signs include direct visualization of renal artery stenosis on B-mode images, increased peak systolic velocity greater than 200 cm/s, and increased renal-to-aorta peak systolic velocity greater than 3.5 (although cutoffs may differ between institutions).[55,61] If peak aortic velocity is less than 40 cm/s or greater than 100 cm/s due to decreased cardiac function or atherosclerosis, however, the renal-to-aortic ratio may be artificially elevated or depressed. In these cases, an absolute peak systolic velocity in the renal artery of greater than 200 cm/s should be used (**Fig. 34**).[61] Higher cutoffs should be used when evaluating stented renal arteries, due to the "theoretical concern that stents decreased vessel wall compliance, leading to false-positive elevation of peak systolic velocity."[55] These suggested cutoffs are for the main renal artery, because ultrasound has low sensitivity for detecting accessory renal arteries.[56]

Indirect signs of renovascular hypertension on ultrasound include tardus parvus waveform distal

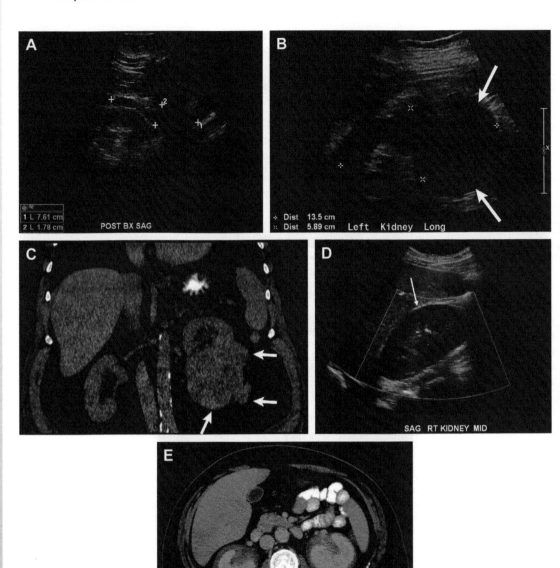

Fig. 33. Perirenal processes. (*A*) Longitudinal gray-scale ultrasound of the lower pole of the kidney in a 68-year-old man immediately after ultrasound-guided renal biopsy demonstrates a hypoechoic collection (within calipers) adjacent to the kidney. This collection was avascular on Doppler ultrasound (not shown) and new compared with prebiopsy ultrasound, consistent with acute perirenal hematoma. (*B*) Longitudinal gray-scale ultrasound demonstrates a hypoechoic mass (*arrows*) arising from the lower pole of the kidney and extending into the perirenal space. Coronal contrast-enhanced CT (*C*) also depicts the lesion (*arrows*) spreading from the kidney into the adjacent fat and thickening of the left perirenal fascia. This was pathologically confirmed to be renal cell carcinoma. (*D*) Longitudinal color Doppler ultrasound of the right kidney demonstrates a hypoechoic rind of tissue (*arrow*) surrounding the kidney. There is no internal vascularity. (*E*) Axial contrast-enhanced CT demonstrates bilateral perirenal rind of enhancing soft tissue (*arrows*). Biopsy was performed due to concern for lymphoma, but demonstrated numerous histiocytes and the patient was later diagnosed with Erdheim-Chester disease, a rare non–Langerhans type histiocytosis.

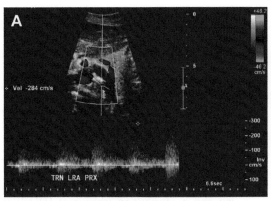
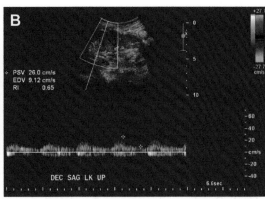

Fig. 34. Renovascular hypertension in an 84-year-old woman. (*A*) Spectral Doppler image in the proximal left renal artery demonstrates increased peak systolic velocity to 284 cm/s (aortic velocity 114 cm/s). (*B*) Doppler spectrum from the upper pole intrarenal artery shows a tardus parvus waveform. Similar waveforms were present in the mid- and lower pole consistent with renovascular hypertension, likely due to atherosclerotic renal artery stenosis.

to the stenosis, including prolonged acceleration time or slow acceleration index on spectral Doppler. Tardus parvus waveforms do not, however, always occur distal to stenosis if increased upstream resistance is present, such as atherosclerosis or decreased vascular compliance.[55] There is currently no consensus on the utility of resistive indices in renovascular hypertension; resistive indices above 0.8 are associated with decreased renal function but not with response to endovascular therapy.[62]

Renal vein thrombosis may occur as a result of trauma or medical renal disease (most commonly nephrotic syndrome). B-mode ultrasound may demonstrate an enlarged kidney and an echogenic filling defect in the renal vein. Doppler imaging of the renal vein may show decreased or absent flow in the renal vein; collateral vessels may be present depending on the acuity of onset. Spectral imaging of the renal artery may show an abnormal high-resistance waveform, diastolic flow reversal, and increased resistive indices.

Arteriovenous fistulas and pseudoaneurysms are most commonly the result of penetrating trauma, such as renal biopsy. *Arteriovenous fistulas* are best evaluated with spectral Doppler ultrasound; findings include increased flow velocity in the feeding artery and draining vein, decreased resistance waveform in the feeding artery, and spectral broadening (**Fig. 35**). Renal *pseudoaneurysms* appear as cystic structures on B-mode ultrasound. Doppler ultrasound may demonstrate a yin-yang pattern of swirling blood with to-and-fro flow within the neck.

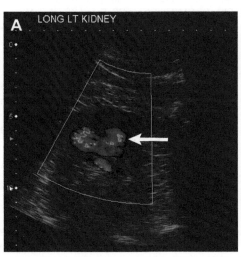
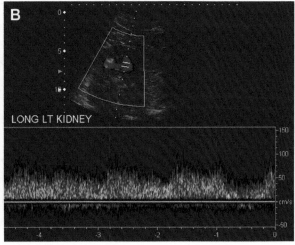

Fig. 35. Renal arteriovenous fistula. (*A*) Longitudinal color Doppler ultrasound image through the left kidney demonstrates a large highly vascular region (*arrow*) in the hilum. (*B*) Spectral Doppler waveform shows arterialized venous, low resistance waveform, consistent with arteriovenous fistula.

Pseudoaneurysms and arteriovenous fistulas may occur together.

SUMMARY

Ultrasound may be used for the detection and assessment of a wide variety of renal pathology. Familiarization with the appearance of common renal pseudotumors is key for differentiating these mimics from renal neoplasms. Ultrasound is useful in the setting of medical renal disease for excluding obstructive uropathy, with identification of obstructing calculi aided by creating the twinkle artifact. Renal neoplasms may be detected on renal ultrasound, which is particularly good at demonstrating renal vein involvement. Although CT and MR imaging are often used to characterize lesions, contrast-enhanced ultrasound is emerging as an alternative imaging modality. Lastly, Doppler ultrasound is useful for the identification of renovascular disease.

REFERENCES

1. American Institute of Ultrasound in Medicine. Clinically oriented anatomy. 5th North American edition. Baltimore (MD): Lippincott Williams & Wilkins; 2006.
2. AIUM practice guideline for the performance of an ultrasound examination of the abdomen and/or retroperitoneum. J Ultrasound Med 2012;31:1301–12.
3. Bhatt S, MacLennan G, Dogra V. Renal pseudotumors. AJR Am J Roentgenol 2007;188:1380–7.
4. Lafortune M, Constantin A, Breton G, et al. Sonography of the hypertrophied column of Bertin. AJR Am J Roentgenol 1986;146:53–6.
5. Yeh HC, Halton KP, Shapiro RS, et al. Junctional parenchyma: revised definition of hypertrophic column of Bertin. Radiology 1992;185:725–32.
6. Carter AR, Horgan JG, Jennings TA, et al. The junctional parenchymal defect: a sonographic variant of renal anatomy. Radiology 1985;154:499–502.
7. Weizer AZ, Silverstein AD, Auge BK, et al. Determining the incidence of horseshoe kidney from radiographic data at a single institution. J Urol 2003;170:1722–6.
8. Muttarak M, Sriburi T. Congenital renal anomalies detected in adulthood. Biomed Imaging Interv J 2012;8:e7.
9. Hammond NA, Nikolaidis P, Miller FH. Infectious and inflammatory diseases of the kidney. Radiol Clin North Am 2012;50:259–70.
10. Vourganti SA, Agarwal PK, Bodner DR. Ultrasonographic evaluation of renal infections. Ultrasound Clin 2010;5:355–66.
11. Rosenfield AT, Siegel NJ. Renal parenchymal disease: histopathologic-sonographic correlation. AJR Am J Roentgenol 1981;137:793–8.
12. Farmer KD, Gellett LR, Dubbins PA. The sonographic appearance of acute focal pyelonephritis 8 years experience. Clin Radiol 2002;57:483–7.
13. Huang JJ, Tseng CC. Emphysematous pyelonephritis: clinicoradiological classification, management, prognosis, and pathogenesis. Arch Intern Med 2000;160:797–805.
14. Kawashima A, Sandler CM, Goldman SM, et al. CT of renal inflammatory disease. Radiographics 1997;17:851–66 [discussion: 867–8].
15. Vijayaraghavan SB. Ultrasonography of genitourinary tuberculosis. Ultrasound Clin 2010;5:367–78.
16. Symeonidou C, Standish R, Sahdev A, et al. Imaging and histopathologic features of HIV-related renal disease. Radiographics 2008;28:1339–54.
17. Roling J, Schmid H, Fischereder M, et al. HIV-associated renal diseases and highly active antiretroviral therapy-induced nephropathy. Clin Infect Dis 2006;42:1488–95.
18. Schwartz BF, Schenkman N, Armenakas NA, et al. Imaging characteristics of indinavir calculi. J Urol 1999;161:1085–7.
19. Lin EP, Shweta B, Dogra VS, et al. Sonography of urolithiasis and hydronephrosis. Ultrasound Clin 2007;2:1–16.
20. Scales CD Jr, Smith AC, Hanley JM, et al, Urologic Diseases in America Project. Prevalence of kidney stones in the United States. Eur Urol 2012;62:160–5.
21. Romero V, Akpinar H, Assimos DG. Kidney stones: a global picture of prevalence, incidence, and associated risk factors. Rev Urol 2010;12:e86–96.
22. Smith RC, Levine J, Dalrymple NC, et al. Acute flank pain: a modern approach to diagnosis and management. Semin Ultrasound CT MR 1999;20:108–35.
23. Fowler KA, Locken JA, Duchesne JH, et al. US for detecting renal calculi with nonenhanced CT as a reference standard. Radiology 2002;222:109–13.
24. Sheafor DH, Hertzberg BS, Freed KS, et al. Nonenhanced helical CT and US in the emergency evaluation of patients with renal colic: prospective comparison. Radiology 2000;217:792–7.
25. Jindal G, Ramchandani P. Acute flank pain secondary to urolithiasis: radiologic evaluation and alternate diagnoses. Radiol Clin North Am 2007;45: 395–410, vii.
26. King W 3rd, Kimme-Smith C, Winter J. Renal stone shadowing: an investigation of contributing factors. Radiology 1985;154:191–6.
27. Vallone G, Napolitano G, Fonio P, et al. US detection of renal and ureteral calculi in patients with suspected renal colic. Crit Ultrasound J 2013; 5(Suppl 1):S3.
28. Kielar AZ, Shabana W, Vakili M, et al. Prospective evaluation of Doppler sonography to detect the twinkling artifact versus unenhanced computed tomography for identifying urinary tract calculi. J Ultrasound Med 2012;31:1619–25.

29. Jandaghi AB, Falahatkar S, Alizadeh A, et al. Assessment of ureterovesical jet dynamics in obstructed ureter by urinary stone with color Doppler and duplex Doppler examinations. Urolithiasis 2013;41:159–63.

30. Delair SM, Kurzrock EA. Clinical utility of ureteral jets: disparate opinions. J Endourol 2006;20:111–4.

31. Sidhu R, Bhatt S, Dogra VS. Renal colic. Ultrasound Clin 2008;3:159–70.

32. Park JM, Bloom DA. The pathophysiology of UPJ obstruction. Current concepts. Urol Clin North Am 1998;25:161–9.

33. Chavhan G, Daneman A, Moineddin R, et al. Renal pyramid echogenicity in ureteropelvic junction obstruction: correlation between altered echogenicity and differential renal function. Pediatr Radiol 2008;38:1068–73.

34. Callahan MJ. The drooping lily sign. Radiology 2001;219:226–8.

35. Garel L. Renal cystic disease. Ultrasound Clin 2010;5:15–59.

36. Avni FE, Garel C, Cassart M, et al. Imaging and classification of congenital cystic renal diseases. AJR Am J Roentgenol 2012;198:1004–13.

37. Terada N, Ichioka K, Matsuta Y, et al. The natural history of simple renal cysts. J Urol 2002;167:21–3.

38. Grantham JJ. Pathogenesis of renal cyst expansion: opportunities for therapy. Am J Kidney Dis 1994;23:210–8.

39. Quaia E, Bertolotto M, Cioffi V, et al. Comparison of contrast-enhanced sonography with unenhanced sonography and contrast-enhanced CT in the diagnosis of malignancy in complex cystic renal masses. AJR Am J Roentgenol 2008;191:1239–49.

40. Loftus H, Ong AC. Cystic kidney diseases: many ways to form a cyst. Pediatr Nephrol 2013;28: 33–49.

41. Fabris A, Lupo A, Ferraro PM, et al. Familial clustering of medullary sponge kidney is autosomal dominant with reduced penetrance and variable expressivity. Kidney Int 2013;83:272–7.

42. Cho JJ, Strickland M. Lithium-induced microcysts. Ultrasound Q 2012;28:179–80.

43. Paspulati RM, Bhatt S. Sonography in benign and malignant renal masses. Radiol Clin North Am 2006;44:787–803.

44. Choyke PL, Glenn GM, Walther MM, et al. Hereditary renal cancers. Radiology 2003;226:33–46.

45. Hartman DS, Davis CJ Jr, Johns T, et al. Cystic renal cell carcinoma. Urology 1986;28:145–53.

46. Siegel CL, Middleton WD, Teefey SA, et al. Angiomyolipoma and renal cell carcinoma: US differentiation. Radiology 1996;198:789–93.

47. Lee HY, Kim SH, Jung SI, et al. Renal cell carcinoma in an end-stage kidney: evaluation with spectral Doppler ultrasound. J Med Ultrasound 2004;12:91–4.

48. Kim SH, Cho JY, Kim SY, et al. Ultrasound evaluation of renal masses. Ultrasound Clin 2013;8:565–79.

49. Margolis NE, Shaver CM, Rosenkrantz AB. Indeterminate liver and renal lesions: comparison of computed tomography and magnetic resonance imaging in providing a definitive diagnosis and impact on recommendations for additional imaging. J Comput Assist Tomogr 2013;37:882–6.

50. Bertolotto MD, Derchi LE, Cicero C, et al. Renal masses as characterized by ultrasound contrast. Ultrasound Clin 2013;8:581–92.

51. Yamakado K, Tanaka N, Nakagawa T, et al. Renal angiomyolipoma: relationships between tumor size, aneurysm formation, and rupture. Radiology 2002;225:78–82.

52. McGahan JP, Richards JR, Jones CD, et al. Use of ultrasonography in the patient with acute renal trauma. J Ultrasound Med 1999;18:207–13 [quiz: 215–6].

53. Zhang JQ, Fielding JR, Zou KH. Etiology of spontaneous perirenal hemorrhage: a meta-analysis. J Urol 2002;167:1593–6.

54. Surabhi VR, Menias C, Prasad SR, et al. Neoplastic and non-neoplastic proliferative disorders of the perirenal space: cross-sectional imaging findings. Radiographics 2008;28:1005–17.

55. Wang SY, Scoutt LM. Ultrasound evaluation of renovascular hypertension. Ultrasound Clin 2011; 6:491–511.

56. White CJ, Olin JW. Diagnosis and management of atherosclerotic renal artery stenosis: improving patient selection and outcomes. Nat Clin Pract Cardiovasc Med 2009;6:176–90.

57. Simon N, Franklin SS, Bleifer KH, et al. Clinical characteristics of renovascular hypertension. JAMA 1972;220:1209–18.

58. Slovut DP, Olin JW. Fibromuscular dysplasia. N Engl J Med 2004;350:1862–71.

59. Cheung CM, Hegarty J, Kalra PA. Dilemmas in the management of renal artery stenosis. Br Med Bull 2005;73–74:35–55.

60. Jain S, Kumari S, Ganguly NK, et al. Current status of Takayasu arteritis in India. Int J Cardiol 1996; 54(Suppl):S111–6.

61. Soares GM, Murphy TP, Singha MS, et al. Renal artery duplex ultrasonography as a screening and surveillance tool to detect renal artery stenosis: a comparison with current reference standard imaging. J Ultrasound Med 2006;25:293–8.

62. Crutchley TA, Pearce JD, Craven TE, et al. Clinical utility of the resistive index in atherosclerotic renovascular disease. J Vasc Surg 2009;49:148–55, 55.e1–3; [discussion: 55].

Ultrasonography of the Renal Transplant

Jessica G. Zarzour, MD[a],*, Mark E. Lockhart, MD, MPH[b]

KEYWORDS

- Renal transplant ultrasonography • Graft dysfunction • Renal artery stenosis
- Renal vein thrombosis • Arteriovenous fistulas • Pseudoaneurysms • Peritransplant fluid collections

KEY POINTS

- Signs of renal artery stenosis include color Doppler showing turbulent flow with aliasing at the site of stenosis, peak systolic velocity (PSV) greater than 2.5 m/s in the main renal artery, the ratio of the PSV in the main renal artery to the external iliac artery greater than 1.8, and segmental artery parvus-tardus waveform morphology.
- The differential diagnosis for reversed diastolic flow includes rejection, acute tubular necrosis, renal vein thrombosis, and extrarenal compression.
- Power Doppler should be used when evaluating for graft perfusion and segmental infarcts.
- Acute rejection, acute tubular necrosis, and drug toxicity are the most common causes of early graft failure and are indistinguishable by ultrasonography.
- The time of onset of peritransplant fluid collections can aid in their diagnosis. Hematomas and seromas most frequently occur in the first week. Urinomas occur 1 week to 1 month after transplantation. Lymphoceles and abscess are more common after 1 month.
- Renal transplant patients are at increased risk of developing malignancies, such as lymphoma, renal cell carcinoma, and lung cancer.

ULTRASOUND EXAMINATION OF THE RENAL TRANSPLANT

The routine examination of the transplanted kidney includes grayscale, color Doppler, and spectral Doppler images. Longitudinal and transverse grayscale images of the allograft are obtained to evaluate for peritransplant fluid collections, hydronephrosis, masses, and cortical thickness. Grayscale images of the urinary bladder are obtained. Color Doppler is used to evaluate the patency and flow direction of the main renal artery, at the anastomosis, renal vein, adjacent iliac artery and vein, and intrarenal arteries. Spectral Doppler images are used to measure the peak systolic velocity (PSV) at the arterial anastomosis, any region of aliasing in the main renal artery, and peak velocity in the iliac artery cranial to the anastomosis (**Fig. 1**).[1]

The Doppler resistive index (RI) (= [PSV – end diastolic velocity]/PSV) is a tool for quantifying the alterations in renal blood flow that may occur with renal disease.[1] Duplex images taken of the upper, mid, and lower poles of the kidney within the intrarenal arteries central to the junction of the cortex and medulla are performed routinely

Funding sources: none (Dr J. Zarzour); Deputy Editor, *Journal of Ultrasound in Medicine*, Member, Board of the American Institute of Ultrasound in Medicine, Member, American College of Radiology Commission on Ultrasound (Dr M.E. Lockhart).
Conflict of interest: none.
a Department of Radiology, University of Alabama at Birmingham, 619 19th Street South, JT N348, Birmingham, AL 35249-6830, USA; b Body Imaging, Department of Radiology, University of Alabama at Birmingham, 619 19th Street South, JT N348, Birmingham, AL 35249-6830, USA
* Corresponding author.
E-mail address: jgzarzour@uabmc.edu

ultrasound.theclinics.com

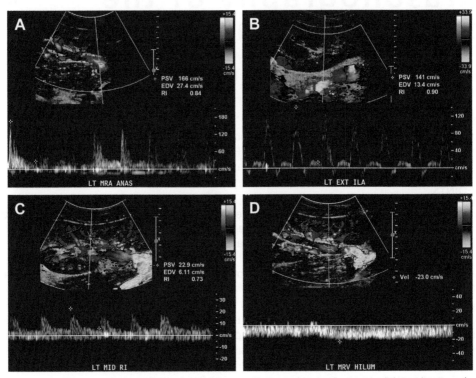

Fig. 1. Normal appearance of renal artery anastomosis without evidence of stenosis. (*A*) Duplex Doppler of the main renal artery shows laminar flow without aliasing and normal velocity lower than 250 cm/s on spectral analysis. (*B*) PSV of the external iliac artery is included to allow calculation of renal artery/iliac artery ratio lower than 1.8. (*C*) Indirect evaluation of the segmental artery shows no abnormal resistance or delayed systolic acceleration. Note that the early systolic peaks in this patient may not always be present even in a normal transplant. (*D*) Main renal vein has normal phasic flow.

for RI measurements.[2] An RI between 0.5 and 0.8 is considered to be within normal limits. Care must be taken to not compress the kidney when scanning the patient, because RI can be artificially increased if too much pressure is used.[3] Although resistive indices are useful in a binary fashion (normal vs abnormal), it is nonspecific in determining the underlying abnormality.

VASCULAR ABNORMALITIES

Vascular complications are uncommon after renal transplantation but are an important cause of early graft loss. A recent review of 1945 live related renal transplants showed vascular complications in 1.29% of patients, with renal artery stenosis representing the most common complication.[4] Although older studies reported a higher prevalence of stenosis, other more recent series have shown the incidence of renal artery stenosis to range from 1% to 3%.[5–8] Renal artery thrombosis is the least common, but most dreaded, vascular complication. Other vascular complications include infarct and renal vein thrombosis. After intervention of a renal allograft, arteriovenous fistula (AVF) and pseudoaneurysm (PSA) may occur.

ANATOMY

The transplanted allograft is routinely placed in the iliac fossa in the extraperitoneal pelvis, most commonly on the right. For cadaveric allografts, the main renal artery and Carrel patch are anastomosed to the recipient external iliac artery in an end to side anastomosis.[9] The Carrel patch is a small cuff of the donor aorta included to reduce the development of transplant renal artery stenosis. For living donor allografts, the main renal artery is most commonly anastomosed to the external iliac or common iliac artery in an end to side manner, but may be anastomosed to the internal iliac artery (hypogastric) in an end to end manner.[9,10] A prospective study[9] with half of the patients having an end to end anastomosis and half having end to side anastomosis showed no difference in graft survival or complications with a 2-year follow-up. In allografts with multiple renal arteries, each individual artery may be anastomosed to the external, internal, or common iliac arteries.[10] Alternatively, the 2 arteries may be anastomosed side to side (ex vivo), resulting in a common stem, which is then anastomosed to the recipient internal iliac artery using an end to end technique.[10,11] Multiple recent studies[12,13] have reported no significant difference in complications, survival, or rate of renal artery stenosis in patients who received kidneys with 1 or more than 1 renal arteries. The main renal vein is commonly anastomosed to the external iliac vein in an end to side anastomosis.

RENAL ARTERY STENOSIS

Renal artery stenosis most commonly presents as hypertension or allograft dysfunction. Renal artery stenosis most commonly occurs at the site of anastomosis. Donor artery stenosis results from intimal injury caused during organ retrieval or perfusion with localized ischemia leading to stricture. Recipient arterial stenosis may be caused by clamp injuries or atherosclerotic disease. Stenosis can be mimicked by kinking of the renal artery, most commonly when the right kidney is used (short renal vein and long renal artery). Renal artery stenosis is usually diagnosed between 3 and 12 months after transplantation.[14] Renal artery stenosis morphology at ultrasonography that is discovered greater than a year after transplant is often secondary to atherosclerosis in the recipient common iliac artery (pseudostenosis).[12,15]

Pseudostenosis has an equally negative effect on survival of the allograft as does renal artery stenosis and may be seen in almost half of the patients with findings suggestive of renal artery stenosis.[12] Risk factors for pseudostenosis include diabetes, age, weight, and panel reactive antibodies.[12]

Color Doppler can show turbulent flow with aliasing at the site of stenosis. This finding may be heard as a bruit on physical examination. Spectral Doppler evaluation suggests a hemodynamically significant stenosis when a PSV of greater than 250 cm/s is identified in the main renal artery or the ratio of the PSV in the main renal artery to the external iliac artery of greater than 1.8 (**Fig. 2**A, B).[16–18] One study of 106 patients[16] showed a 100% sensitivity and 95% specificity for diagnosis of renal artery stenosis when using a PSV of 250 cm/s as a threshold. There is no universally accepted PSV threshold as a criterion of the diagnosis of renal artery stenosis, and other centers use lower and higher thresholds.[19–21] However, the use of a lower PSV threshold less than 200 cm/s may lead to increased numbers of false-positive examinations and undermine referring physician confidence. Secondary signs of renal artery stenosis include delayed systolic

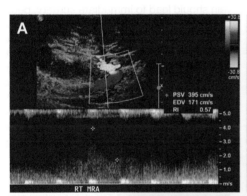
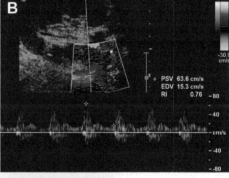
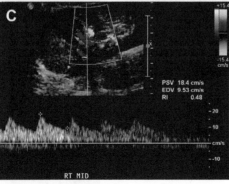

Fig. 2. Renal artery stenosis. (*A*) Duplex Doppler examination of the main renal artery shows color aliasing with a PSV of 395 cm/s. (*B*) There is a PSV 63.6 cm/s in the ipsilateral external iliac artery. This situation results in a main renal artery/external iliac artery ratio of 6.2, consistent with renal artery stenosis. (*C*) Indirect evaluation of the segmental renal artery shows delayed systolic acceleration with low RI.

acceleration, parvus-tardus waveforms, and decreased resistive indices within the intrarenal segmental arteries (see **Fig. 2**C). Caution is warranted in the use of sonographic velocity criteria in the perioperative period, because transient edema may simulate a fibrotic renal artery stricture. One study of 22 patients in the perioperative period[22] showed that all patients with an increased PSV immediately after transplantation surgery (and otherwise normal appearing graft) resolved to normal values during a follow-up period of 3 months. Another recent study of 128 patients[23] showed 57 patients (44.5%) to have severely increased PSV (>400 cm/s) in the immediate postoperative period, and only 3 of those patients had persistently increased PSV on follow-up. The increased PSV may spontaneously regress and normalize over time in these cases, so follow-up for the finding of increased PSV is advised.[22,24] If the allograft function is compromised soon after surgery, reexploration is sometimes considered. Other causes of increased PSV include vessel size mismatch and difficulty optimizing Doppler scanning technique.[24] Percutaneous transluminal angioplasty with stenting is the initial treatment of choice in cases of true renal artery stenosis beyond the perioperative period.[14]

RENAL ARTERY THROMBOSIS/INFARCT

Renal artery thrombosis can range from involvement of the main renal artery to occlusion of small subsegmental arteries. Complete thrombosis of the main renal artery is a devastating complication after renal transplantation, which usually leads to graft loss. On color Doppler, no parenchymal flow is visualized. Optimization of power Doppler has been shown to improve detection of areas of decreased blood flow when compared with color Doppler and should be used (**Fig. 3**).[25,26]

In areas of subsegmental infarcts, grayscale images show normal or increased echogenicity, and color Doppler shows decreased flow (**Fig. 4**).[27] Power Doppler should be used to increase sensitivity for small amounts of flow. Also, a recent study of 186 kidneys in the immediate postoperative setting[28] showed improved visualization of renal allograft parenchymal defects by using contrast-enhanced ultrasonography. The addition of contrast-enhanced ultrasonography allowed for clear visualization of segmental infarctions caused by occlusion of small arteries.[28]

RENAL VEIN THROMBOSIS

Direct visualization of the entire length of the renal vein is possible because of the superficial location

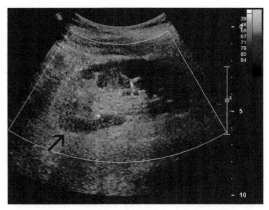

Fig. 3. Renal artery thrombosis. Power Doppler image in patient with renal failure perioperatively after transplantation shows no blood flow to the allograft (*arrows*), secondary to renal artery thrombosis.

of the transplant kidney. Renal vein thrombosis is rare and most often occurs in the first 2 weeks after transplantation. It is more prevalent in left iliac fossa transplants secondary to compression of the left common iliac vein between the right common iliac artery and the sacrum.[29] On grayscale images, the kidney may appear swollen and enlarged. Visualization of the thrombus in the renal vein should lead to immediate surgery, because of the high rate of allograft loss.[30] Indirect signs of renal vein thrombosis include reversal of diastolic flow in the renal vein (**Fig. 5**).[31] Visualization of reversed diastolic flow is not specific to renal vein thrombosis and is seen more commonly in acute rejection, acute tubular necrosis (ATN), and extrarenal compression.[18,30,32,33] Reversal of diastolic flow should be used in combination with identification of absent venous flow for diagnosis of renal vein thrombosis.

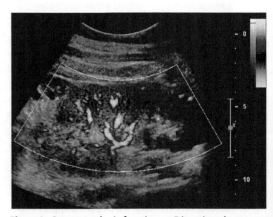

Fig. 4. Segmental infarction. Directional power Doppler image shows a segmental infarct with lack of flow at the lower pole of the transplanted kidney.

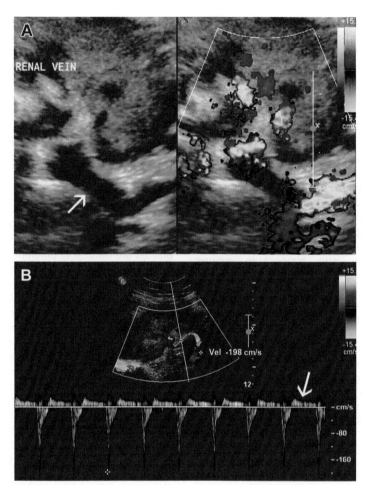

Fig. 5. Renal vein thrombosis. (*A*) Split screen image shows mildly echogenic material within the transplant renal vein (*arrow*) on grayscale portion. On the color Doppler portion, there is lack of flow in this same region. (*B*) Spectral Doppler evaluation of the transplant segmental artery shows reversal of diastolic flow (*arrow*).

VASCULAR ABNORMALITIES AFTER INTERVENTIONAL PROCEDURES
AVF

AVF occurs most commonly after percutaneous biopsy and has been reported to occur at an incidence of 16%.[34] Greater than 70% spontaneously regress.[35] However, large or persistent fistulas may cause hematuria, transplant dysfunction, vascular ischemia, and high-output heart failure caused by a steal phenomenon.[36,37] High flow rates within the fistula result in local tissue reverberation, seen as color encoding on Doppler images (**Fig. 6**).[38,39] In the area of reverberation, no hypoechoic pocket is visualized when color Doppler is turned off, which helps distinguish AVF from a PSA. Spectral Doppler images show low resistance flow (high proportion of diastolic flow relative to systole) caused by bypass of the glomerular resistance, and arterialization of the flow in the renal vein may be present.[38,39] Careful

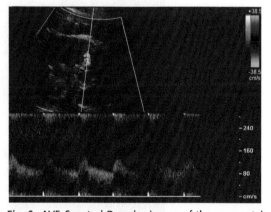

Fig. 6. AVF. Spectral Doppler image of the segmental renal artery shows turbulent high velocity and low resistive waveforms with tissue reverberation artifact in the cortex at the site of previous biopsy (Doppler gate).

examination of each segmental artery at the upper, mid, and lower (most commonly chosen region for biopsy) pole should be performed, because the low resistance flow may be limited to a single segmental artery.[40]

PSA

PSA may occur within the allograft after biopsy or other intervention. They may also occur in an extrarenal location such as at the arterial anastomosis or at site of perioperative infection.[41] Diagnosis is important, because PSAs are often clinically silent until they rupture. Rupture of an intrarenal PSA causes hematuria.[42] On ultrasonography, a PSA appears as a round or oval anechoic structure on grayscale images and may be heterogeneous with hypoechoic regions caused by intramural thrombus, but color Doppler images show their vascular nature.[41] The number of compartments (lobes) in the sac, the connection of the sac to the artery, and the length and width of the PSA neck should be assessed with grayscale ultrasonography.[43] Color Doppler establishes the diagnosis by showing the typical swirling motion (yin-yang sign) (**Fig. 7**).[43] The spectral Doppler to and fro waveform at the neck between the sac and the feeding artery may be difficult to visualize in the intrarenal PSA.[43]

COMPARTMENT SYNDROME

Retroperitoneal compartment syndrome is a rare transplant complication, with reported incidences ranging from 1.2% to 2%.[44,45] The increased intra-abdominal pressures result in organ dysfunction, leading to organ ischemia and severe allograft dysfunction, which leads to global infarction if left untreated. If recognized early, the kidney can be repositioned in the peritoneum to salvage the transplant.[45] The ultrasonographic findings of compartment syndrome are variable, reflecting the timing of the study and how compromised the arterial flow has become. There may be poor parenchymal flow, increased PSV, and parvustardus flow as signs of compartment syndrome, whereas others have reported absent or reversed diastolic flow.[44,45]

GRAFT DYSFUNCTION

Acute rejection, ATN, and drug toxicity are the most common causes of early graft failure. These entities are difficult to differentiate with ultrasonographic findings alone, and biopsy is often necessary. Grayscale ultrasonographic images are nonspecific but may show enlarged kidney with either decreased or increased cortical echogenicity (**Fig. 8**). Swelling of the pyramids resulting in loss of cortical/medullary differentiation or obliteration of the sinus echo complex may also be noted. However, the grayscale sonographic findings may be completely normal as well.

Resistive indices are often high (>0.80) in the setting of graft dysfunction, and are nonspecific in differentiating the cause of graft dysfunction.[1,46] There is a wide variation in sensitivity and specificity for detection of rejection. One study showed that sensitivity varied from 54% to 75% and specificity varied from 33% to 90%. There was initial hope that power Doppler would improve detection of rejection, but this was also shown to have wide variation in sensitivity and specificity.[47,48]

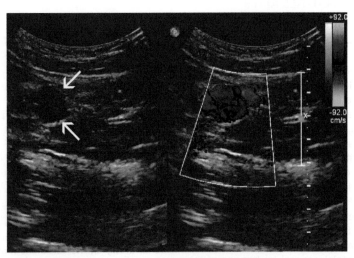

Fig. 7. PSA. On split screen image, grayscale portion shows a round anechoic structure (*arrows*) near the transplant hilum. Color Doppler portion shows circular flow of a PSA in this region within the renal allograft, described as the yin-yang sign.

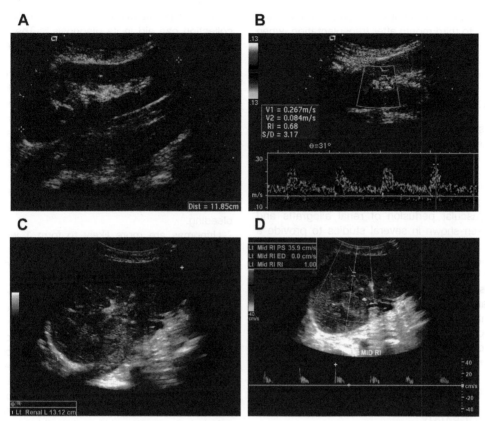

Fig. 8. Rejection. (*A*) Baseline grayscale of the transplant shows normal size and echotexture. (*B*) On baseline Doppler, there is normal waveform morphology, with RI 0.68. (*C*) During an episode of transplant dysfunction, the kidney appears echogenic and enlarged, measuring 13.1 cm. (*D*) Duplex Doppler during this episode shows that a high-resistance waveform, RI 1.0, is present within an interpolar segmental artery (Doppler gate).

Although data suggest that intrarenal RIs partial reflect the intrinsic state of the allograft, the RI is a reflection of the combination of central hemodynamics, the arterial wall compliance, pulsatility of flow, and peripheral resistance.[49–51] Increased RIs have been shown to be an independent marker of future graft loss, but are nonspecific for the cause of graft loss.[52] However, a more recent prospective study[51] evaluated the prognostic performance of RIs with regard to graft function and patient and allograft survival. In a follow-up period of 2 years, the RIs were found to be associated with central hemodynamic factors and recipient age, thus correlated with recipient survival but not with graft survival.

In hyperacute rejection, the allograft immediately fails at the vascular anastomosis and has to be removed. Acute rejection occurs in the few postoperative months, most commonly 1 to 3 weeks after surgery. Acute rejection is indistinguishable from ATN and drug toxicity by ultrasonography. The incidence of acute rejection ranges from 10% to 37%.[53] Ultrasonography may show graft edema, hypoechoic pyramids,

and prominence of the papilla.[54] Because of the interstitial swelling, resistive indices may increase and diastolic flow may even be reversed.[32]

Chronic rejection occurs in the months to years after the transplantation. Chronic rejection is caused by antibodies directed to the graft endothelium as a consequence of repeated episodes of acute rejection, which leads to progressive vascular compromise of the graft as well as extensive interstitial fibrosis.[55] Findings of chronic rejection include corticomedullary thinning, echogenic cortex, mild pelvocaliectasis, and increased RIs.[38]

ATN is caused by reversible ischemic damage to the renal tubular cells before engraftment. It is the most frequent complication in the first 48 hours after transplantation. Although the graft dysfunction may be severe, it is usually fully reversible and requires only supportive therapy. Risk factors for ATN include cadaveric allograft, hypotension in the donor before implantation, prolonged warm (> 30 minutes) and cold (> 24 hours) ischemic times.[56]

Cyclosporine toxicity results from the direct nephrotoxic effect of high serum levels of cyclosporine A. It most commonly occurs in the second to third month after transplantation, when drug doses are being titrated. Sonographic findings can include increased resistive indices but are nonspecific and often normal.[56,57]

CONTRAST-ENHANCED ULTRASONOGRAPHY

The usefulness of contrast-enhanced ultrasonography in differentiating causes of allograft dysfunction is still being investigated and has not yet been approved for routine clinical use in transplants in the United States. Contrast-enhanced ultrasonography provides quantitative information about the microvascular perfusion of renal allografts and has been shown in several studies to provide a diagnostic tool for determining the cause of graft dysfunction. Quantification of arterial inflow in the transplanted kidney using microbubbles has been shown to predict chronic allograft nephropathy earlier than color Doppler sonography.[58] Use of contrast-enhanced ultrasonography in the early postoperative period may be helpful in distinguishing acute rejection and ATN. A recent study showed that there is greater delay in the time of inflow to the cortex and renal pyramids in patients with acute rejection than in recipients with ATN.[59]

ELASTOGRAPHY

Elastography is another new tool in investigation of chronic allograft failure. Transient elastography devices were initially developed to assess liver stiffness and are now being used to assess renal allograft fibrosis. Although renal transplant biopsy is a common method of evaluating the interstitial fibrosis and tubular atrophy, it is invasive and has associated complications. Elastography based on ultrasonography has been described as a method to noninvasively assess renal allograft fibrosis.[60] In 1 methodology, elastography uses acoustic radiation force impulse (ARFI) quantification to measure graft stiffness. During imaging, the region of interest in the renal cortex is mechanically excited by short acoustic pulses to generate localized tissue displacement.[61] In more fibrotic tissue, displacement is attenuated.[61] ARFI has been found to positively correlate with the grade of fibrosis in kidney allografts.[62,63] Although preliminary results are encouraging, many factors must be considered, including area of region of interest, transducer pressure, incident angle, and depth of target.[61]

PERITRANSPLANT FLUID COLLECTIONS

Peritransplant fluid collections may include seroma, hematoma, urinoma, lymphocele, and abscess. The time of onset of a peritransplant fluid collection can aid in its diagnosis.[64] The clinical significance of the collection can vary depending on its size and location.

In the first week after transplantation, hematomas and seromas occur most commonly. The incidence of postoperative hematoma varies from 4% to 8%.[65] A hematoma may be subcapsular or perinephric. If it is subcapsular (**Fig. 9**), it is more likely to cause allograft dysfunction as a result of mass effect. Hematomas appear echogenic in the acute phase and become less echogenic over time as clot lysis occurs.[65] Hematomas usually spontaneously resolve, unless there is active bleeding.

Urinomas are more likely to form 1 week to 1 month after transplantation and usually show rapid growth (see further discussion of urinomas in urologic complication section).

Lymphoceles are more likely to occur after 1 month after surgery but can occur weeks to years after transplantation. Lymphoceles have a prevalence of 0.5% to 20%.[66] Risk factors for lymphoceles include inadequate ligation of the lymphatic channels across the iliac vessels, administration of heparin, and increased lymphatic flow secondary to edema of the lower extremities.[66] The most common location of a lymphocele is between the graft and the bladder. They often have loculations and septations (**Fig. 10**) and are the most common peritransplant fluid collection to cause hydronephrosis. Percutaneous drainage is usually required for treatment if the patient is symptomatic.

Bacterial seeding of a peritransplant collection can result in abscess formation. Abscess may also form as a complication of surgery or progression of pyelonephritis.

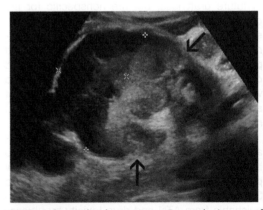

Fig. 9. Subcapsular hematoma. Grayscale image of transplanted kidney shows a subcapsular hematoma (*calipers*). Note the distortion of the adjacent renal cortex (*arrows*).

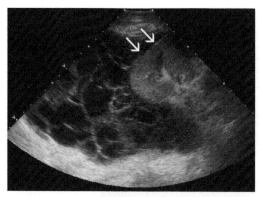

Fig. 10. Lymphocele. On grayscale image, there is a complex fluid collection containing loculations and septations encapsulating the adjacent kidney (*arrows*).

UROLOGIC COMPLICATIONS

The current prevalence of urologic complications ranges from 4% to 8%, with a low mortality.[66–68] Urologic complications include urine leak, obstruction, urolithiasis, and vesicoureteral reflux. The urinary tract is anastomosed either by an ureteroureterostomy or ureteroneocystostomy. The ureteroneocystostomy reconstructive technique is now favored, because it has been shown to have a lower incidence of urine leak or obstruction.[66–68] Urine leak and obstruction are normally discovered in the first month after transplantation.[68]

URINE LEAK AND URINOMAS

Extravasation of urine most often occurs at the ureteroneocystostomy.[69] Leak may also occur anywhere along the collecting system from arterial insufficiency, leading to necrosis. In the setting of obstruction and increased urinary pressures, calyceal rupture may result. Calyceal leakage may also occur at a site of previous segmental infarction.[66] On ultrasonography, urinoma appears as an anechoic structure and can vary widely in size. It typically has no septations and can rapidly increase in size. Large urinomas may result in urinary ascites.[66] Occasionally, urinomas can become infected and form abscesses. Urinomas are typically drained to reduce the risk of infection and extrinsic ureteral obstruction. The site of leak is typically managed by placing a ureteral stent.

OBSTRUCTION

Urinary obstruction occurs in approximately 2% of transplantations and almost always within the first 6 months.[68] Because the kidney is devascularized, the patient may not experience typical renal colic. Increased creatinine levels may be the only early sign. More commonly, dilatation of the transplant collecting system occurs secondary to reflux of urine from the urinary bladder, rather than mechanical obstruction. Mild to moderate pelvocaliectasis may even be normal in the transplanted kidney in the setting of a full bladder. If transplant hydronephrosis is discovered, the patient's bladder should be emptied, and then, repeated scan of the kidney should be performed.

If mechanical ureteral obstruction occurs, the most common site is a stricture at the ureterovesical anastomosis. Strictures occur in the distal third of the ureter greater than 90% of the time.[66,70] Strictures may form as a result of ureteral devascularization during graft manipulation, kinking, or errors in surgical technique.[66] Less common causes of obstruction include a peritransplant collection, pelvic fibrosis, fungal balls, stones, and clots.[66,69,70] Ultrasonography is used to confirm the diagnosis of hydronephrosis. However, the transplanted kidney may not show the expected hydronephrotic response because of intrarenal edema and fibrosis.[66]

STONES

Renal lithiasis is typically a late complication of renal transplants, with a reported incidence of less than 1%.[71,72] Stones may be gifted with the donated kidney or may form in the recipient after transplantation. Renal transplants are more prone to stone formation for a variety of reasons, including urinary stasis, recurrent urinary tract infections (especially with *Proteus mirabilis*), renal tubular acidosis, pH changes, nonabsorbable suture material that acts as a nidus, tertiary hyperparathyroidism, hypercalcemia, hyperuricosuria caused by calcineurin inhibitors, and hypercalciuria.[71] If the stone results in obstruction, ultrasonography is helpful to show hydronephrosis (**Fig. 11**). Occasionally, the stone may be directly identified in the

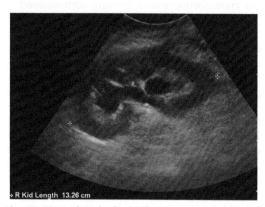

Fig. 11. Transplant hydronephrosis. Grayscale ultrasonography shows moderate pelvocaliectasis of the transplant graft with calyceal blunting.

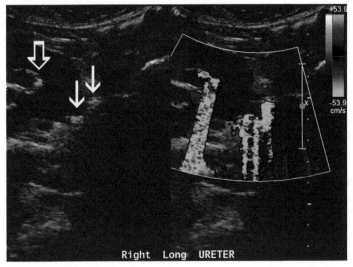

Fig. 12. Transplant ureteral calculus. On split screen, the grayscale shows echogenic foci adjacent to the allograft (*arrows*) and within the lower pole calyceal region (*open arrow*). The color Doppler portion shows twinkle artifact, highlighting the stones.

transplant ureter near its insertion into the urinary bladder. In the case of nonobstructing stones, ultrasonography is insensitive and computed tomography is advantageous. If ultrasonography is performed, use of color Doppler technique can assist in finding twinkle artifact, which may be suggestive of a stone (**Fig. 12**). However, a recent study[73] showed use of twinkle artifact to have a high false-positive rate (51%) when 5 mm unenhanced CT images were used as the reference standard. Another recent study[74] suggested the use of a lower color Doppler carrier frequency to improve the sensitivity for detection of renal calculi.

NEOPLASTIC COMPLICATIONS

Transplant outcomes have improved over time, but there continues to be morbidity as a result of the immunosuppressive therapy administered to prevent graft rejection. Studies[75] have shown a 2-fold to 4-fold increased risk of developing cancer in transplant recipients. The prevalence of malignancies caused by viral infections is particularly high, such as Hodgkin and non-Hodgkin lymphoma (Epstein-Barr virus), Kaposi sarcoma (human herpes virus 8), anogenital cancers (human papillomavirus), and liver cancer (hepatitis C and B viruses). In a recent data analysis of 175,732 solid organ transplants, 54.7% of the patients were kidney transplant recipients. There was a 6.05-fold risk of non-Hodgkin lymphoma, a 6.66-fold risk of renal cell carcinoma, and a 1.46-fold risk of lung cancer in renal transplant patients.[75]

Renal cell carcinoma can occur in the native or transplanted kidney (**Fig. 13**). It more commonly

occurs in the native kidney because of acquired renal cystic disease in patients who have previously been on hemodialysis.[76] Patients with a history of exposure to cyclophosphamide are also at increased risk of developing urothelial cancers. Although cyclophosphamide is not commonly used because of the availability of cyclosporine A, renal transplant patients may have a history of cyclophosphamide exposure.[77]

Posttransplantation lymphoproliferative disorder (PTLD) occurs because of an abnormal proliferation of T or B cells as a response to primary or reactivated Epstein-Barr virus. It can manifest as diffuse adenopathy or as an extranodal mass in solid organs (ie, liver, kidney, lungs, gastrointestinal tract, and central nervous system).[78,79] The

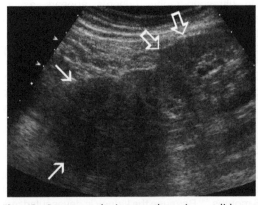

Fig. 13. On grayscale image, there is a solid mass (*arrows*) arising from the transplanted kidney (*open arrows*). The mass was subsequently proved to represent renal cell carcinoma.

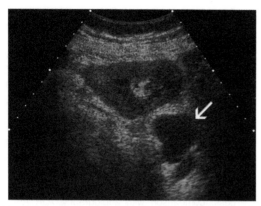

Fig. 14. Posttransplantation lymphoproliferative disease. On grayscale ultrasonography, a solid mass at the renal hilum (*arrow*) is detected between the transplant kidney and urinary bladder, later shown to represent PTLD.

most common site of involvement in renal transplant patients is at the hilum of the allograft **(Fig. 14)**.[80] Sonography is useful to measure the size of the hilar mass as the immunosuppression is adjusted. PTLD may also affect the parenchyma of the graft itself.

SUMMARY

Renal transplantation is a life-changing operation for patients with end-stage renal disease. Knowledge of complications that occur in the early postoperative stage as well as years after the transplant is important for short-term and long-term survival of the renal allograft. Ultrasonography is often the first-line imaging modality in evaluating transplant complications, and knowledge of the sonographic criteria can aid in successful diagnosis.

REFERENCES

1. Tublin ME, Bude RO, Platt JF. The resistive index in renal Doppler sonography: where do we stand? [review]. AJR Am J Roentgenol 2003;180(4):885–92.
2. Dighe M, Remer E, Casalino D, et al. ACR appropriateness criteria renal transplant dysfunction. 2012. Accessed February 21, 2014.
3. Krumme B. Renal Doppler sonography–update in clinical nephrology. Nephron Clin Pract 2006; 103(2):c24–8.
4. Srivastava A, Kumar J, Sharma S, et al. Vascular complication in live related renal transplant: an experience of 1945 cases. Indian J Urol 2013; 29(1):42–7.
5. Polak WG, Jezior D, Garcarek J, et al. Incidence and outcome of transplant renal artery stenosis: single center experience. Transplant Proc 2006; 38(1):131–2.
6. Patel NH, Jindal RM, Wilkin T, et al. Renal arterial stenosis in renal allografts: retrospective study of predisposing factors and outcome after percutaneous transluminal angioplasty. Radiology 2001; 219(3):663–7.
7. Salehipour M, Salahi H, Jalaeian H, et al. Vascular complications following 1500 consecutive living and cadaveric donor renal transplantations: a single center study. Saudi J Kidney Dis Transpl 2009;20(4):570–2.
8. Bruno S, Remuzzi G, Ruggenenti P. Transplant renal artery stenosis. J Am Soc Nephrol 2004; 15(1):134–41.
9. Matheus WE, Reis LO, Ferreira U, et al. Kidney transplant anastomosis: internal or external iliac artery? Urology 2009;6(4):260–6.
10. Ali-El-Dein B, Osman Y, Shokeir AA, et al. Multiple arteries in live donor renal transplantation: surgical aspects and outcomes. J Urol 2003;169(6):2013–7.
11. Novick AC. Microvascular reconstruction of complex branch renal artery disease. Urol Clin North Am 1984;11(3):465–75.
12. Saidi R, Kawai T, Kennealey P, et al. Living donor kidney transplantation with multiple arteries: recent increase in modern era of laparoscopic donor nephrectomy. Arch Surg 2009;144(5):472–5.
13. Rizzari MD, Suszynski TM, Gillingham KJ, et al. Outcome of living kidney donors left with multiple renal arteries. Clin Transplant 2012;26(1):E7–11.
14. Gang S, Rajapurkar M. Vascular complications following renal transplantation. J Nephrol Ren Transplant 2009;2(1):122–32.
15. Aslam S, Salifu MO, Ghali H, et al. Common iliac artery stenosis presenting as renal allograft dysfunction in two diabetic recipients. Transplantation 2001;71(6):814–7.
16. Baxter GM, Ireland H, Moss JG, et al. Colour Doppler ultrasound in renal transplant artery stenosis: which Doppler index? Clin Radiol 1995;50(9): 618–22.
17. de Morais RH, Muglia VF, Mamere AE, et al. Duplex Doppler sonography of transplant renal artery stenosis. J Clin Ultrasound 2003;31(3):135–41.
18. Baxter GM. Ultrasound of renal transplantation. Clin Radiol 2001;56(10):802–18.
19. Gottlieb RH, Lieberman JL, Pabico RC, et al. Diagnosis of renal artery stenosis in transplanted kidneys: value of Doppler waveform analysis of the intrarenal arteries. Am J Roentgenol 1995;165(6):1441–6.
20. Patel U, Khaw KK, Hughes NC. Doppler ultrasound for detection of renal transplant artery stenosis-threshold peak systolic velocity needs to be higher in a low-risk or surveillance population. Clin Radiol 2003;58(10):772–7.
21. Snider JF, Hunter DW, Moradian GP, et al. Transplant renal artery stenosis: evaluation with duplex sonography. Radiology 1989;172(3 Pt 2):1027–30.

22. Thalhammer C, Aschwanden M, Mayr M, et al. Duplex sonography after living donor kidney transplantation: new insights in the early postoperative phase. Ultraschall Med 2006;27(2):141–5.

23. Siskind E, Lombardi P, Blum M, et al. Significance of elevated transplant renal artery velocities in the postoperative renal transplant patient. Clin Transplant 2013;27(2):E157–60.

24. Brabrand K, Holdaas H, Gunther A, et al. Spontaneous regression of initially elevated peak systolic velocity in renal transplant artery. Transpl Int 2011;24(6):555–9.

25. Hamper UM, DeJong MR, Caskey CI, et al. Power Doppler imaging: clinical experience and correlation with color Doppler US and other imaging modalities. Radiographics 1997;17(2):499–513.

26. Albrecht T, Lotzof K, Hussain HK, et al. Power Doppler US of the normal prepubertal testis: does it live up to its promises? Radiology 1997;203(1):227–31.

27. Grenier N, Douws C, Morel D, et al. Detection of vascular complications in renal allografts with color Doppler flow imaging. Radiology 1991;178(1):217–23.

28. Grzelak P, Kurnatowska I, Nowicki M, et al. Perfusion disturbances of kidney graft parenchyma evaluated with contrast-enhanced ultrasonography in the immediate period following kidney transplantation. Nephron Clin Pract 2013;124(3–4):173–8.

29. Jordan ML, Cook GT, Cardella CJ. Ten years of experience with vascular complications in renal transplantation. J Urol 1982;128(4):689–92.

30. Saarinen O, Salmela K, Ahonen J, et al. Reversed diastolic blood flow at duplex Doppler. A sign of poor prognosis in renal transplants. Acta Radiol 1994;35(1):10–4.

31. Reuther G, Wanjura D, Bauer H. Acute renal vein thrombosis in renal allografts: detection with duplex Doppler US. Radiology 1989;170(2):557–8.

32. Lockhart ME, Wells CG, Morgan DE, et al. Reversed diastolic flow in the renal transplant: perioperative implications versus transplants older than 1 month. AJR Am J Roentgenol 2008;190(3):650–5.

33. Warshauer DM, Taylor KJ, Bia MJ, et al. Unusual causes of increased vascular impedance in renal transplants: duplex Doppler evaluation. Radiology 1988;169(2):367–70.

34. Diaz-Buxo JA, Kopen DF, Donadio JV Jr. Renal allograft arteriovenous fistula following percutaneous biopsy. J Urol 1974;112(5):577–80.

35. Benoit G, Charpentier B, Roche A, et al. Arteriocalyceal fistula after grafted kidney biopsy. Successful management by selective catheter embolization. Urology 1984;24(5):487–90.

36. Laberge JM. Interventional management of renal transplant arteriovenous fistula. Semin Intervent Radiol 2004;21(4):239–46.

37. Rajiah P, Lim YY, Taylor P. Renal transplant imaging and complications. Abdom Imaging 2006;31(6):735–46.

38. Brown ED, Chen MY, Wolfman NT, et al. Complications of renal transplantation: evaluation with US and radionuclide imaging. Radiographics 2000;20(3):607–22.

39. Middleton WD, Kellman GM, Melson GL, et al. Postbiopsy renal transplant arteriovenous fistulas: color Doppler US characteristics. Radiology 1989;171(1):253–7.

40. Middleton WD, Picus DD, Marx MV, et al. Color Doppler sonography of hemodialysis vascular access: comparison with angiography. AJR Am J Roentgenol 1989;152(3):633–9.

41. Renigers SA, Spigos DG. Pseudoaneurysm of the arterial anastomosis in a renal transplant. AJR Am J Roentgenol 1978;131(3):525–6.

42. Low G, Crockett AM, Leung K, et al. Imaging of vascular complications and their consequences following transplantation in the abdomen. Radiographics 2013;33(3):633–52.

43. Saad NE, Saad WE, Davies MG, et al. Pseudoaneurysms and the role of minimally invasive techniques in their management. Radiographics 2005;25(Suppl 1):S173–89.

44. Ball CG, Kirkpatrick AW, Yilmaz S, et al. Renal allograft compartment syndrome: an underappreciated postoperative complication. Am J Surg 2006;191(5):619–24.

45. Horrow MM, Parsikia A, Zaki R, et al. Immediate postoperative sonography of renal transplants: vascular findings and outcomes. AJR Am J Roentgenol 2013;201(3):W479–86.

46. Rifkin MD, Needleman L, Pasto ME, et al. Evaluation of renal transplant rejection by duplex Doppler examination: value of the resistive index. AJR Am J Roentgenol 1987;148(4):759–62.

47. Datta R, Sandhu M, Saxena AK, et al. Role of duplex Doppler and power Doppler sonography in transplanted kidneys with acute renal parenchymal dysfunction. Australas Radiol 2005;49(1):15–20.

48. Rigsby CM, Burns PN, Weltin GG, et al. Doppler signal quantitation in renal allografts: comparison in normal and rejecting transplants, with pathologic correlation. Radiology 1987;162(1 Pt 1):39–42.

49. Bude RO, Rubin JM. Relationship between the resistive index and vascular compliance and resistance. Radiology 1999;211(2):411–7.

50. Kolonko A, Szotowska M, Kuczera P, et al. Extrarenal factors influencing resistance index in stable kidney transplant recipients. Transplantation 2013;96(4):406–12.

51. Naesens M, Heylen L, Lerut E, et al. Intrarenal resistive index after renal transplantation. N Engl J Med 2013;369(19):1797–806.

52. Radermacher J, Mengel M, Ellis S, et al. The renal arterial resistance index and renal allograft survival. N Engl J Med 2003;349(2):115–24.

53. Irshad A, Ackerman S, Sosnouski D, et al. A review of sonographic evaluation of renal transplant complications. Curr Probl Diagn Radiol 2008; 37(2):67–79.

54. Venz S, Kahl A, Hierholzer J, et al. Contribution of color and power Doppler sonography to the differential diagnosis of acute and chronic rejection, and tacrolimus nephrotoxicity in renal allografts. Transpl Int 1999;12(2):127–34.

55. Ozkan F, Yavuz YC, Inci MF, et al. Interobserver variability of ultrasound elastography in transplant kidneys: correlations with clinical-Doppler parameters. Ultrasound Med Biol 2013;39(1):4–9.

56. Zwirewich C. Renal transplant imaging and intervention: practical aspects. Vancouver Hospital & Health Sciences Center 2007;1–27.

57. Buckley AR, Cooperberg PL, Reeve CE, et al. The distinction between acute renal transplant rejection and cyclosporine nephrotoxicity: value of duplex sonography. AJR Am J Roentgenol 1987;149(3): 521–5.

58. Schwenger V, Hinkel UP, Nahm AM, et al. Real-time contrast-enhanced sonography in renal transplant recipients. Clin Transplant 2006;20(Suppl 17):51–4.

59. Grzelak P, Szymczyk K, Strzelczyk J, et al. Perfusion of kidney graft pyramids and cortex in contrast-enhanced ultrasonography in the determination of the cause of delayed graft function. Ann Transplant 2011;16(1):48–53.

60. Sommerer C, Scharf M, Seitz C, et al. Assessment of renal allograft fibrosis by transient elastography. Transpl Int 2013;26(5):545–51.

61. He WY, Jin YJ, Wang WP, et al. Tissue elasticity quantification by acoustic radiation force impulse for the assessment of renal allograft function. Ultrasound Med Biol 2014;40(2):322–9.

62. Stock KF, Klein BS, Vo Cong MT, et al. ARFI-based tissue elasticity quantification in comparison to histology for the diagnosis of renal transplant fibrosis. Clin Hemorheol Microcirc 2010;46(2-3):139–48.

63. Syversveen T, Brabrand K, Midtvedt K, et al. Assessment of renal allograft fibrosis by acoustic radiation force impulse quantification–a pilot study. Transpl Int 2011;24(1):100–5.

64. Silver TM, Campbell D, Wicks JD, et al. Peritransplant fluid collections. Ultrasound evaluation and clinical significance. Radiology 1981;138(1):145–51.

65. Dimitroulis D, Bokos J, Zavos G, et al. Vascular complications in renal transplantation: a single-center experience in 1367 renal transplantations and review of the literature. Transplant Proc 2009; 41(5):1609–14.

66. Akbar SA, Jafri SZ, Amendola MA, et al. Complications of renal transplantation. Radiographics 2005; 25(5):1335–56.

67. Gogus C, Yaman O, Soygur T, et al. Urological complications in renal transplantation: long-term follow-up of the Woodruff ureteroneocystostomy procedure in 433 patients. Urol Int 2002;69(2):99–101.

68. Kocak T, Nane I, Ander H, et al. Urological and surgical complications in 362 consecutive living related donor kidney transplantations. Urol Int 2004;72(3):252–6.

69. Duty BD, Conlin MJ, Fuchs EF, et al. The current role of endourologic management of renal transplantation complications. Adv Urol 2013;2013: 246520.

70. Mundy AR, Podesta ML, Bewick M, et al. The urological complications of 1000 renal transplants. Br J Urol 1981;53(5):397–402.

71. Stravodimos KG, Adamis S, Tyritzis S, et al. Renal transplant lithiasis: analysis of our series and review of the literature. J Endourol 2012;26(1):38–44.

72. Capocasale E, Busi N, Mazzoni MP, et al. Donor graft lithiasis in kidney transplantation. Transplant Proc 2002;34(4):1191–2.

73. Dillman JR, Kappil M, Weadock WJ, et al. Sonographic twinkling artifact for renal calculus detection: correlation with CT. Radiology 2011;259(3):911–6.

74. Gao J, Hentel K, Rubin JM. Correlation between twinkling artifact and color Doppler carrier frequency: preliminary observations in renal calculi. Ultrasound Med Biol 2012;38(9):1534–9.

75. Engels EA, Pfeiffer RM, Fraumeni JF Jr, et al. Spectrum of cancer risk among US solid organ transplant recipients. JAMA 2011;306(17):1891–901.

76. Bretan PN Jr, Busch MP, Hricak H, et al. Chronic renal failure: a significant risk factor in the development of acquired renal cysts and renal cell carcinoma. Case reports and review of the literature. Cancer 1986;57(9):1871–9.

77. Levine LA, Richie JP. Urological complications of cyclophosphamide. J Urol 1989;141(5):1063–9.

78. Hanto DW, Gajl-Peczalska KJ, Frizzera G, et al. Epstein-Barr virus (EBV) induced polyclonal and monoclonal B-cell lymphoproliferative diseases occurring after renal transplantation. Clinical, pathologic, and virologic findings and implications for therapy. Ann Surg 1983;198(3):356–69.

79. Sola-Valls N, Rodriguez CN, Arcal C, et al. Primary brain lymphomas after kidney transplantation: an under-recognized problem? J Nephrol 2014;27(1): 95–102.

80. Lopez-Ben R, Smith JK, Kew CE 2nd, et al. Focal posttransplantation lymphoproliferative disorder at the renal allograft hilum. AJR Am J Roentgenol 2000;175(5):1417–22.

Sonography of the Retroperitoneum

Barton F. Lane, MD*, Jade J. Wong-You-Cheong, MD

KEYWORDS

- Ultrasonography • Retroperitoneum • Abdominal imaging • Adrenal glands • Pancreas

KEY POINTS

- As a readily available, inexpensive, and non–radiation-producing imaging modality, ultrasonography is an important tool for the initial evaluation of the retroperitoneum.
- It is important to understand the sonographic appearance of normal retroperitoneal anatomy and structures, to avoid false-positive diagnosis of disease.
- Ultrasonography plays a complementary role to computed tomography and magnetic resonance imaging in characterizing the origin and location of retroperitoneal masses and fluid collections.
- There is significant overlap in the ultrasonographic appearance of retroperitoneal disease, and definitive diagnosis is often not possible solely with ultrasonography.

ANATOMY OF THE RETROPERITONEUM

The retroperitoneum is in the posterior abdomen, separated from the peritoneal cavity by the following structures:

- Anteriorly: posterior parietal peritoneal fascia
- Posteriorly: transversalis fascia
- Laterally: lateral conal fascia

Along the lateral flanks extending anteriorly, the retroperitoneum is continuous with the properitoneal fat. The retroperitoneal space extends from the level of the diaphragms superiorly to the pelvic brim inferiorly. Below this point, it is continuous with the extraperitoneal space of the pelvis.[1]

The retroperitoneum is divided into 3 compartments (**Fig. 1, Table 1**). A fourth compartment, the retrofascial space, lies in the midline posterior to the retroperitoneum and contains the psoas and quadratus lumborum muscles and is surrounded by its own fascia, although often these structures are included in the retroperitoneum.

The superior borders of the perirenal space may not be intact in some individuals, in which case fluid can potentially track from the perirenal space into the subdiaphragmatic space on the left or the bare area of the liver on the right.[2,3]

The great vessels are frequently included in discussions of the retroperitoneum; however, they may lie within a separate fascial plane between the medial borders of the bilateral posterior pararenal spaces.[4] The great vessels are addressed in the article on ultrasonographic assessment of the aorta and mesenteric arteries by Drs Pellerito and Revzin elsewhere in this issue.

SCANNING TECHNIQUE

Imaging should be obtained with a curved or vector transducer at the highest available frequency, typically up to 5 MHz in adults. Tissue penetration is a limiting factor at higher frequencies; however, technological advances on newer scanners allow for high-resolution imaging at up to 9 MHz without

The authors have nothing to disclose.
Department of Diagnostic Radiology and Nuclear Medicine, University of Maryland School of Medicine, 22 South Greene Street, Baltimore, MD 21201, USA
* Corresponding author.
E-mail address: blane@umm.edu

ultrasound.theclinics.com

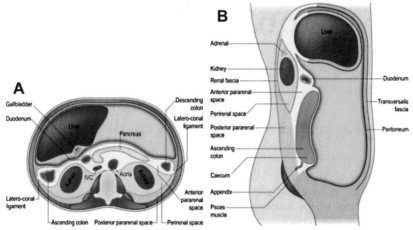

Fig. 1. The retroperitoneal spaces. Diagrammatic sections through the kidneys ([A] transverse, [B] parasagittal) to show the perirenal and pararenal spaces and the lateroconal ligaments. (*Adapted from* Meyer MA. Dynamic radiology of the abdomen. Normal and pathologic anatomy. 3rd edition. New York: Springer-Verlag; 2000.)

loss of penetration. Enabling tissue harmonics and compound imaging can increase image quality.[5,6] For large masses, extended field of view scans may be helpful.

Patient fasting before the ultrasonographic examination may be helpful and should be encouraged but is not necessarily required. Imaging is obtained traditionally in the longitudinal and transverse planes, with the patient in the supine position, with additional left or right posterolateral positions sometimes helpful to visualize the great vessels and retrofascial structures. This procedure can be aided by imaging in an oblique coronal plane to obtain greater portions of the great vessels and psoas muscles, iliac arteries, and renal arteries, as well as delineating retroperitoneal lymph nodes.[7,8]

Oral contrast agents are available and can improve visualization of the stomach, duodenum, and pancreas but are not widely used.[9,10] Intravascular microbubble contrast agents are not approved for use in the United States for imaging of the abdomen and are not further discussed in this review.

To improve the detection and localization of retroperitoneal lesions, a standardized approach is beneficial (**Box 1**).

NORMAL STRUCTURES VISIBLE WITH ULTRASONOGRAPHY

On the right side, the liver and kidney act as acoustic windows, allowing for visualization of deeper structures and the great vessels. Imaging the left

Table 1
Contents and borders of the retroperitoneal spaces

	Contents	Borders
Anterior pararenal space	Pancreas Duodenum (second– fourth segments) Ascending colon Descending colon	Anterior: posterior parietal peritoneum Posterior: anterior perirenal (Gerota) fascia Lateral: fusion of the lateral conal fascia and parietal peritoneum Inferior: communicates with the posterior pararenal space
Perirenal space	Adrenal glands Kidneys Ureters	Anterior/posterior/lateral: perirenal (Gerota) fascia Superior: layers fuse and attach to diaphragm Inferior: layers fuse
Posterior pararenal space	No organs Fat	Anterior: posterior perirenal fascia Posterior: transversalis fascia Lateral: communicates with properitoneal space Inferior: communicates with pelvic extraperitoneal space, anterior pararenal space

---

Box 1
Diagnostic algorithm for ultrasonographic evaluation of retroperitoneal lesions

1. Confirm that the finding is real. Mimics of tumors include true lesions (such as fluid collections) and pseudolesions (such as hypoechoic fat or aperistaltic bowel) **(Fig. 2)**. It is important to scan in 2 orthogonal planes, with cine clips if possible.

2. Assess internal structure. Does the mass contain air or calcium? Is it solid or cystic? What is the internal vascularity?

3. Determine origin.

   a. Is the organ retroperitoneal in location? Clues include anterior displacement of the kidneys, pancreas, great vessels, or ascending or descending colon. On the right side, adrenal tumors displace the right upper quadrant retroperitoneal fat reflection anteriorly, which can help distinguish them from masses originating from the liver.[11]

   b. Does the mass arise from or involve one of the organs of the retroperitoneum? Assess for the beak sign or embedded organ sign **(Fig. 3)**.[12]

4. Which retroperitoneal compartment contains the mass? This factor can be difficult to assess with ultrasonography, and may be better determined with computed tomography (CT) or magnetic resonance (MR) imaging.

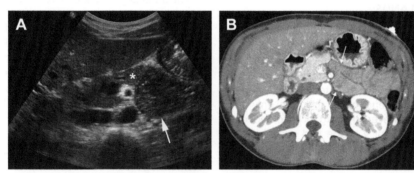

Fig. 2. Pseudolesion. Transverse ultrasonography (*A*) through the upper abdomen in a young woman with right upper quadrant pain. A hypoechoic, nonperistalsing mass (*arrow*) is noted adjacent to the stomach and abutting the pancreatic body (*asterisk*), concerning for a pancreatic mass. Contrast-enhanced CT (*B*) obtained for further evaluation fails to identify a mass but shows loops of jejunum (*arrows*), corresponding to the ultrasonography finding.

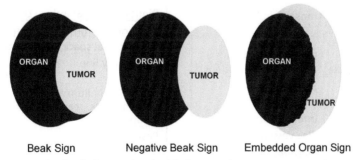

Beak Sign   Negative Beak Sign   Embedded Organ Sign

Fig. 3. The beak sign, negative beak sign, and embedded organ sign. An organ creating acute angles around a tumor (the beak sign) suggests that the tumor arises from that organ. Obtuse angles between the organ and tumor (the negative beak sign) occur when the tumor compresses but does not arise from the organ. When an organ appears embedded within a tumor (the embedded organ sign), this is also a sign that the tumor likely arises from that organ. In this situation, the interface between the tumor and organ is often irregular.

side can be more challenging, because the spleen provides a smaller acoustic window than the liver. The presence of gas within the descending colon and small bowel in the left upper abdomen can further impede acoustic penetration. Visualization of the retroperitoneal structures is more likely with favorable conditions, such as in thinner patients and when there is minimal bowel gas (**Table 2**).

The diaphragmatic crura provide anatomic landmarks superiorly. The right crus is larger and more lobular than the left and is more often visible.[13] The crura appear as hypoechoic linear structures surrounded by echogenic fat and fibrous tissue (**Fig. 4**). It is important not to confuse the crura with pathologic structures.

The aorta, iliac vessels, psoas, kidneys, and inferior vena cava (IVC) serve as useful anatomic landmarks. If the imager becomes lost during the course of a scan, these structures are easily identified for the purpose of becoming reoriented.

ADRENAL GLANDS
Anatomy and Imaging Techniques

Visualization of the normal adrenal glands in adults is challenging, because of their small size and location anterior and medial to the kidneys, which requires imaging via an intercostal approach (**Table 3**). The adrenal gland tissue is only 2 to 6 mm thick; however, the organ is folded over into an inverted Y or V shape and overall is 2 to 3 cm wide and 3 to 6 cm long. The right adrenal gland is positioned slightly more caudal than the left and is more often visible. The normal right adrenal gland can be visualized in up to 92% of patients, and the left in up to 71%, with a high frequency transducer, although in routine clinical practice, they are identified with less frequency.[14,15]

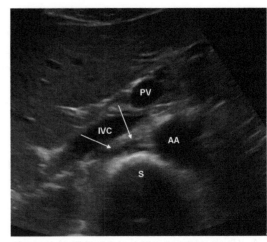

Fig. 4. Transverse ultrasonography through the epigastrium. A segment of the right crus (*arrows*) is visible as a hypoechoic linear structure anterior to the spine (S) and between the abdominal aorta (AA) and inferior vena cava (IVC). PV, portal vein.

The adrenal glands are more readily visualized in neonates, secondary to their proportionally large size (up to one-third renal size at birth), the small amount of perirenal fat, and the small size of the patient, allowing for higher-frequency (and thus higher-resolution) imaging. The gland is hypoechoic relative to the surrounding fat, and rarely, the central medulla may be visible as a thin echogenic line (**Fig. 5**).[15]

Hemorrhage

Hemorrhage can be secondary to a variety of causes, with trauma being most common. Hemorrhage is typically associated with other injuries of the thorax, abdomen, or retroperitoneum and is generally diagnosed with CT (**Fig. 6**).[16] Other

Table 2
Structures visible with transabdominal ultrasonography

Nearly Always Visible	Potentially Visible (Favorable Conditions)
Pancreas (head and body)	Adrenal glands
Kidneys	Inferior aorta
Duodenum	Iliac vessels
Psoas (abdominal portion)	Iliopsoas muscle
Great vessels (aorta and IVC)	Quadratus lumborum muscle
Diaphragmatic crura	Lymph nodes

Table 3
Scanning for the adrenal glands

Right Adrenal Gland	Left Adrenal Gland
Right 9th or 10th intercostal space	Left 8th or 9th intercostal space
Midaxillary line	Posterior to midaxillary line
Using renal hilum as a landmark, scan superiorly	Use upper pole of kidney as landmark, scan anteriorly
Posterior to IVC, superior to the kidney, and adjacent to the right crus	Between kidney, spleen, and left crus

Data from Dewbury K, Rutherford EE. Adrenals. In: Allan PL, Baxter GM, Weston MJ, editors. Clinical ultrasound. 3rd edition. Churchill Livingstone Elsevier: 2011. p. 632–42.

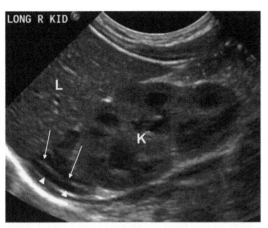

Fig. 5. Longitudinal right upper quadrant ultrasonography in a 1-day-old neonate. One limb of the right adrenal gland is clearly visible superior to the kidney (K) and posterior to the liver (L). The central echogenic medulla (*arrows*) is clearly distinct from the hypoechoic cortex (*arrowheads*).

Box 2
Ultrasonographic features of hematoma

- Acute phase: anechoic
- Subacute phase: echogenic, equal to adjacent fat or organs (eg, kidney)
- Internal septations secondary to retracting clots
- Internal echogenic masslike lesions and debris, secondary to retracting clots; the appearance can overlap that of an abscess
- Lack of internal Doppler signal
- Change in appearance or decrease in size on subsequent scans
- Chronic: resolution, residual cyst, or calcification

---

causes include hyperplasia as a result of adrenocorticotrophic hormone (ACTH) therapy or severe stress, sepsis, and anticoagulation therapy. Surgical disruption of the adrenal vein has also been reported as a cause, associated with orthotopic liver transplant.[17] The ultrasonographic appearance is variable (**Box 2, Fig. 7**).

Cysts

Adrenal cysts are rare, usually asymptomatic, benign, and incidentally discovered. They tend to occur more frequently in females and are usually unilateral. Approximately half are endothelial in origin, either lymphangiomas or angiomas. Pseudocysts related to hemorrhage, either spontaneous or related to a tumor, are the next most common, with epithelial and parasitic (echinococcal) being less common.[18] The imaging appearance is typical as with any cyst, with a thin wall, anechoic interior, and increased through transmission. Calcification of the wall is occasionally present, as are internal echogenic foci.

Adrenal tumors
There are several benign and malignant adrenal tumors that a sonographer can expect to encounter during their career. However, there is considerable overlap in the ultrasonographic appearance of these lesions, and a definitive diagnosis is often not possible with ultrasonographic features alone (**Tables 4** and **5**). Ultrasonographic findings in conjunction with the patient's clinical information (including history of malignancy, serum electrolytes, and serum/urine hormonal assays) may enable a reasonable differential diagnosis and guide

A 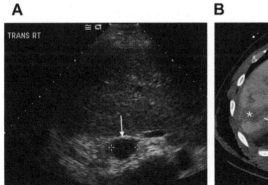 **B**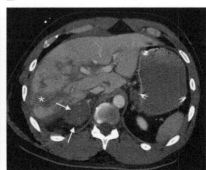

Fig. 6. Adrenal hematoma. Transverse ultrasonography through the right upper quadrant (*A*) shows a hypoechoic suprarenal lesion (*white arrow*) in a patient who sustained a motor vehicle collision. No internal color flow is shown. Corresponding contrast-enhanced CT (*B*) shows the right adrenal hematoma (*white arrows*). Linear hypoenhancement in the liver (*asterisk*) denotes an associated hepatic laceration.

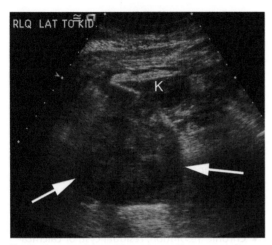

Fig. 7. Retroperitoneal hematoma. Transverse ultrasonography through the right flank. A mixed echogenicity collection (*arrows*) displaces the right kidney (K) anteriorly.

additional imaging or biopsy. Adrenal mass size is used in the triage of indeterminate adrenal masses; lesions greater than 4 to 6 cm in patients who have no known malignancy are resected, because the risk of malignancy is increased.[19,20]

Adrenal tumors: benign

Adenoma Adenomas are usually nonfunctioning and incidentally discovered on CT imaging, rarely on ultrasonography, unless large. Hyperfunctioning adenomas may give rise to symptoms, most commonly Cushing syndrome (excessive cortisol secretion) or Conn disease (excessive aldosterone secretion). Cushing syndrome most commonly results from adrenal hyperplasia but can result from an adenoma and, less commonly, carcinoma. When secondary to hyperplasia resulting from excessive pituitary ACTH production, it is termed Cushing disease. Conn disease similarly results from hyperplasia more often than from an adenoma, with carcinoma a rare cause. CT and MR imaging are the standard for diagnosis (**Fig. 8**).

Myelolipoma Myelolipomas are nonfunctioning tumors consisting of fat and bone marrow elements, arising from the cortex of the adrenal gland. They are usually discovered incidentally but can cause symptoms if large or in the setting of internal hemorrhage. Extra-adrenal myelolipomas are rarely encountered.[21] CT or MR imaging are diagnostic for showing the presence of fat, which in an adrenal mass is nearly pathognomonic for myelolipoma (**Fig. 9**).

Pheochromocytoma Adrenal pheochromocytomas are hyperfunctioning tumors arising from the adrenal medulla that secrete norepinephrine and epinephrine. This catecholamine secretion leads to the typical symptoms of hypertension, headache, palpitations, and excessive perspiration. There are many associated disorders, including multiple endocrine neoplasia (MEN) IIa and IIb, neurofibromatosis, and von Hippel-Lindau disease.

Table 4
Typical ultrasonographic appearance of benign adrenal tumors

	Typical Appearance	Clinical	Differential Diagnosis

Adenoma	<5 cm
	Solid
	Well-circumscribed
	Small
	Homogenous
		3% of adults
		Usually asymptomatic
		Cushing syndrome or
		  Conn disease if
		  hyperfunctioning
			Metastasis
			Pheochromocytoma
			Hemorrhage

Myelolipoma	<5 cm
	Echogenic if
	  predominantly fat
	Isoechoic or hypoechoic
	  if predominantly
	  myeloid components
	May have hemorrhage
	  or calcifications
		Fifth–sixth decades
		Usually asymptomatic
		Symptoms if
		  hemorrhage or large
		  (mass effect)
			Fat-containing lesions
			Lipoma
			Liposarcoma
			Lymphangioma
			Teratoma

Pheochromocytoma	>4 cm
	Well-encapsulated
	Homogeneous if solid
	Heterogeneous if
	  hemorrhage and
	  necrosis
	May have calcifications
		Fourth–sixth decades
		Catecholamine
		  secretion
		10% bilateral
		10% malignant
		Associations: MEN, von
		  Hippel-Lindau
			Metastasis
			Hemorrhage
			Adenoma

Table 5
Typical ultrasonographic appearance of malignant adrenal tumors

	Typical Appearance	Clinical	Differential Diagnosis
Metastasis	Homogeneous if small Can be heterogeneous if larger Rarely calcify	Correlate with history of malignancy	Adenoma Pheochromocytoma Hemorrhage
Adrenal cortical carcinoma	Homogeneous if small Heterogeneous if large: hemorrhage, necrosis, calcification Vascular invasion: Doppler is helpful Well-delineated borders Echogenic capsule in some	~50% are hyperfunctioning (smaller tumors) Larger tumors tend to be nonfunctioning	Metastasis Pheochromocytoma Neuroblastoma Hemorrhage
Neuroblastoma Ganglioneuroblastoma	Heterogeneous with coarse calcifications Irregular contour Ill-defined borders Invasion of adjacent organs Encasement of vessels	Children: 80% in <5 y Second most common abdominal tumor of childhood Two-thirds occur in the abdomen: adrenal gland most common location	Wilms tumor Hemorrhage Adrenal cortical carcinoma

The diagnosis can be made biochemically by ascertaining the levels of urinary catecholamines and metabolites. Imaging serves to determine the location (adrenal vs extra-adrenal) and whether bilateral lesions are present. Although CT and MR imaging are typically requested to evaluate for the presence of pheochromocytoma, large masses may be detected by ultrasonography (**Fig. 10**).[22]

Uncommon adrenal tumors
- Hemangioma
- Ganglioneuroma
- Teratoma
- Lipoma
- Leiomyoma
- Fibroma
- Neurofibroma
- Osteoma

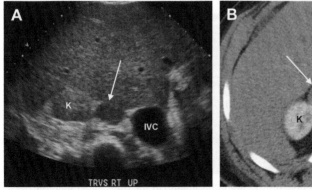

Fig. 8. (A) Transverse ultrasonography through the right upper quadrant. A nonspecific solid homogeneous mass (*arrow*) is noted lateral posterior to the liver, between the upper pole of the right kidney (K) and the IVC. Corresponding contrast-enhanced CT (B) shows a hypodense adrenal mass (*arrow*), with attenuation values confirming this to be an adenoma.

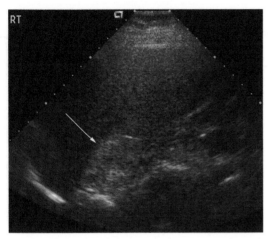

Fig. 9. Transverse ultrasonographic image through the right upper quadrant shows an echogenic liver consistent with steatosis, and an echogenic right adrenal mass (*arrow*). This mass was confirmed to contain fat on CT, consistent with a myelolipoma.

Adrenal tumors: malignant

Metastases The adrenal glands are the fourth most common site of metastases after the lung, liver, and bones. The most common primary tumors are lung, breast, renal, colon, and melanoma. Non-Hodgkin lymphoma can also involve the adrenal glands. Because benign adrenal adenomas are common, even in a patient with a known primary malignancy, the likelihood of a lesion being benign remains high.

In a patient with known extra-adrenal malignancy, the distinction of a metastasis from adenoma cannot be reliably made with ultrasonography, particularly when small. However, an irregular border favors metastasis, as does size greater than 3 cm.[23] CT or MR imaging can reliably characterize most adenomas (**Fig. 11**).

Adrenal cortical carcinoma Adrenal cortical carcinomas are rare aggressive malignant tumors, which can arise from any of the layers of the adrenal cortex. Approximately half are hyperfunctioning, which can present as Cushing disease, adrenogenital syndrome, or precocious puberty. They range in size at presentation but are often large, particularly if nonfunctioning. Adrenal cortical carcinoma is aggressive and is one of the tumors that directly invades the vasculature; invasion of the adrenal vein, IVC, and even the right atrium can be present at diagnosis. Doppler ultrasonography is helpful in evaluating for intravascular involvement.[24]

Neuroblastoma and ganglioneuroblastoma These malignant tumors are found almost exclusively in children. Neuroblastoma is second only to Wilms tumor as the most common abdominal tumor in childhood. Neuroblastomas can be nonfunctioning or secrete catecholamines. Most have metastasized by the time of diagnosis, usually to the bone marrow, lymph nodes, liver, and skin (**Fig. 12**).

Ganglioneuroblastomas contain elements of both benign ganglioma and neuroblastoma. Ganglioneuroblastomas are less aggressive than neuroblastomas, with a more favorable prognosis. As with neuroblastoma, they are rare in adults. The imaging appearance depends on the degree of differentiation; they can range from solid to predominantly cystic.[25]

PANCREAS
Anatomy and Imaging Techniques

The major role of sonography is to evaluate pancreatitis or malignancy.[26] Contrast-enhanced CT is the initial modality of choice if there is a high clinical suspicion of pancreatic disease, with

A   **B**

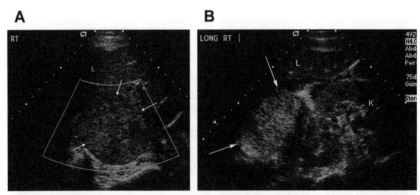

Fig. 10. (*A*) Transverse and (*B*) longitudinal ultrasonographic images in the right upper quadrant of a 25-year-old woman with headaches and hypertensive crisis. A large, circumscribed mass is noted posterior to the liver (L) and superior to the right kidney (K). Minimal internal vascularity is evident with color Doppler (*arrows*). The lack of significant internal flow suggests internal hemorrhage. Blood and urine analysis were consistent with pheochromocytoma.

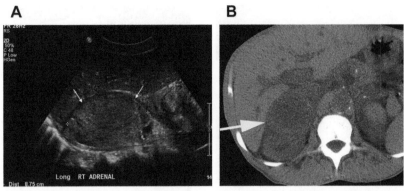

Fig. 11. (*A*) Transverse ultrasonography through the right upper quadrant in a man with non–small cell lung cancer. There is a large solid right adrenal mass (*white arrows*). (*B*) Corresponding CT without contrast (secondary to renal insufficiency) confirms the mixed attenuation right adrenal metastasis (*arrow*).

ultrasonography typically used to detect gallstones or bile duct stones as potential causes of pancreatitis.

Imaging can be facilitated by the patient's fasting before the examination. Water or oral contrast can improve imaging of the tail.[9] Continual graded transducer pressure aids in collapsing bowel loops and the gastric antrum and can improve visualization during the course of the examination, although this may be limited by focal tenderness.[27] The normal pancreas should be homogeneous and isoechoic to, or greater in echogenicity than, the liver (**Fig. 13, Table 6**). The presence of hepatic steatosis may alter this relationship.

Acute Pancreatitis

Acute pancreatitis is diagnosed by clinical presentation, laboratory abnormalities, and imaging characteristics. Imaging is usually accomplished with contrast-enhanced CT, which can readily show the extent of pancreatic and peripancreatic inflammation, as well as the complications of necrosis, fluid collections, splenic vein thrombosis, and pancreatic ductal dilatation. Ultrasonography is limited in evaluating the pancreas in the acute inflammatory phase (**Figs. 14** and **15, Table 7**). The pancreas may appear normal; alternatively, focal enlargement of the gland or peripancreatic inflammation can mimic a mass. Fluid collections can develop in the early (1st week) and late (weeks to months) phases.

Chronic Pancreatitis

Repeated occurrences of mild or subclinical pancreatitis lead to progressive destruction of the gland, resulting in chronic pancreatitis. With alcoholic pancreatitis, there is increased protein secretion into the ducts, with development of ductal obstruction and intraductal calcifications. There is fibrous proliferation around the pancreatic

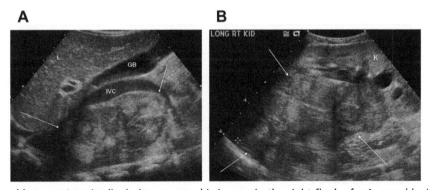

Fig. 12. Neuroblastoma. Longitudinal ultrasonographic images in the right flank of a 4-year-old with palpable abdominal mass, show a heterogeneous, mixed echogenicity mass (*arrows*) posterior and lateral to the liver and IVC (*A*). The adrenal gland is not identified, and the mass (*arrows*) is inseparable from the right kidney (*B*). At surgery, the mass entirely encompassed the adrenal gland, and invaded the right kidney. GB, gallbladder; K, kidney; L, liver.

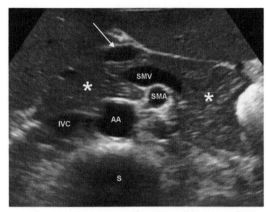

Fig. 13. Normal pancreas. Transverse ultrasonographic image through the upper abdomen in a 54-year-old man. The pancreatic parenchyma (*asterisks*) appears isoechoic to the liver. Typical structures visible at this level are the spine (S), abdominal aorta (AA), superior mesenteric artery (SMA), superior mesenteric vein (SMV), and the IVC. The gastroduodenal artery (*arrow*) can also occasionally be visualized along the anterior margin of the head/neck, as in this patient.

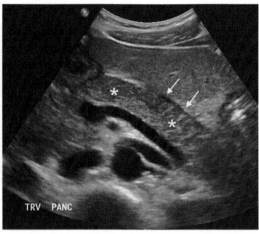

Fig. 14. Acute pancreatitis. Transverse ultrasonography through the upper abdomen in a patient with abdominal pain, and increased amylase and lipase levels. The pancreas (*asterisks*) is enlarged and hypoechoic relative to the left lobe of the liver, visible anteriorly. Peripancreatic linear hypoechoic fluid is present anterior to the pancreatic body (*arrows*).

ducts and within the parenchyma, leading to a lobular appearance of the gland (**Table 8**). As with acute pancreatitis, ultrasonography is not sensitive for diagnosing chronic pancreatitis; however, the presence of ductal and parenchymal calcification is highly suggestive (**Fig. 16**). A normal ultrasonogram does not exclude this clinical diagnosis.

Pseudocyst

Pseudocysts are walled-off collections of pancreatic fluid that develop after pancreatitis. They develop over time as pancreatic fluid, containing amylase and lipase, leaks from the pancreatic

duct, and develops a fibrous capsule, organizing into a well-circumscribed fluid collection (**Fig. 17**, **Table 9**). This process typically occurs within 4 weeks after the initial episode of pancreatitis.

According to the revised Atlanta classification system of acute pancreatitis, the term pseudocyst is reserved for those collections occurring greater than 4 weeks after the initial onset of pancreatitis, without internal debris or nonliquefied material.

As would be expected, pseudocysts most frequently occur in the anterior pararenal space, although they can spread to and develop in remote sites in the abdomen. Sonographically, they appear as anechoic collections with increased through transmission. The presence of gas should

---

Table 6
Anatomic landmarks and structures of the pancreas

Segment	Anatomic Landmarks	Visible Anatomy
Head	Most caudal Anterior to IVC Inferior to PV	GDA anteriorly CBD posteriorly PD may be visible
Uncinate	Extends inferior, posterior, and medial from head Posterior to mesenteric vessels	If present, a replaced RHA may be visible arising from the right margin of the SMA
Neck	Anterior to SMV/PV	
Body/tail	Lateral to the SMV/PV No anatomic distinction between body/tail	PD usually visible SV visible along posterior margin

Abbreviations: CBD, common bile duct; GDA, gastroduodenal artery; PD, pancreatic duct; PV, portal vein; RHA, right hepatic artery; SMA, superior mesenteric artery; SMV, superior mesenteric vein; SV, splenic vein.

A B

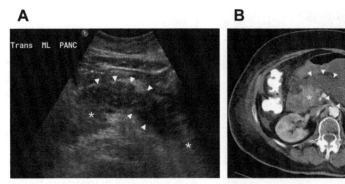

Fig. 15. Necrotizing pancreatitis. (*A*) Transverse ultrasonography through the upper abdomen in a patient with acute pancreatitis shows a markedly hypoechoic pancreatic body (*arrowheads*), with normal echogenicity pancreatic parenchyma in the head and tail (*asterisks*). (*B*) Contrast-enhanced CT scan at approximately the same level shows pancreatic necrosis (*arrowheads*) involving the body, corresponding to the hypoechoic region on ultrasonography, with sparing of the head and tail (*asterisks*).

raise concern for infection. Because pseudocysts are often large and can traverse multiple retroperitoneal spaces, CT is most useful in evaluating the full extent (**Fig. 18**). Ultrasonography is helpful in guiding percutaneous aspiration and drainage catheter placement.

Autoimmune Pancreatitis

Autoimmune pancreatitis (AIP) is a variant of chronic pancreatitis, which is recognized with increasing frequency. There is an association with other autoimmune conditions, most commonly sclerosing cholangiopathy. Others include retroperitoneal fibrosis, interstitial pneumonitis, sialadenitis, thyroiditis, and interstitial nephritis.

The diagnosis is made by a combination of the imaging features (**Table 10**), in conjunction with increased serum γ-globulin or IgG levels or pancreatic histology showing fibrosis and infiltration with lymphocytes and plasmacytes.[28]

Pancreatic tumors

Adenocarcinoma is the most common tumor of the pancreas, accounting for up to 90% of pancreatic neoplasms. Cystic neoplasms and neuroendocrine (islet cell) tumors comprise nearly all of the remaining lesions (**Table 11**). Lymphoma and metastatic lesions rarely involve the pancreas.[29]

Adenocarcinoma

Although a rare malignancy, pancreatic adenocarcinoma is the fourth leading cause of death from cancer in the United States. Less than 20% are resectable at the time of diagnosis. Even if operable, if the resected margins remain positive, the prognosis is similar to nonoperative management. Median survival is 10 to 12 months for locally

Table 7
Ultrasonographic appearance of acute pancreatitis

Pancreatic Findings	Peripancreatic Findings
Decreased echogenicity	Linear hypoechoic or anechoic regions
Poor delineation of the anterior margin	Thrombosis of splenic or portal vein
Enlargement: should be <23 mm anteroposterior diameter anterior to the superior mesenteric vein	Splenic artery pseudoaneurysm Fluid collection

Data from Tchelepi H, Ralls PW. Ultrasound of acute pancreatitis. Ultrasound Clin 2007;2:415–22.

Table 8
Ultrasonographic findings in chronic pancreatitis

Finding	Significance
Lobular and heterogeneous	~50%; secondary to fibrosis and atrophy
Focal enlargement	~40% of cases; can mimic a mass
Ductal dilatation	May mimic obstruction from tumor or biliary stone
Echogenic foci	~40%; secondary to calcifications and fibrosis
Intraductal calcifications	Highly specific for pancreatitis; rare in tumors
Pseudocyst	May require drainage if large or infected

Data from Alpern MB, Sandler MA, Kellman GM, et al. Chronic pancreatitis: ultrasonic features. Radiology 1985;155:215–9.

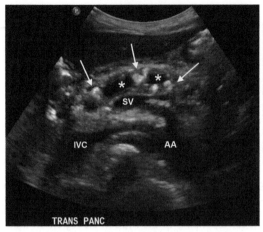

Fig. 16. Transverse ultrasonography through the epigastrium in a patient with chronic pancreatitis. Multiple calcifications (*arrows*) are seen in the pancreatic head and within the dilated pancreatic duct (*asterisks*). AA, abdominal aorta; SV, splenic vein.

advanced disease, 4 to 6 months in the setting of metastatic disease.

Adenocarcinoma most commonly arises in the head of the pancreas, with symptoms related to bile duct obstruction (**Fig. 19**). Tumors arising in the body and tail do not cause early symptoms and therefore tend to be larger and more advanced at diagnosis. From these lesions, symptoms result either from metastatic disease or local invasion into the gastrointestinal tract. Contrast-enhanced CT is the modality of choice; however, ultrasonography has been reported to be from

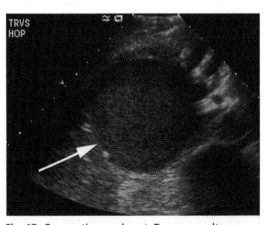

Fig. 17. Pancreatic pseudocyst. Transverse ultrasonography through the head of pancreas in a patient with chronic pancreatitis, showing a unilocular cyst with internal debris (*arrow*). Color Doppler (not shown) confirms the absence of internal vascularity. In conjunction with the clinical history, this finding helps distinguish this cyst from a cystic neoplasm.

Table 9 Fluid collections in pancreatitis		
Type of Pancreatitis	**<4 wk from Onset**	**>4 wk from Onset**
Interstitial edematous pancreatitis	Acute peripancreatic fluid collection	Pancreatic pseudocyst
Necrotizing pancreatitis	Acute necrotic collection	Walled-off necrosis

Data from Thoeni RF. The revised Atlanta classification of acute pancreatitis: its importance for the radiologist and its effect on treatment. Radiology 2012;262:751–64.

72% to 98% sensitive and up to 90% specific for tumor detection (**Fig. 20**).[30]

Cystic Neoplasms

Cystic neoplasms represent 10% to 15% of pancreatic tumors and include serous cystadenoma, mucinous cystic neoplasm, intraductal papillary mucinous neoplasm (IPMN), and less commonly, solid papillary mucinous neoplasm. Serous cystadenomas are benign and can be managed conservatively when classic imaging findings are present (**Table 12**). Mucinous cystadenomas, as malignant or premalignant neoplasms, require surgical resection. Ultrasonographic findings can assist in distinguishing these 2 entities; however, CT or MR imaging is typically necessary for accurate classification (**Fig. 21**).

IPMN is a benign or low-grade malignant lesion, which arises from ductal epithelium of either the main pancreatic duct, side branch, or both. Evidence of the ductal communication is diagnostic but generally not possible with ultrasonography; MR cholangiopancreatography or endoscopic retrograde cholangiopancreatography is necessary. Main-branch type IPMN are typically resected; side-branch type are typically managed conservatively if they are less than 3 cm in size and without solid components.

Solid pseudopapillary neoplasm is a rare low-grade malignant tumor occurring almost exclusively in young women (**Fig. 22**). Patient demographics and typical imaging findings assist in the diagnosis. These patients have a favorable prognosis after resection.[31]

Neuroendocrine Tumors

Arising from the pancreatic islet cells, approximately 85% are functioning, with secretion of a variety of hormones. Insulinomas are the most common, followed by gastrinomas. These tumors arise both sporadically as well as in association

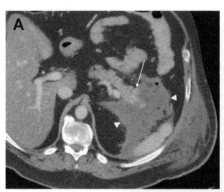
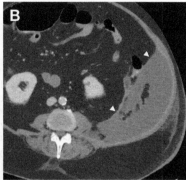
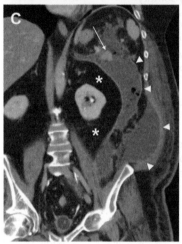

Fig. 18. (*A, B*) Axial and (*C*) coronal contrast-enhanced CT images in a patient with acute pancreatitis and disruption of the distal pancreatic duct. A loculated pseudocyst (*arrowheads*) surrounds the pancreatic tail (*arrows*), extends inferiorly from the anterior pararenal space into the posterior pararenal space of the left flank, but spares the perirenal space (*asterisks*). Note the well-delineated fascial borders of the perirenal space.

with MEN syndrome. Glucagonoma, vipoma, somatostatinoma, and carcinoid make up the remainder of islet cell tumors. Most are clinically apparent as a result of the hormone secretion and are therefore small when evaluated with imaging. Transabdominal ultrasonography is limited in sensitivity.

Retroperitoneal Tumors (Extraorgan)

Most retroperitoneal tumors arise from the solid organs, namely the kidneys, adrenal glands, and pancreas. Of the tumors not arising from the solid organs, most are of mesenchymal origin, and most are malignant (**Table 13**). In addition, lymphadenopathy can involve the retroperitoneal spaces.

Lesions are generally divided into 5 main categories:

- Primary retroperitoneal tumors
- Secondary tumors
- Fluid collections
- Infection
- Pseudolesions

Definitive diagnosis of retroperitoneal masses is often not possible with ultrasonographic imaging alone, and the distinction between benign

Table 10
Ultrasonographic appearance of AIP

Finding	Significance
Focal or diffuse enlargement	May mimic a pancreatic tumor
Narrowed pancreatic duct	Helps distinguish from obstructing tumor, chronic pancreatitis
Lack of calcifications	Helps distinguish from other chronic pancreatitis
Lack of fluid collections	Helps distinguish from other acute and chronic pancreatitis

Table 11
Solid tumors of the pancreas

	Typical Appearance	Clinical

Adenocarcinoma	Usually head of pancreas
	Hypoechoic, poorly defined mass
	Pancreatic duct and common bile duct,
	  dilatation, double duct sign
	Parenchymal atrophy
	Margins may be obscured if the pancreas is
	  low in echogenicity
		Seventh decade and older
		Rare before fifth decade
		Jaundice
		Weight loss
		Pain if large

Neuroendocrine tumor: insulinoma (60%)	Usually body and tail Usually solitary Round, most <2 cm Hypoechoic Well-defined	Fourth–sixth decades Hypoglycemic symptoms 90% benign

Neuroendocrine tumor:
  gastrinoma (20%)
	Usually multiple
	15% extrapancreatic: duodenum
	Small
		Mean age 50 y
		Gastric acid and peptic ulcers,
		  Zollinger-Ellison syndrome
		≤60% are malignant

and malignant lesions is rarely possible. However, important diagnostic clues can be obtained by using a standard diagnostic approach (see **Box 1**).

Primary neoplasms; malignant
Primary tumors of the retroperitoneum are uncommon, accounting for less than 0.2% of all malignancies.[32] Approximately 70% to 90% are malignant.[33] By definition, these tumors arise within the retroperitoneal spaces, without (at least initially) attachment to the retroperitoneal organs. They frequently lack early presenting symptoms

and are discovered only when they have reached considerable size. Abdominal pain is the most frequent presenting symptom.

Although CT and MR imaging are typically better able to show the overall size and extent of tumors, ultrasonography can sometimes provide a better evaluation of invasion of local tissues. The sonographic imaging features are variable and have considerable overlap between tumor types (**Table 14**).

An important clinical consideration is the extent of invasion of adjacent organs of the abdominal wall, which can have surgical implications and

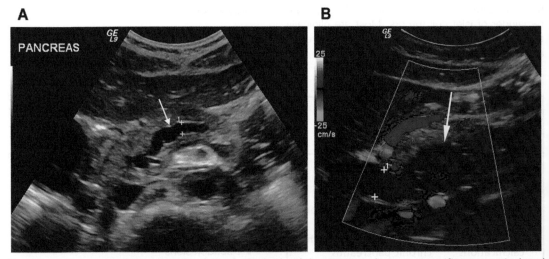

Fig. 19. (*A*) Transverse ultrasonography through the body of the pancreas shows nonspecific pancreatic ductal dilatation (*arrow, calipers*). (*B*) Imaging inferiorly through the pancreatic head shows a hypoechoic mass (*arrow*) as the cause of obstruction. In addition, the common bile duct is dilated (*calipers*); along with the dilated pancreatic duct, this is the double duct sign. Endoscopic biopsy confirmed pancreatic adenocarcinoma.

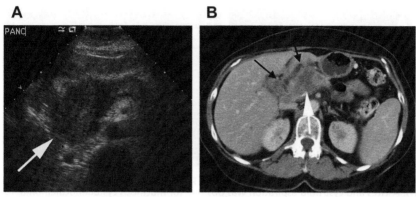

Fig. 20. (*A*) Transverse ultrasonography through the epigastrium shows a hypoechoic, lobular mass (*arrow*) enlarging and replacing the pancreatic head. (*B*) Corresponding contrast-enhanced CT demonstrates the poorly defined, hypoenhancing mass (*white arrow*). CT is better for staging; note the peripancreatic infiltration (*black arrows*). Endoscopic biopsy confirmed pancreatic adenocarcinoma.

portend a worse prognosis. It is also important to assess the internal vascularity, not only for surgical planning but also to guide potential percutaneous ultrasound-guided biopsy of nonnecrotic areas (**Fig. 23**).

Liposarcoma

Liposarcoma is the most common primary retroperitoneal neoplasm. There are 3 histologic subtypes: well-differentiated, myxoid and round-cell, and pleomorphic; and more than 1 subtype may be present within the same tumor.[34] The most common subtype is well-differentiated.

Well-differentiated liposarcomas are slow growing and typically large at diagnosis, with presenting symptoms secondary to compression of adjacent structures.[32] Well-differentiated tumors do not metastasize but frequently recur locally after resection. Dedifferentiation of the tumor

Table 12
Cystic neoplasms of the pancreas

	Typical Appearance	Clinical
Serous cystadenoma (previously microcystic adenoma)	Usually head of pancreas Tiny cysts <20 mm Central scar in 15%: echogenic, calcifications Thin septations, radiate from central scar	≥Sixth decade Strong female predominance Benign
Mucinous cystadenoma (previously macrocystic adenoma)	Usually body and tail of pancreas Larger cysts >20 mm, less numerous than in serous cystadenoma Thick walls Occasional peripheral calcification Papillary projections	Fourth–sixth decade Female predominance Premalignant/malignant
IPMN	Dilatation of main pancreatic duct or side branches Occasional cyst formation Papillary projections indicate dysplasia	Seventh decade Slight male predominance Premalignant
Solid pseudopapillary neoplasm	Usually head of pancreas Solid and cystic components Encapsulated (rare in other pancreatic tumors) Internal hemorrhage (rare in other pancreatic tumors)	Second–fourth decades Strong female predominance Low malignant potential

Data from Martínez-Noguera A, D'Onofrio M. Ultrasonography of the pancreas. 1. Conventional imaging. Abdom Imaging 2006;32:136–49; and Sohn TA, Yeo CJ, Cameron JL, et al. Intraductal papillary mucinous neoplasms of the pancreas: an updated experience. Ann Surg 2004;239:788–97.

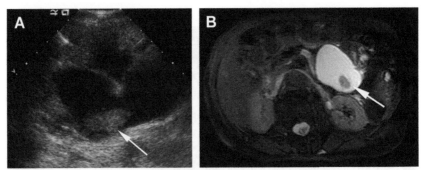

Fig. 21. (*A*) Transverse ultrasonography through the tail of pancreas shows a bilobed cystic structure with a mural nodule (*arrow*). Ascites and cyst fluid aspiration was positive for mucinous cystadenocarcinoma. (*B*) Corresponding axial fat-suppressed T2-weighted MR imaging confirms the hypointense mural nodule (*arrow*) within the cystic mass.

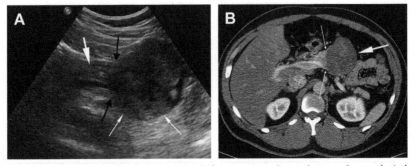

Fig. 22. (*A*) Transverse ultrasonographic image in the left upper quadrant shows a hypoechoic heterogeneous mass (*thin arrows*), abutting the distal pancreatic body (*large arrow*). The beak sign is present (*black arrows*), suggesting a pancreatic origin. (*B*) Corresponding contrast-enhanced CT scan confirms the origin of the mass (*large arrow*) from the distal pancreas. The beak sign is again shown (*thin arrows*). Pathology at surgery confirmed a solid pseudopapillary pancreatic tumor.

Table 13
Primary retroperitoneal tumors

	Malignant	Benign
Mesenchymal	Liposarcoma Leiomyosarcoma Pleomorphic undifferentiated sarcoma Rhabdomyosarcoma Fibrosarcoma	Lipoma Leiomyoma Rhabdomyoma Fibroma
Neurogenic	Neuroblastoma Ganglioneuroblastoma Paraganglioma Malignant nerve sheath tumor	Ganglioneuroma Paraganglioneuroma Neurofibroma
Vascular	Angiosarcoma Lymphangiosarcoma Hemangiopericytoma	Lymphangioma Hemangioma
Germ cell	Malignant teratoma Embryonal carcinoma	Mature teratoma

Table 14
Ultrasonographic appearance of the most common malignant primary retroperitoneal tumors

Malignant Tumors	Typical Appearance	Clinical
Liposarcoma	Well-differentiated: may not be visible Poorly differentiated: solid components, rare calcification	Sixth–eighth decades
Leiomyosarcoma	Large Hemorrhage Cystic change: necrosis Calcification uncommon Vascular invasion, especially IVC	Fifth–sixth decades Female predominance

Undifferentiated
  pleomorphic
  sarcoma
	Large
	Hemorrhage
	Cystic change: necrosis
	Calcification in 20%
		Sixth–seventh decades
		Male predominance

imparts metastatic potential. On imaging, this tumor can be evident as internal heterogeneity, with increased solid components with poor delineation from fat components, and occasionally, calcifications. These findings are more readily apparent on CT or MR imaging and may not be evident sonographically.

Leiomyosarcoma

Leiomyosarcoma is the second most common primary retroperitoneal neoplasm and arises from smooth muscle, blood vessel wall, or Wolffian duct remnants.[35] The 3 major growth patterns are extrinsic to the vasculature (62%), mixed intravascular and extravascular (33%) (**Fig. 24**), and entirely intravascular (5%). The rare intravascular-only tumors tend to arise within the IVC between the diaphragm and renal veins.

Undifferentiated Pleomorphic Sarcoma

Previously referred to as malignant fibrous histiocytoma, undifferentiated pleomorphic sarcoma (or pleomorphic undifferentiated sarcoma) is the third most common primary retroperitoneal malignancy, but overall, it is the most common soft tissue sarcoma.

Primary neoplasms: benign

As outlined earlier, it is more likely that a discovered primary retroperitoneal mass is malignant than benign. However, it should not be assumed that all lesions are malignant until full characterization with imaging and potential biopsy has been completed. Ultrasonographic features of the most common benign retroperitoneal tumors are listed in **Table 15**.

Lipoma/Lipomatosis

Lipomatosis is the overgrowth of mature unencapsulated fat cells. Symptoms, if present, are generally vague and may be secondary to mass effect on adjacent structures such as the ureters or iliac veins. It is more common in males than in females. On CT or MR imaging, lipomatosis is shown by

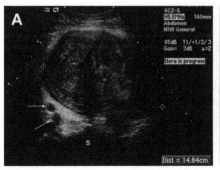
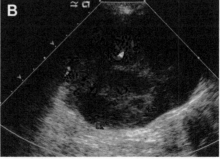

Fig. 23. (*A*) Transverse ultrasonography through the pelvis in a 55-year-old man with a pelvic mass shows a heterogeneous, mixed echogenicity mass anterior to the spine (S), displacing the right iliac vessels (*arrows*). (*B*) Color Doppler image obtained immediately before percutaneous biopsy shows internal vascularity, localizing a nonnecrotic site for biopsy, which confirmed high-grade leiomyosarcoma.

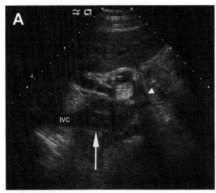 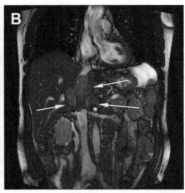

Fig. 24. (*A*) Longitudinal ultrasonography through the right upper abdomen shows a heterogeneous mass (*arrow*) expanding the lumen of the IVC, extending anteriorly and contiguous with an upper retroperitoneal mass (*arrowhead*). (*B*) Corresponding true fast imaging with steady state precession (balanced sequence) MR imaging confirms the lobular tumor in the IVC (*arrows*). Vascular invasion is consistent with the diagnosis of leiomyosarcoma.

excess fat, usually in the pelvis, with separation and crowding of other anatomic structures. Other than a few thin fibrous strands, there is no soft tissue or masslike component. Ultrasonography is unlikely to establish the diagnosis.

Retroperitoneal Fibrosis

There is a long list of potential causes of retroperitoneal fibrosis, but in approximately 70% of cases, the cause is idiopathic. Associations include:

- Drugs (most frequently methysergide)
- Inflammatory disorders
- Malignancy
- Autoimmune; retroperitoneal fibrosis is occasionally associated with Riedel thyroiditis, sclerosing cholangitis, fibrotic pseudotumor of the orbit, and AIP

Table 15
Ultrasonographic appearance of the most common benign primary retroperitoneal tumors

Benign Tumors	Typical Appearance	Clinical
Lipoma/lipomatosis	Likely not visible	
Retroperitoneal fibrosis	Homogeneous Smoothly marginated Hypoechoic or anechoic Surrounds aorta and proximal iliac vessels	Fifth–seventh decades Male predominance
Angiomyolipoma	Homogeneous if small Echogenic: a fat-containing mass arising from the kidney is nearly pathognomonic If large internal vessels, aneurysm, and hemorrhage, may distinguish from liposarcoma	Nearly always renal in origin Extra-adrenal rare
Teratoma	Mixed solid and cystic spaces Echogenic fat Calcification in >50% ~80% have a soft tissue nodule Rokitansky nodule or Dermoid plug: echogenic with posterior shadowing Left suprarenal space (adult teratoma)	Most common <6 mo of age Second peak early adulthood
Paraganglioma	>4 cm Well-encapsulated Homogeneous if solid Heterogeneous if hemorrhage and necrosis May have calcifications	Fourth–sixth decades Catecholamine secretion

Data from Lepor H, Walsh PC. Idiopathic retroperitoneal fibrosis. J Urol 1979;122:1–6.

Retroperitoneal fibrosis can mimic a soft tissue mass or adenopathy. Pathologically, it consists of fibrous plaquelike tissue, which proliferates around the aorta, IVC, iliac arteries, and ureters. In the early stages, it may be asymptomatic, but as the fibrosis progresses, symptoms develop secondary to the compressive effects. These symptoms include:

- Pain
- Lower extremity edema
- Hydronephrosis
- Testicular swelling

Ultrasonography is insensitive in detecting retroperitoneal fibrosis; the diagnosis is typically made with CT. Sonographically, the appearance is nonspecific, with plaquelike soft tissue typically surrounding the aorta and vena cava (**Fig. 25**). The findings overlap with malignancy and lymphoma, which tend to be more nodular.[36] Ultrasonography can be useful in providing imaging guidance for biopsy and for the follow-up of associated complications such as hydronephrosis.[1]

Angiomyolipoma

Extrarenal angiomyolipomas are rare, with fewer than 60 cases reported.[37] Angiomyolipomas most commonly arise in the kidneys and represent approximately 1% of renal tumors. They are composed of varying amounts of blood vessels, smooth muscle, and fat, but predominantly fat. They are typically asymptomatic but can hemorrhage. Exophytic angiomyolipomas can mimic a fat-containing retroperitoneal mass.

Teratoma

After Wilms tumor and neuroblastoma, teratoma is the third most common retroperitoneal tumor in children. These tumors originate from pluripotent germ cells and contain tissues from at least 2 germ cell layers, although usually, all 3 layers are present: ectoderm universally present, mesoderm in 90%, and endoderm in most.[32] Overall, less than 10% of teratomas occur in the retroperitoneum (**Fig. 26**). These tumors are most common in infancy (<6 months), with a second peak in early adulthood. An interesting characteristic of adult teratomas is the propensity to occur in the left suprarenal space.[38]

Most teratomas are benign, mature teratomas. Less than 3% of mature teratomas harbor internal malignant tissue. Immature or malignant teratomas are also rare (<1%). Malignancy associated with a teratoma is more common in children than adults. The presence of malignancy, and the distinction of mature from immature, can rarely be made with imaging, unless there is obvious invasion of adjacent organs or vessels.

Paraganglioma (Extra-Adrenal Pheochromocytoma)

Ten percent of pheochromocytomas are extra-adrenal in location and are termed paragangliomas. The most common location is the organs of Zuckerkandl, which are located anterior to the inferior aorta, near the iliac arterial bifurcation. These tumors are more difficult to identify with ultrasonography, in which case CT or MR imaging is more useful. Alternatively, iodine[131]-MIBG (meta-iodobenzylguanidine) scintigraphy can be used for localization of the primary lesion or metastatic disease in the setting of malignant pheochromocytoma. The appearance is similar to pheochromocytomas occurring in the adrenal gland (see earlier discussion); however, compared with those of adrenal origin, paragangliomas are more

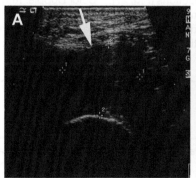
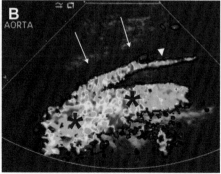

Fig. 25. (*A*) Transverse ultrasonography image at the level of the common iliac arteries. There is an ovoid hypoechoic mass (*arrow*) encasing the arteries, without evidence of vascular invasion. (*B*) Longitudinal image with color Doppler shows the mass (*arrows*) anterior to the abdominal aorta (*asterisks*) and encasing but not occluding the inferior mesenteric artery (*arrowhead*). Percutaneous image-guided biopsy confirmed retroperitoneal fibrosis.

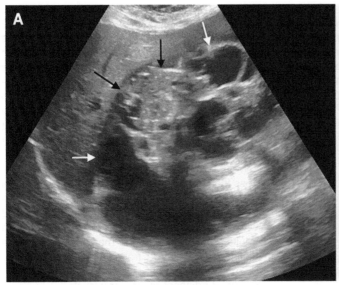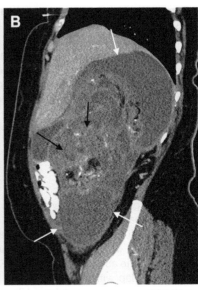

Fig. 26. (*A*) Longitudinal ultrasonographic image in the right flank of a recently pregnant 36-year-old woman. There is a large complex mass, with cystic (*white arrows*) and solid (*black arrows*) components. Additional punctuate echogenic foci within the central solid component correlate with calcifications. The liver is compressed superiorly but appears separate from the mass. (*B*) Sagittal CT image through the mass confirms the presence of calcifications and fat (*black arrows*), as well as the cystic components (*white arrows*). (The density anterior is a segment of the ascending colon containing contrast.) Ultrasound-guided biopsy confirmed the diagnosis of mature cystic teratoma.

aggressive, with up to 50% being metastatic at presentation.[32]

Other Neoplasms

Neurogenic tumors
Neurogenic tumors occur in a younger age group than the sarcomas and are more likely to be benign. These tumors can be grouped into 3 categories based on their cell origin (**Table 16**). The imaging features overlap with those of other retroperitoneal tumors.

Lymphadenopathy
Lymphadenopathy that is visible with ultrasonography is most likely to be secondary to lymphoma, with non-Hodgkin lymphoma more likely to

manifest as retroperitoneal disease than Hodgkin lymphoma. Lymph nodes associated with metastatic disease are less common and, when present, are likely to be related to a primary urologic or gynecologic malignancy. In contrast to lymphoma, metastatic nodes may be more heterogeneous and echogenic in appearance; however, this is not specific and histologic distinction is not possible solely with ultrasonography.

Discrete nodes are typically hypoechoic, but without increased through transmission, which can help distinguish them from cysts or fluid collections (**Fig. 27**).[39] Color Doppler may show internal vascularity, although this is not specific for distinguishing malignant from benign nodes. Additional diagnostic clues for malignancy are round

Table 16
Neurogenic tumor classification

	Malignant	Benign
Nerve sheath	Malignant schwannoma Neurofibrosarcoma	Schwannoma Neurofibroma
Ganglion	Neuroblastoma	Ganglioneuroma Ganglioneuroblastoma
Paraganglion	Malignant pheochromocytoma Malignant paraganglioma	Pheochromocytoma Paraganglioma

Data from Rajiah P, Sinha R, Cuevas C, et al. Imaging of uncommon retroperitoneal masses. Radiographics 2011;31:949–76.

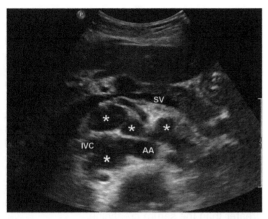

Fig. 27. Transverse ultrasonography at the level of the pancreas in an immunocompromised patient with disseminated mycobacterial infection, showing multiple hypoechoic, well-circumscribed round and ovoid lymph nodes (*asterisks*). The lack of increased through transmission distinguishes these nodes from cystic lesions or fluid collections. AA, abdominal aorta; SV, splenic vein.

nodes with a longitudinal/transverse ratio of less than 2 and effacement of the normal echogenic vascular hilum.[40] Size is the most frequently used criterion in distinguishing malignant from benign nodes in the abdomen (**Table 17**); however, normal-size nodes can infrequently harbor malignancy, such as in some cases of lymphoma.[41] Nodes can fuse to form confluent para-aortic masses (**Fig. 28**).

FLUID COLLECTIONS

In contrast to primary tumors, fluid collections within the retroperitoneum are common. Many of these fluid collections have a similar imaging appearance, and localization within the retroperitoneum and the pattern of spread can be helpful in determining the diagnosis. Ultrasonography is

Table 17 Upper limit size criteria for normal lymph nodes in the abdomen (mm)	
Retrocrural	6
Paracardiac	8
Gastrohepatic ligament	8
Upper para-aortic	9
Lower para-aortic	11
Porta hepatis	7
Portacaval	10

Data from Dorfman RE, Alpern MB, Gross BH, et al. Upper abdominal lymph nodes: criteria for normal size determined with CT. Radiology 1991;180:319–22.

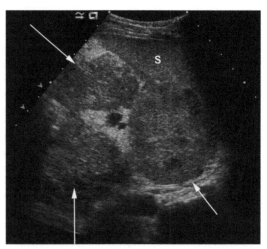

Fig. 28. Transverse ultrasonography through left upper quadrant in a patient with lymphoma shows multiple soft tissue masses (*arrows*) posterior to the spleen (S). Splenic lesions were also present.

often unable to determine the cause of a fluid collection based on imaging appearance alone. The most frequently encountered are:

- Hematoma
- Pseudocysts/pancreatitis-related fluid collections
- Abscess
- Urinoma
- Lymphocele
- Lymphangioma/lymphangiomatosis

Hematoma

Causes of retroperitoneal hemorrhage include:

- Hypercoaguable state
- Blunt or penetrating trauma
- Diagnostic or medical procedure (eg, biopsy, lithotripsy)
- Spontaneous vascular rupture
- Tumor hemorrhage

The most common locations for hemorrhage are in the perirenal space or within the psoas muscles (retrofascial space), which can be more difficult to identify with ultrasonography. In general, CT is the modality of choice if a retroperitoneal bleed is suspected.

The sonographic appearance is variable (see **Box 2**). Hematomas can be indistinguishable from abscess and can mimic a solid tumor (see **Figs. 6** and **7**).

Pseudocyst

Refer to pancreas section.

Abscess

Abscesses in the retroperitoneum are usually postsurgical, or the result of direct extension of infection involving the kidneys or retrofascial compartment (psoas or paraspinal). Inflammatory conditions of the bowel such as diverticulitis and Crohn disease can also extend into the retroperitoneum.[41]

The ultrasonographic appearance overlaps with other fluid collections. Abscesses typically have thick walls, internal septations, and debris (**Fig. 29**). When present, gas within a collection increases the diagnostic confidence but may not be visible sonographically. Large amounts of gas may obscure the kidney or other structures and confound the ultrasonographic appearance, in which case CT imaging may be more helpful. As with other fluid collections, aspiration is often necessary for definitive diagnosis. Percutaneous catheter drainage is the treatment of choice.

Urinoma

Urinomas occur after renal transplantation, surgery or trauma to the native kidneys, or as the result of obstruction. Hydronephrosis is usually present.[42] At ultrasonography, urinomas appear as well-defined anechoic fluid collections. Internal septations are uncommon, the presence of which should alternatively raise the possibility of a hematoma.[43] Postcontrast CT scanning with delayed imaging can confirm the diagnosis, because extravasated contrast fills the cavity. Alternatively, a radionuclide study shows progressive uptake in the cavity. In renal transplant patients with renal dysfunction, or when intravenous contrast is otherwise contraindicated, ultrasound-guided aspiration can be obtained. The diagnosis is confirmed when the creatinine level of the fluid is greater than the serum creatinine.

Lymphocele

Lymphoceles are collections of lymph that occur after 15% of renal transplants and up to 24% of lymphadenectomy patients.[43,44] Most are asymptomatic; however, if they become large enough, they can cause compression of adjacent structures such as the ureter or vessels, leading to clinical symptoms.

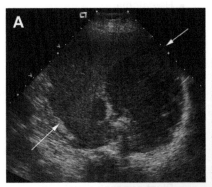
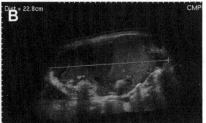
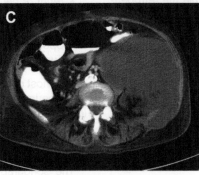

Fig. 29. (*A*) Transverse ultrasonography through the left flank in a 57-year-old woman with a fever and a brain abscess. There is a complex heterogeneous mass, with both echogenic and hypoechoic components (*arrows*). Increased through transmission suggests a fluid collection. (*B*) Extended field of view image in the sagittal plane better shows the size and craniocaudal extent of the collection. The hypoechoic component was confirmed to be pus on aspiration. A fistula from the colon was confirmed as the cause. (*C*) Corresponding contrast-enhanced CT better localizes the abscess. Note that the CT appearance is homogeneous, with the internal complexity better depicted with ultrasonography.

On ultrasonography, these are anechoic collections with through transmission, resembling a simple cyst. Occasionally, they can have internal septations and debris, making differentiation from urinoma or abscess difficult (**Fig. 30**).

Lymphangioma/Lymphangiomatosis

Lymphangiomas result from a congenital malformation of the lymphatic system, in which the retroperitoneal lymphatics fail to properly communicate with the main lymphatic ducts. Although lymphangiomas can present in the first 2 years of life, they occur in all age groups and are slightly more prevalent in males. On ultrasonography, they are thin-walled, well-circumscribed unilocular or multilocular cysts. They tend to be elongated and can occur in the perirenal, pararenal, or pelvic extraperitoneal spaces.[45]

Lymphangiomatosis, or cystic angiomatosis, is an uncommon condition characterized by the widespread involvement of bony and soft tissue with locally infiltrative lymphangiomas. It frequently involves the bones, mediastinum, spleen, liver, lungs, neck, and pleura. Symptoms are related to the site and extent of invasion, such as with pathologic fractures from bone involvement or respiratory difficulty related to pleural involvement.[44]

PSEUDOLESIONS

There are multiple benign lesions and normal structures that can mimic masses and collections in the retroperitoneal space. Some of these entities can be distinguished during the course of the ultrasonographic examination by altering the technique; however, some may require correlation

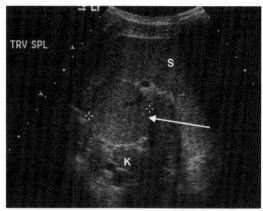

Fig. 31. Transverse image in the left upper quadrant showing a homogeneous round mass (*arrow*) between the kidney (K) and spleen (S). The appearance overlaps that of an adrenal mass; additional cross-sectional imaging (*not shown*) confirmed the lesion to be a splenule.

with other cross-sectional imaging. Some examples are aperistaltic bowel (see **Fig. 2**), horseshoe kidney, splenule/splenosis (**Fig. 31**), and occasionally, varices.[46]

SUMMARY

Ultrasonography is a primary imaging tool for evaluating the retroperitoneum, although there is significant overlap in the sonographic appearance of benign and malignant processes. It is therefore important to have knowledge of the broad range of potential abnormalities and of the strengths and limitations of ultrasonography, to make proper use of this technique.

REFERENCES

1. Meyers MA, Charnsangavej C, Oliphant M. The extraperitoneal spaces: normal and pathologic anatomy. In: Meyers MA, Charnsangavej C, Oliphant M, editors. Meyers' dynamic radiology of the abdomen: normal and pathologic anatomy. 6th edition. New York: Springer Science + Business Media; 2011. p. 109–202.
2. Lim JH, Kim B, Auh YH. Anatomical communications of the perirenal space. Br J Radiol 1998;71:450–6.
3. Thornton FJ, Kandiah SS, Monkhouse WS, et al. Helical CT evaluation of the perirenal space and its boundaries: a cadaveric study. Radiology 2001; 218:659–63.
4. Simons GW, Sty JR, Starshak RJ. Retroperitoneal and retrofascial abscesses: a review. J Bone Joint Surg Am 1983;65:1041–58.
5. Oktar SO, Yücel C, Özdemir H, et al. Comparison of conventional sonography, real-time compound

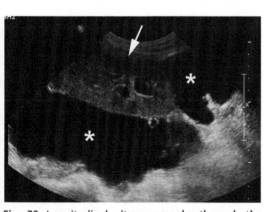

Fig. 30. Longitudinal ultrasonography through the right lower quadrant shows a renal transplant (*arrow*). A large simple fluid collection (*asterisks*) surrounds the transplant and is associated with mild hydronephrosis. A lymphocele was confirmed with percutaneous image-guided aspiration.

sonography, tissue harmonic sonography, and tissue harmonic compound sonography of abdominal and pelvic lesions. AJR Am J Roentgenol 2003; 181:1341–7.

6. Yücel C, Özdemir H, Aşik E, et al. Benefits of tissue harmonic imaging in the evaluation of abdominal and pelvic lesions. Abdom Imaging 2003;28: 103–9.

7. Pardes JG, Auh YH, Kneeland JB, et al. The oblique coronal view in sonography of the retroperitoneum. AJR Am J Roentgenol 1985;144:1241–7.

8. Bradley MJ, Cosgrove DO. The abdominal wall, peritoneum and retroperitoneum. In: Allan PL, Baxter GM, Weston MJ, editors. Clinical ultrasound. 3rd edition. Churchill Livingstone Elsevier; 2011. p. 798–827.

9. Abu-Yousef MM, El-Zein Y. Improved US visualization of the pancreatic tail with simethicone, water, and patient rotation. Radiology 2000;217:780–5.

10. Lev-Toaff AS, Langer JE, Rubin DL, et al. Safety and efficacy of a new oral contrast agent for sonography: a phase II trial. AJR Am J Roentgenol 1999; 173:431–6.

11. Gore RM, Callen PW, Filly RA. Displaced retroperitoneal fat: sonographic guide to right upper quadrant mass localization. Radiology 1982;142:701–5.

12. Nishino M, Hayakawa K, Minami M, et al. Primary retroperitoneal neoplasms: CT and MR imaging findings with anatomic and pathologic diagnostic clues. Radiographics 2003;23:45–57.

13. Callen PW, Filly RA, Sarti DA, et al. Ultrasonography of the diaphragmatic crura. Radiology 1979;130: 721–4.

14. Yeh H. Sonography of the adrenal glands: normal glands and small masses. AJR Am J Roentgenol 1980;135:1167–77.

15. Marchal G, Gelin J, Verbeken E, et al. High resolution real time sonography of the adrenal glands: a routine examination? J Ultrasound Med 1986;5:65–8.

16. Burks DW, Mirvis SE, Shanmuganathan K, et al. Acute adrenal injury after blunt abdominal trauma: CT findings. AJR Am J Roentgenol 1992;158:503–7.

17. Bowen AD, Keslar PJ, Newman B, et al. Adrenal haemorrhage after liver transplantation. Radiology 1990;176:85–8.

18. Foster DG. Adrenal cysts: review of literature and report of case. Arch Surg 1986;92:131–43.

19. Remer EM, Casalino DD, Bishoff JT, et al. ACR Appropriateness Criteria incidentally discovered adrenal mass. American College of Radiology. Available at: http://www.acr.org/~/media/ACR/Documents/ AppCriteria/Diagnostic/IncidentallyDiscoveredAdrenal Mass.pdf. Accessed February 1, 2014.

20. NIH State-of-the-Science Statement on management of the clinically inapparent adrenal mass ("incidentaloma"). NIH Consens State Sci Statements 2002;19(2):1–23.

21. Musante F, Derchi LE, Zappasodi F, et al. Myelolipoma of the adrenal gland: sonographic and CT features. AJR Am J Roentgenol 1988;151:961–4.

22. Bowerman RA, Silver TM, Jaffe MH, et al. Sonography of adrenal pheochromocytomas. AJR Am J Roentgenol 1981;137:1227–31.

23. Candel AG, Gattuso P, Reyes CV, et al. Fine-needle aspiration biopsy of adrenal masses in patients with extraadrenal malignancy. Surgery 1993;114:1132–6 [discussion: 1136–7].

24. Hamper UM, Fishman EK, Harman DS, et al. Primary adrenocortical carcinoma: sonographic evaluation with clinical and pathologic correlation in 26 patients. AJR Am J Roentgenol 1987;148:915–9.

25. Rha SE, Byun JY, Jung SE, et al. Neurogenic tumors in the abdomen: tumor types and imaging characteristics. Radiographics 2003;23:29–43.

26. Atri M, Finnegan PW. The pancreas. In: Rumack CM, Wilson SR, Charboneau JW, editors. Diagnostic ultrasound. 3rd edition. St Louis (MO): Mosby; 2005. p. 213–67.

27. Amin Z. Pancreas. In: Allan PL, Baxter GM, Weston MJ, editors. Clinical ultrasound. 3rd edition. Churchill Livingstone Elsevier; 2011. p. 285–323.

28. Okazaki K, Uchida K, Matsushita M, et al. How to diagnose autoimmune pancreatitis by the revised Japanese clinical criteria. J Gastroenterol 2007; 42(Suppl XVIII):32–8.

29. Nichols MT, Russ PD, Chen YK. Pancreatic imaging: current and emerging technologies. Pancreas 2006; 33:211–20.

30. Martínez-Noguera A, D'Onofrio M. Ultrasonography of the pancreas. 1. Conventional imaging. Abdom Imaging 2006;32:136–49.

31. Choi JY, Kim MJ, Kim JH, et al. Solid pseudopapillary tumor of the pancreas: typical and atypical manifestations. AJR Am J Roentgenol 2006;187: W178–86.

32. Rajiah P, Sinha R, Cuevas C, et al. Imaging of uncommon retroperitoneal masses. Radiographics 2011;31:949–76.

33. Solla JA, Reed K. Primary retroperitoneal sarcomas. Am J Surg 1986;152:496–8.

34. Craig WD, Fanburg-Smith JC, Henry LR, et al. Fat-containing lesions of the retroperitoneum: radiologic-pathologic correlation. Radiographics 2009;29:261–90.

35. Hartman DS, Hayes WS, Choyke PL, et al. Leiomyosarcoma of the retroperitoneum and inferior vena cava: radiologic-pathologic correlation. Radiographics 1992;12:1203–20.

36. Cronin CG, Lohan DG, Blake MA, et al. Retroperitoneal fibrosis: a review of clinical features and imaging findings. AJR Am J Roentgenol 2008;191: 423–31.

37. Minja E, Pellerin M, Saviano N, et al. Retroperitoneal extrarenal angiomyolipomas: an evidence-based

approach to a rare clinical entity. Case Rep Nephrol 2012;2012:374107.

38. Gatcombe HG, Assikis V, Kooby D, et al. Primary retroperitoneal teratomas: a review of the literature. J Surg Oncol 2004;86:107–13.

39. Jing BS. Diagnostic imaging of abdominal and pelvic lymph nodes in lymphoma. Radiol Clin North Am 1990;28:801–31.

40. Vassallo P, Wernecke K, Roos N, et al. Differentiation of benign from malignant superficial lymphadenopathy: the role of high-resolution US. Radiology 1992;183:215–20.

41. Downey DB. The retroperitoneum and great vessels. In: Rumack CM, Wilson SR, Charboneau JW, editors. Diagnostic ultrasound. 3rd edition. St Louis (MO): Mosby; 2005. p. 443–87.

42. Healy ME, Teng SS, Moss AA. Uriniferous pseudocyst: computed tomographic findings. Radiology 1984;153:757–62.

43. Brown ED, Chen MY, Wolfman NT, et al. Complications of renal transplantation: evaluation with US and radionuclide imaging. Radiographics 2000;20:607–22.

44. Yang DH, Goo HW. Generalized lymphangiomatosis: radiologic findings in three pediatric patients. Korean J Radiol 2006;7:287–91.

45. Davidson AJ, Harman DS. Lymphangioma of the retroperitoneum: CT and sonographic characteristics. Radiology 1990;175:507–10.

46. Kedar RP, Cosgrove DO. Case report: retroperitoneal varices mimicking a mass: diagnosis on color Doppler. Br J Radiol 1994;67:661–2.

Ultrasonography Assessment of the Aorta and Mesenteric Arteries

Margarita V. Revzin, MD, MS[a],*, John S. Pellerito, MD[b]

KEYWORDS

- Ultrasonography • Aorta • Mesenteric arteries • AAA • Chronic mesenteric ischemia

KEY POINTS

- A basic knowledge of the anatomy of the abdominal aorta and its major branches is essential for proper interpretation of sonographic findings and for understanding the pathologic disease states that affect these vessels.
- An understanding of relevant anatomy and hemodynamics for normal vessels as well as for multiple disease states, including abdominal aortic aneurysm, vascular stenosis, dissection, and occlusion, is important for correct diagnosis.
- There are various Doppler techniques, protocols, and diagnostic criteria used in the evaluation of the aorta and mesenteric arteries.

INTRODUCTION

This article discusses the sonographic evaluation of the abdominal aorta and mesenteric arteries. Relevant anatomy and hemodynamics are reviewed for normal vessels as well as for multiple disease states, including abdominal aortic aneurysm (AAA), vascular stenosis, dissection, and occlusion. Doppler techniques, protocols, and diagnostic criteria are presented for evaluation of the aorta and mesenteric arteries. The learner is presented with essential information for correct diagnosis and recognition of potential pitfalls to avoid.

ANATOMY OF THE ABDOMINAL AORTA AND ITS MAJOR BRANCHES

A basic knowledge of the anatomy of the abdominal aorta and its major branches is essential for proper interpretation of sonographic findings and for understanding the pathologic disease states that affect these vessels.

Abdominal Aorta

The abdominal aorta is a continuation of the thoracic aorta. It begins at the aortic hiatus of the diaphragm, at the T12 level, and ends at approximately the L4 level by dividing into the right and left common iliac arteries. The common iliac arteries diverge and run inferolaterally along the psoas musculature. The abdominal aorta is approximately 13 cm in length, and its major branches may be described as both paired and unpaired, and parietal and visceral. Among its unpaired branches are the celiac trunk, superior mesenteric artery (SMA), and inferior mesenteric artery (IMA), and among paired branches are the renal and gonadal arteries. The lumbar arteries are parietal paired vessels that are located on both sides of the posterior aorta. There are normally 4 pairs of lumbar branches, with the inferior vessels on occasion arising from iliac artery branches. The abdominal aorta lies anterior to the spine, posterior to the pancreas and stomach, and to the left of the inferior vena cava.

Disclosure: None.
[a] Department of Diagnostic Radiology, Yale University School of Medicine, Box 208042, Tompkin's East 2, New Haven, CT 06520-8042, USA; [b] Department of Radiology, North Shore University Hospital, 300 Community Drive, Manhasset, NY 11030, USA
* Corresponding author.
E-mail address: ritarevzin@hotmail.com

Ultrasound Clin 9 (2014) 723–749
http://dx.doi.org/10.1016/j.cult.2014.07.010
1556-858X/14/$ – see front matter © 2014 Elsevier Inc. All rights reserved.

ultrasound.theclinics.com

Anatomy of the Mesenteric Arteries and Collateral Pathways

Mesenteric arteries arise from the abdominal aorta. The celiac trunk is the first branch, measuring approximately 3 cm in length and arising from the anterior aspect of the aorta approximately at the level of the T12 and L1 vertebral bodies. It subsequently branches into the splenic, hepatic, and left gastric arteries. The SMA arises from the anterior aspect of the abdominal aorta and usually takes off 1 cm inferior to the celiac trunk, at the L1 level. The vessel courses caudally along the aorta surrounded by retroperitoneal fat, following the mesentery of the small bowel into the right lower quadrant. SMA gives off multiple branches including the inferior pancreaticoduodenal artery; 4 to 6 jejunal branches; 9 to 13 ileal branches; and the ileocolic, right colic, and middle colic arteries. In addition, the IMA originates from the anterolateral aspect of the aorta at the level of the L3 vertebral body, approximately 4 cm above the aortic bifurcation. It divides into the ascending left colic artery and 2 descending branches: the sigmoid and superior hemorrhoidal arteries (**Fig. 1**).

There is a rich collateral circulation between all three of the mesenteric arteries, ensuring blood supply to the essential organs and bowel if one or more of the vessels get compromised. Communication between the celiac and the superior mesenteric systems occurs by way of the gastroduodenal artery. The gastroduodenal artery is formed from the superior pancreaticoduodenal artery, a branch from the celiac system, and the inferior pancreaticoduodenal artery, a branch from the SMA. The SMA and IMA systems are joined by the arc of Riolan, connecting the middle colic branch of the SMA with the left colic branch of the IMA. It forms a short loop that runs close to the root of the mesentery. In addition, SMA and IMA are anastomosed by means of the marginal artery of Drummond, which is a continuous arterial circle or arcade along the inner margin of the colon, formed by anastomoses of the terminal branches of the ileocolic, right colic, and middle colic arteries (from the SMA) with the left colic and sigmoid branches of the IMA. In addition, there is communication of the IMA and internal iliac systems via anastomoses of the superior hemorrhoidal arteries (IMA branches) with the inferior hemorrhoidal arteries (internal iliac artery branches).

There is significant variation in the anatomy of the collateral circulation, with weak or absent connection between the mesenteric arteries in up to 30% of the population.[1]

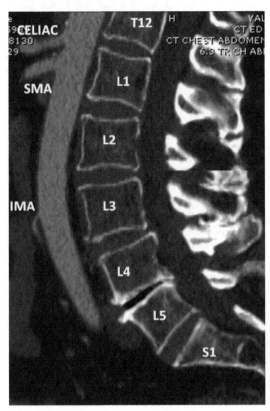

Fig. 1. Aortic branches. Contrast-enhanced sagittal computed tomography (CT) view of the aorta and its major branches. Relationship of the branches to the spine: celiac (T12–L1), SMA (L1), IMA (L3).

HEMODYNAMICS OF THE ABDOMINAL AORTA AND MESENTERIC ARTERIES
Hemodynamics of the Aorta

The abdominal aorta is an elastic structure that propagates moving blood peripherally during the cardiac cycle by means of distention in systole and elastic recoil of its walls in diastole. This physiology is reflected in pulsatile changes that are observed in the waveform during the cardiac cycle. Waveforms obtained in the proximal abdominal aorta differ from the ones obtained in the distal aorta. Although both segments show triphasic waveforms, the proximal abdominal aorta waveform patterns have more continuous blood flow during diastole (**Fig. 2A**).[2] This phenomenon is caused by the presence of several major branches of the abdominal aorta that supply the liver, spleen, and kidneys. These organs have low-resistance blood flow patterns and require continuous forward flow throughout systole and diastole for their function. Below the renal arteries, the abdominal aorta waveform pattern mimics that of a peripheral artery, showing a characteristic

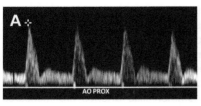

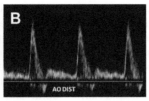

Fig. 2. Aortic waveforms. (A) Pulsed Doppler of the proximal aorta showing low-resistance waveform with presence of flow in diastole. (B) Distal aortic waveforms showing a characteristic peripheral triphasic waveform.

triphasic waveform with minimal diastolic flow and more prominent flow reversal in early diastole (see **Fig. 2**B).[2,3] The average peak systolic velocity (PSV) in the abdominal aorta is 110 cm/s in the population with an average age of 12 years old.[4] With increasing age, the PSV decreases, ranging from 70 to 100 cm/s.

Hemodynamics of the Mesenteric Vessels

There is a difference in normal flow patterns between the celiac arterial system and the mesenteric

arteries (SMA and IMA). The celiac trunk supplies blood to the low-resistance vascular beds of the liver and spleen, and therefore shows continuous forward flow in both systole and diastole to supply the high oxygen demands of the liver and spleen throughout the cardiac cycle (**Fig. 3**A). There is no significant change in the waveform appearance of the celiac system in the preprandial and postprandial states.[5,6]

The SMA and IMA supply variable-resistance vascular beds of the small intestine and colon and show variable flow patterns, from high

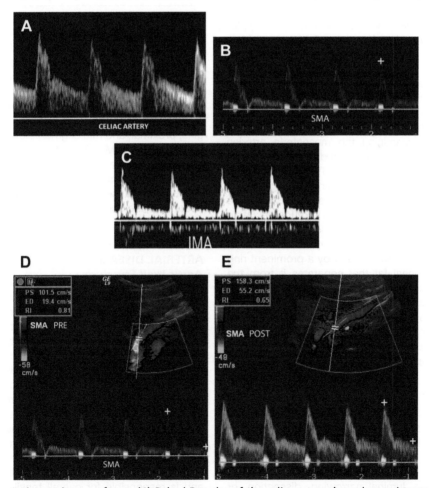

Fig. 3. Mesenteric arteries waveforms. (A) Pulsed Doppler of the celiac artery shows low-resistance waveforms with high diastolic velocity. (B, C) Preprandial pulsed Doppler of the SMA and IMA show high-resistance waveforms with minimal flow in diastole. (D, E) Preprandial and postprandial pulsed Doppler of the SMA show variable flow pattern with increase in the diastolic velocity in the SMA after a meal.

resistance in the preprandial state to lower resistance flow in the postprandial state (see **Fig. 3**B–E). This pattern is attributable to vasodilatation of mesenteric branches in response to the increased oxygen demands of the bowel following a meal. As a result, both peak systolic and end-diastolic velocities increase after a lipid-rich meal. The average PSVs in the mesenteric arteries are as follows: in the celiac artery, PSV ranges from 98 to 105 cm/s; in SMA, 97 to 142 cm/s; and in IMA, 93 to 189 cm/s.[7]

Technique

Sonographic assessment of the abdominal aorta and splanchnic vessels is preferentially performed after 8 to 12 hours of fasting to reduce bowel gas. No medications are given before the evaluation. Modern ultrasonography equipment is used, with high-quality color and power Doppler imaging and sensitive pulsed Doppler capabilities. Given that the aorta and mesenteric branches are situated deep in the abdomen, a Doppler scanner with a low-frequency 2-MHz to 5-MHz convex (curvilinear) transducer is used in a typical adult.

Different approaches can be used to examine the aorta and mesenteric arteries. The anterior approach is most common, with the transducer placed just below the xiphoid process of the sternum. When examining the mesenteric arteries several landmarks may be used to ensure correct interpretation of the anatomy. The celiac artery in the transverse view has a distinctive appearance with a T-shaped bifurcation (seagull sign). The SMA often serves as a landmark for identification of other major mesenteric vessels because of its unique anatomic location: on the transverse view, the SMA is surrounded by a prominent ring of retroperitoneal fat that separates it from the pancreas. In patients with normal bowel rotation, the SMA lies to the left of the superior mesenteric vein, posterior to the splenic vein and pancreas, and anterior to the left renal vein. Visualization of these structures improves detection of these vessels and helps to detect variant anatomy.

PROTOCOL
Abdominal Aorta

The standard protocol for scanning the abdominal aorta is for the abdominal aorta initially to be surveyed using gray-scale and color Doppler modes for any pathologic conditions such as atherosclerotic disease, luminal narrowing, dissection, or aneurysm. Longitudinal and transverse images of the abdominal aorta are subsequently obtained from the level of the diaphragm to the level of the bifurcation, with visualization of both common iliac arteries. Measurements of vessel diameter should be performed at several levels: proximal, midabdominal and distal abdominal aorta, and proximal segments of both common iliac arteries. On the longitudinal and transverse views, the aorta and common iliac arteries are measured outer diameter to outer diameter in the anteroposterior and transverse planes. The measurement calipers should be placed along the outside edge of the wall of the aorta. The transverse dimension of the aorta can also be evaluated in the coronal plane. Both common iliac arteries are particularly well visualized in the coronal plane with the patient in the left lateral decubitus position. Color Doppler scanning through the midaorta is subsequently performed and spectral waveforms are traced.

Mesenteric Arteries

The standard protocol for scanning the splanchnic vessels is for the evaluation to begin with gray-scale and color Doppler evaluation of the abdominal aorta, followed by pulsed Doppler samples from the aorta at the level of the mesenteric arteries. These measurements serve as baseline velocities for comparison with the mesenteric artery PSVs. PSVs are subsequently obtained at the origins, proximal, and mid segments of the celiac artery, SMA, and IMA. The distal segments of the mesenteric arteries are not seen with ultrasonography, although this is not considered a significant limitation because most atherosclerotic lesions occur near the origins of these vessels.

ATHEROSCLEROSIS AND OCCLUSIVE ARTERIAL DISEASE
Aortic Wall Structure

To understand the pathophysiology of a developing atherosclerotic plaque in the abdominal aorta, clinicians should have a clear understanding of the structure of the aortic wall. The innermost layer is termed the intima and is composed of endothelial cells with minimal underlying subendothelial connective tissue. Its normal functions include prevention of platelet aggregation and thrombosis, regulation of smooth muscle tone in the deeper layer, modulation of smooth muscle cell growth and migration, and control of entry of lipoproteins into the vessel wall. The outermost layer of the aortic wall is termed the adventitia and is responsible for overall tensile strength of the aorta as a vessel. The vasa vasorum and small nerves course through this layer. Between the intima and adventitia lies the media, which is composed of discrete bundles of smooth muscle cells, elastic fibers, and collagen. The muscular component maintains the tone of the wall. The internal and external elastic laminae separate the intima from the media and the media from the adventitial layers, respectively.[8]

Plaque Formation

Atherosclerosis is the most common type of arterial occlusive disease, characterized by the development of a plaque along the wall of an artery with subsequent narrowing of the vascular lumen. This disease is chronic, progressive, and can lead to near-complete or complete occlusion of the vessel. Plaque formation primarily results from damage to the endothelial cells of the intima with deposition of lipids within the wall and development of cellular hypoxia.[9]

The earliest manifestation of atherosclerosis is slow, progressive thickening of the intima caused by increased permeability with subsequent leukocyte migration, inflammatory cell response, and gradual deposition of foam cells within the intima. This process leads to smooth muscle cell migration and development of fatty streaks, which are the areas of initial lipid accumulation. The fatty streaks may progressively develop into fibrous plaques, which are focal lesions on the luminal surface of the artery covered with intact endothelium. Plaques become vulnerable when the fibrous cap ruptures and thrombus forms on the plaque surface. This thrombus is unstable and may lead to embolization.[9]

In contrast, a stable plaque is hyalinized, contains more fibrous tissue, is calcified, and has high lipid content. It has fewer vessels, triggers less inflammation, and has a smooth surface. The rate of embolization from a stable plaque is very low.

Ultrasonography Assessment of the Plaque and Associated Luminal Stenosis

Ultrasonography plays a significant role in the identification of plaques and in the assessment of the degree of stenosis associated with a plaque. On gray-scale imaging, a hemorrhagic plaque is typically hypoechoic and may show surface irregularity, which acts as a nidus for platelet aggregation. In contrast, a stable plaque is typically more hyperechoic on gray-scale imaging because of high calcium deposition and differences in the structural contents of the plaque. Some of the plaques are more heterogeneous in echogenicity,

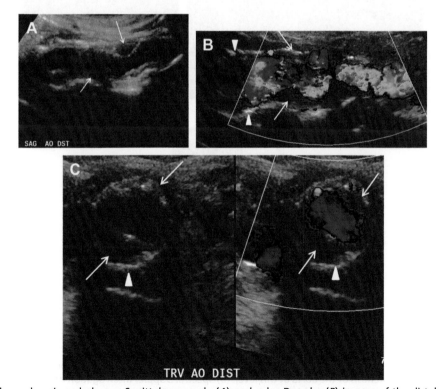

Fig. 4. Atherosclerosis and plaque. Sagittal gray-scale (*A*) and color Doppler (*B*) images of the distal abdominal aorta show significant soft (*arrows*) and calcified (*arrowheads*) plaque with associated mild to moderate irregular luminal narrowing. (*C*) Transverse gray-scale and (*D*) color Doppler images confirm the degree of luminal narrowing by soft (*arrows*) and calcified (*arrowheads*) plaque.

with echogenic and soft tissue (hypoechoic) components that reflect the variability in composition (**Fig. 4**A, B).

In the aorta, the bulk of atherosclerotic plaque arises at the origins of the branch vessels and at the bifurcation. The most common site of atherosclerotic plaque development is the thoracic aorta, and the second most common site of the plaque development is the aortoiliac segment.[10,11] Most atherosclerotic plaques are asymmetric in cross section. These findings are best assessed with thorough examination of a

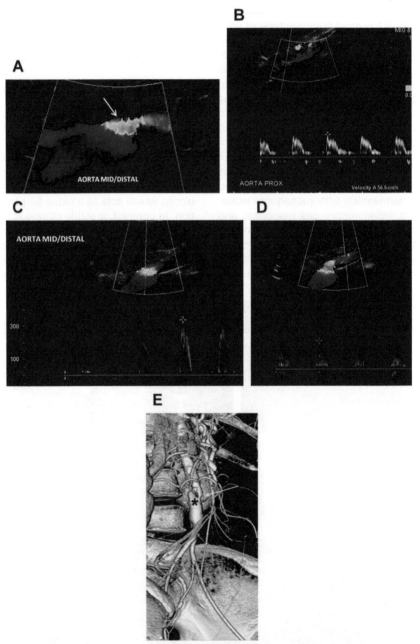

Fig. 5. Aortic stenosis likely caused by a web. (*A*) Color Doppler image of the mid/distal aorta shows focal area of color aliasing (*arrow*) stenosis of the aorta at this level. (*B*) Spectral Doppler interrogation of the proximal abdominal aorta shows low-velocity (57 cm/s) high-resistance waveforms. (*C*) High-velocity flow (>300 cm/s) is seen in the midaorta consistent with stenosis. (*D*) Tardus parvus waveforms are identified distal to the area of stenosis. (*E*) Corresponding volume-rendered CT image of the abdominal aorta shows tight stenosis in the mid/distal aorta (*yellow arrow*) with associated poststenotic dilatation (*asterisk*).

plaque in different planes in order to accurately estimate the degree of stenosis (see **Fig. 4C**).

On ultrasonography, detection of stenosis is enhanced by color Doppler imaging when aliasing is apparent in the stenotic segment (**Fig. 5**). In order to increase sensitivity in the diagnosis of aortic luminal stenosis, clinicians should adjust the color Doppler parameters to laminar flow in the nonaffected segment of the aorta and then look for any focal disturbances of blood flow along the abdominal aorta. Once flow disturbance is detected, a sample volume should be placed in the center of the hemodynamically abnormal vessel. Spectral Doppler waveforms may not only show markedly increased PSVs within the area of stenosis but also may show the presence of tardus parvus waveforms distal to the stenotic segment in both the main and branch vessels (**Figs. 6 and 7**).[12,13]

Occlusion of the Aorta

The development of high-grade stenosis is a slow and progressive process that is usually accompanied by development of collateral blood flow channels.[14] Patients commonly present with worsening lower extremity symptoms, such as claudication, secondary to development of progressive aortic occlusive narrowing. When aortic narrowing is substantial, symptoms may start to occur at rest and also may result in buttock and thigh claudication. Male patients may also present with impotence. The occlusion of the distal aorta accompanied by these symptoms is referred to as Leriche syndrome.

Complete aortic occlusion most commonly occurs in the lower portion of the abdominal aorta (**Fig. 8A–D**). In most cases the thrombus extends upward to the level of renal arteries, without renal artery occlusion. The SMA and its branches serve as a source of collateralization, with reconstitution of the common iliac arteries via communication with colonic branches from the IMA (see **Fig. 8E–G**).[15]

NORMAL SIZES OF THE ABDOMINAL AORTA

The size of the abdominal aorta is gender and age dependent, with men having larger vessels than women and children. The diameter of the aorta increases with age. The average size of the

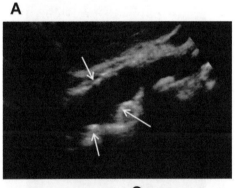

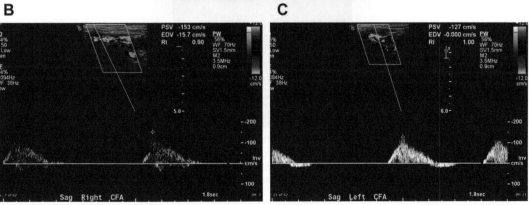

Fig. 6. Aortic stenosis. (*A*) Sagittal gray-scale image of the midabdominal aorta reveals a significant amount of atherosclerotic plaque (*arrows*); however, the degree of stenosis is difficult to assess on this image. (*B, C*) Spectral Doppler interrogation of the bilateral common femoral arteries show tardus parvus waveforms implying the presence of significant inflow disease likely caused by aortic stenosis.

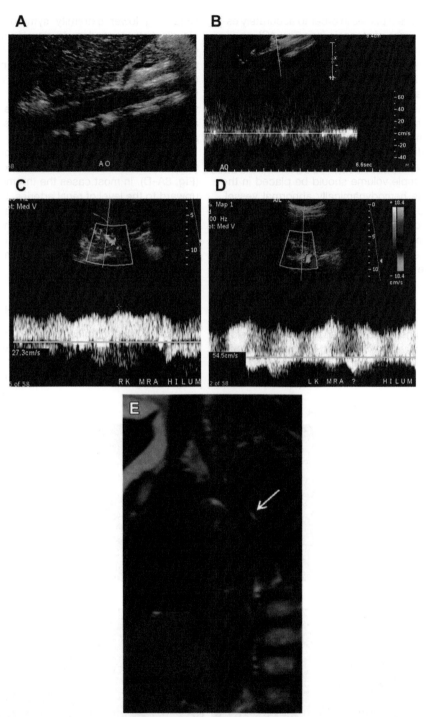

Fig. 7. Coarctation of the aorta. (*A*) Preprocedural sagittal gray-scale images reveal normal caliber of the abdominal aorta. (*B–D*) Preprocedural spectral Doppler interrogation shows tardus parvus waveforms throughout the abdominal aorta and bilateral renal arteries. (*E*) Poststent magnetic resonance (MR) angiogram of the chest shows persistent focal narrowing in the lumen of the descending thoracic aorta (*arrow*) consistent with residual coarctation.

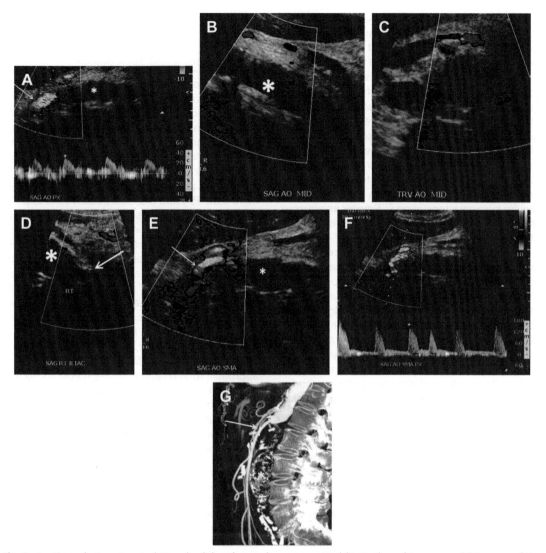

Fig. 8. Aortic occlusion. Spectral Doppler (*A*), color, and power sagittal (*B, D, E*), and transverse (*C*) images of the aorta show flow only in the proximal abdominal aorta (*arrow* in *A*). No flow is seen below the level of the SMA, consistent with aortic (*asterisks* in *A, B, D, E*) and right iliac (*arrow* in *D*) artery occlusion. The SMA serves as a collateral pathway to reconstitute lower extremity arterial systems (*arrow* in *E*). (*F*) High-resistance waveforms are seen in the patent SMA with PSVs up to 180 cm/s. (*G*) Sagittal CT images of the aorta show significant calcified plaque throughout the occluded abdominal aorta (*asterisk*). The patent SMA is enlarged and continues to the pelvis (*arrow*).

abdominal aorta in men is approximately 27 mm in anteroposterior diameter at the level of the diaphragmatic hiatus and gradually tapers to 21 mm at the level of the iliac bifurcation.[16] In women, aortic diameters are smaller by ~3 to 5 mm.[17]

AAA
Natural History of AAAs

AAAs are commonly encountered in the setting of atherosclerotic disease. The most common risk factors are advanced age, history of smoking, and hypertension. Other risk factors include family history, connective tissue diseases, hypercholesterolemia, trauma, and infection.[18,19] AAAs are associated with high mortality caused by aneurysmal rupture, with a ruptured AAA being the 10th leading cause of death in the United States. An AAA is defined as anteroposterior (AP) luminal dimension of more than 30 mm. Most aneurysms range from 30 to 40 mm in AP diameter.

Pathophysiology of AAA and AAA Rupture

Knowledge of the pathophysiology of aneurysms is essential for understanding the mechanism of aneurysmal growth and rupture. AAA formation results from a degenerative process that is characterized by laxity of the wall of the abdominal aorta. At first there is activation of an inflammatory process responsible for production and release of matrix-degrading enzymes, which result in shortening of the half-life of elastin and apoptosis of smooth muscle cells and development of an adherent mural thrombus. Degradation of elastic fiber and collagen results in weakening, laxity, and eventually rupture of the aortic wall.[20] AAAs larger than 5.5 cm are associated with a 10% annual risk of rupture, and these patients usually require surgical intervention.[21] Smaller aneurysms may also rupture, although the annual risk is substantially less (1%/y).[22]

Aneurysm rupture is caused by the presence of uneven stress and strain on an abnormally weakened aneurysmal wall. It has been postulated that intramural thrombi commonly found within the AAA lumen may be responsible for higher rates of rupture, caused by further weakening of the abdominal wall.[23–25] There are several factors that contribute to progression of aneurysmal size and subsequent rupture, including abdominal wall stiffness (the relationship between aortic diameter and pulse pressure), stress and strain on the aneurysmal wall, and tensile strength.[26,27] Irregular distribution of stress on the aortic wall results in focal differences in tensile strength that in turn lead to heterogeneity of the relationship between wall strength and wall stress. An aneurysm ruptures if, in the area of abnormality, wall stress exceeds tensile strength of the vascular tissue.[28] This possibility can be defined by the Laplace law, which states that risk of aneurysm rupture is directly related to aneurysm size because the tension on the wall of the aorta is the product of the radius of the vessel and the blood pressure.

Growth Rate of Aneurysms

Most small AAAs enlarge slowly, but there is high variability in growth rates among different individuals.[29] The size and growth of an AAA depends on patient age and gender.[30] For example, a 3-cm AAA in a male patient has a mean growth rate of 1.28 mm per year. With AAAs up to 5 cm, the growth rate is 3.61 mm/y. In general, for each 0.5-cm increase in AAA diameter, growth rates are increased by 0.59 mm/y and rupture rates are increased by a factor of 1.91.[31] The growth rate is increased in smokers (by 0.35 mm/y), and decreased in patients with diabetes (by 0.51 mm/y). Rupture rates are almost 4-fold higher in women than in men, and are doubled in active smokers.[31,32] There is substantial heterogeneity

in growth rates among studies published in the literature.

AAA Screening and Surveillance

Screening for aneurysms and regular follow-up of known aneurysms is essential, because of the chronic progressive nature of aneurysm growth and the high risk of rupture and subsequent mortality in large aneurysms. Ultrasonography is the most commonly used screening and surveillance modality for AAA, with an accuracy of almost 100%.[33] At present, screening is offered for men more than 65 years old, as well as men with a history of smoking. Various studies have shown a significant reduction in mortality from AAA as a result of screening, ranging from 21% to 68%.[34] The intervals between ultrasonography surveillance examinations depend on the aneurysm size, although currently no consensus exists on the optimal time interval between surveillance ultrasonography examinations.[32,35] AAAs are commonly asymptomatic until the time of rupture.

As mentioned earlier, the rupture risk for small AAAs is low, which favors a watchful waiting approach to management.[36] Exceptions to this approach may include patients with diabetes or heavy smokers, whose risk of rupture is higher. Lower surgical thresholds for women have also been reported, given their higher rates of aneurysm growth and rupture.[31,32]

Types of AAA

AAAs can be categorized by location, morphology, and cause. With regard to location, AAAs can be subcategorized as suprarenal (least common: trauma, infection, iatrogenic causes), juxtarenal, or infrarenal (most common). Morphologic subcategories include saccular, fusiform, or hourglass (2 adjacent but discontinuous aneurysms separated by a normal segment of aorta) types (**Fig. 9**).[14] Causal subtypes are separated into atherosclerotic (most common), inflammatory (incidence <10%; related to retroperitoneal fibrosis and characterized by a thick fibrotic wall),[37] and mycotic (incidence <1%, usually caused by bacterial infection and present in atypical locations with high mortality secondary to rapid growth rate).[38]

Diagnostic Criteria

Ultrasonography criteria for establishing the diagnosis of AAA include:

1. Focal dilatation of the abdominal aorta to greater than 3 cm
2. Increase in the aortic diameter to 1.5 times greater than the adjacent unaffected segment[39,40]

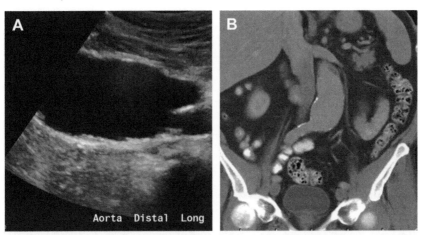

Fig. 9. Fusiform aortic aneurysm. Gray-scale sagittal (*A*) and coronal (*B*) noncontrast CT images through the distal aorta show fusiform dilatation of the aorta.

Suggested follow-up for AAAs includes:

Annual	3–4 cm
Every 6 months	4–4.5 cm
Every 3–6 months	4.5–5 cm
Every 3 months	5–5.5 cm

Focal areas of ectasia or localized bulges of the abdominal aorta may represent early signs of aneurysm formation and should be followed in 2 to 3 years (**Fig. 10**).[14,41–43]

Ultrasonography Assessment of AAA

Ultrasonography evaluation of an aortic aneurysm should include imaging in the longitudinal plane for measurement of the anteroposterior (AP) dimension and perpendicular to the long axis for assessment of the transverse dimension. Both the transverse and AP diameters should be measured outer wall to outer wall (**Fig. 11A–B**). Transverse measurements may also be obtained in the coronal plane. In the presence of aortic ectasia, the measurement of the aneurysm sac may be exaggerated by vessel obliquity. The largest measurement should be reported. A measurement of the length of the aneurysm may be given.

The vessel should also be evaluated with color flow Doppler imaging to assess patency of the lumen and presence of mural thrombus. Color flow disturbances within the aneurysm sac could be attributable to a sudden change in vessel diameter, which results in turbulent flow (see **Fig. 11**). This flow disturbance may result in a pseudo–yin-yang sign, and should not be mistaken for a pseudoaneurysm. The presence of mural thrombus was previously thought to protect from aneurysmal rupture; however, more recent studies have shown otherwise. It is currently postulated that inflammatory changes adjacent to or within the thrombus further damage the aneurysm wall and increase the risk of rupture. Aortic rupture is a life-threatening emergency and should be

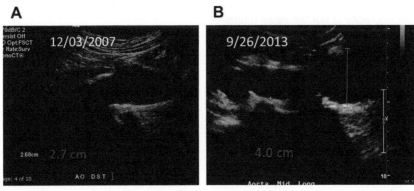

Fig. 10. AAA growth. (*A, B*) Sagittal gray-scale images through the distal abdominal aorta show increase in the size of the aneurysm from 2.7 cm on 12/03/2007 to 4.0 cm on 9/26/2013 with average growth of 2.36 mm/y.

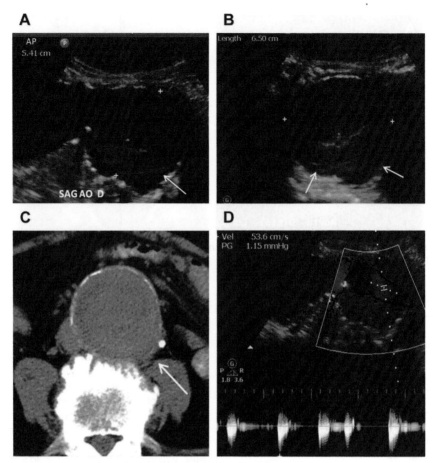

Fig. 11. AAA with intramural thrombus 59-year-old man with abdominal pain and abdominal bruit on physical examination. (*A*, *B*) Sagittal and transverse gray-scale images through the distal abdominal aorta show a 6.5-cm (transverse) by 5.4-cm (AP) aortic aneurysm with posterior wall intramural thrombus (*arrows*). Note that the calibers are placed at the outer wall of the aneurysm. (*C*) Noncontrast axial CT image shows flattening of the posterior aneurysmal wall (*arrow*), raising concern for an impeding rupture. Note calcification within the wall of the aneurysm. Posterior intramural thrombus is less apparent on CT. (*D*) Turbulent flow is seen in the lumen of the aneurysm on the pulsed Doppler display.

suspected in patients with a known AAA who present with abdominal pain.

Ultrasonography Findings of Aortic Rupture

Although ultrasonography is not the usual modality for assessment of AAA rupture, it may be used in patients who present with nonspecific abdominal pain. It is therefore essential that the ultrasonography examiner be familiar with sonographic features of aortic rupture.

The most commonly encountered findings of AAA rupture on ultrasonography are a retroperitoneal hematoma, which appears as an echogenic retroperitoneal fluid collection, usually in a periaortic location, and hemoperitoneum (**Figs. 12** and **13**).[44] Less commonly, ultrasonography examination reveals morphologic deformity of the abdominal aorta, floating thrombus within the aortic lumen, or a break in the continuity of the aortic wall at the site of rupture with or without an adjacent complex fluid collection.[44] Hemorrhage into the psoas muscle has also been described.

AAA REPAIR AND ITS COMPLICATIONS

AAAs are usually treated surgically or with endovascular placement of a stent graft. Elective open AAA repairs are associated with a higher mortality (5%) than endovascular repairs (2%) in the immediate postoperative period.[45] However, because of later complications of endovascular graft repairs, the mortality associated with this procedure increases to 5%, suggesting similar long-term outcomes.

The rupture risk of aneurysms less than 5.5 cm is lower than the risk of a surgical complication;

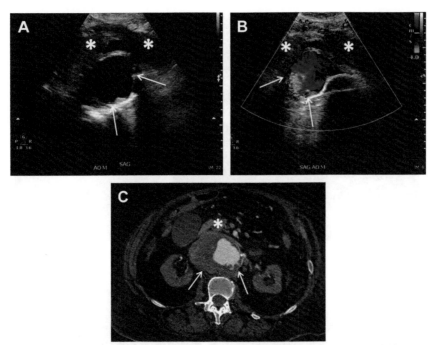

Fig. 12. Ruptured abdominal aorta aneurysm. A 67-year-old woman with known AAA with acute abdominal pain. Gray-scale sagittal (*A*) and color Doppler (*B*) images show an aneurysm of the midabdominal aorta (*arrows*) with complex avascular echogenic material seen anterior to the aneurysm (*asterisks*), consistent with hematoma. (*C*) Corresponding CT shows an irregular aneurysm of the midabdominal aorta (*arrow*) with anterior hematoma (*asterisk*) consistent with AAA rupture.

therefore, for these patients, surveillance is recommended.[36] When endovascular repair is performed, patients are followed with a series of aortic surveillance examinations in order to assess the size of the treated AAA. If the aneurysm sac continues to grow, concern is raised for the presence of an endovascular stent-graft complication. The most frequent complication is an endoleak, which can be divided into 5 subtypes. A type I leak is a result of poor sealing of the proximal or distal segment of the stent with the native arterial wall, thus allowing blood to flow outside the stent and fill the aneurysm sac (**Fig. 14**). A type II endoleak is related to retrograde filling of the aneurysmal sac via a branch of the abdominal aorta (most commonly lumbar, accessory renal, or

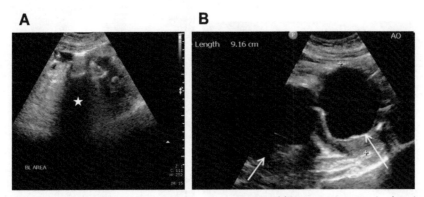

Fig. 13. Ruptured common iliac artery mycotic aneurysm. A 45-year-old immunocompromised patient presented with pyuria and sepsis. (*A*) Gray-scale images in the pelvis show complex heterogeneous tissue (*asterisk*). (*B, C*) Gray-scale image of the left lower quadrant revealed a 9-cm bilobed cystic structure (*arrows* in *B*) with flow on color Doppler (*arrows* in *C*). Concern was for a ruptured aneurysm. (*D*) Coronal CT angiogram of the abdomen demonstrates a left common iliac artery aneurysm (*long arrows*) with associated large amount of retroperitoneal hemorrhage (*asterisk*) and cranial displacement of the left kidney (*short arrow*). Findings are consistent with aneurysmal rupture.

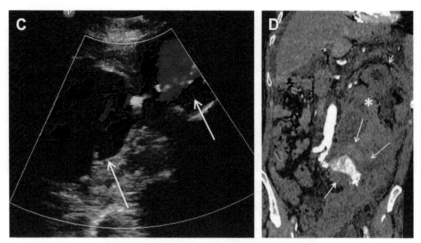

Fig. 13. (*continued*)

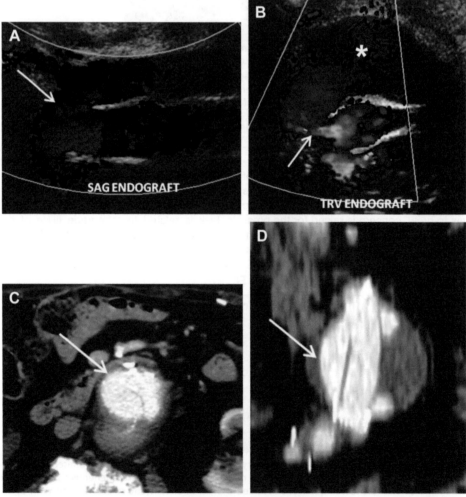

Fig. 14. Type I endoleak. Longitudinal (*A*) and transverse (*B*) color Doppler ultrasonography shows flow (*arrows*) extending from the superior aspect of the aortic endograft into the aneurysm sac (*asterisk*), consistent with a type I endoeak. (*C, D*) The leak is also shown on the axial (*arrow, C*) and coronal (*arrow, D*) contrast-enhanced CT images.

IMA) (**Figs. 15** and **16**). Type III endoleaks are usually seen in multisegmental grafts, with the leak occurring through a defect or tear in the graft (**Fig. 17**). Type IV endoleaks are caused by either the presence of a porous graft that allows seepage of blood into the aneurysm sac, or the presence of small defects in the fabric at the site of sutures or struts (this type of endoleak is best seen with contrast-enhanced computed tomography or angiography and needs to be differentiated from a type III endoleak). A type V endoleak is related to the presence of idiopathic endotension, resulting in significant expansion of the aneurysm sac. It is postulated that this type of endoleak is associated with high pressure in the AAA lumen, and may result in rupture if left untreated.[46–49] Another common complication of endovascular stent grafting is limb occlusion, recognized in 2% to 40% of cases,

depending mostly on the type of graft and duration of follow-up. Approximately one-third of patients with this complication present with acute limb ischemia, whereas most patients present with less severe symptoms or are asymptomatic.[50,51] On color Doppler ultrasonography, no flow is detected in the occluded limb of the stent graft (**Fig. 18**).

DISSECTION OF THE AORTA AND THE MESENTERIC ARTERIES

Aortic dissection is the most common acute aortic condition, associated with high morbidity and mortality and requiring urgent medical or surgical management. It is characterized by a separation of the intimal and medial layers of the aortic wall, with blood subsequently entering the false lumen

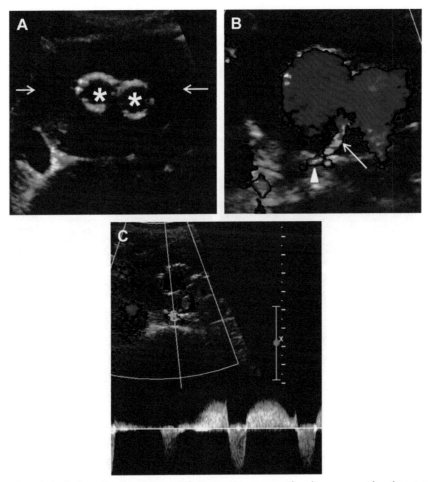

Fig. 15. Type II endoleak from lumbar artery. (*A*) Transverse gray-scale ultrasonography shows an aneurysm (*arrows*) with an endograft within (*asterisks*). (*B*) Color Doppler ultrasonography shows flow within the posterior aspect of the excluded aneurysm (*arrow*) with color Doppler flow within a lumbar artery that is arising posteriorly from the aorta (*arrowhead*). (*C*) Spectral Doppler shows to-and-fro flow within the lumbar artery, consistent with a type 2 endoleak.

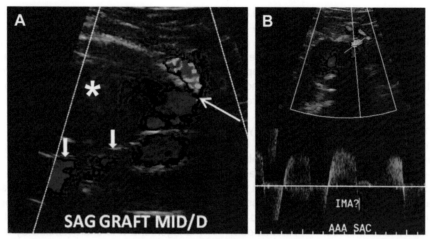

Fig. 16. Type II endoleak from IMA. (*A*) Sagittal color Doppler ultrasonography shows an aneurysm (*asterisk*) with an endograft (*arrows*). Color flow is seen within the anterior aspect of the excluded segment of the aneurysm (*thin arrow*) caused by retrograde flow from the IMA. (*B*) Pulsed Doppler ultrasonography shows to-and-fro flow within the IMA, consistent with a type 2 endoleak.

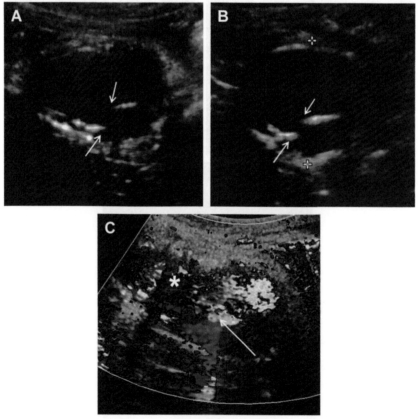

Fig. 17. Type III endoleak. Enlarging aneurysm sac after aortic endograft repair. (*A, B*) Transverse gray-scale ultrasonography images from different phases of the cardiac cycle show a mobile-appearing flap (*arrows*) of endograft material. Note the decreased distance between the arrows in (*B*) compared with (*A*). (*C*) Color Doppler ultrasonography shows flow through this opening (*arrow*) in the endograft into the aneurysm sac (*asterisk*), consistent with a type III endoleak.

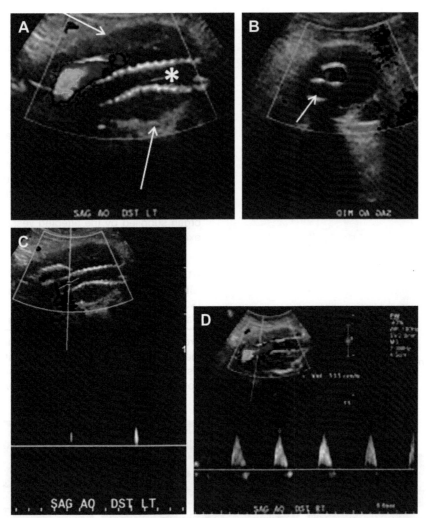

Fig. 18. AAA after repair with occluded limb. A 67-year-old man following endograft placement. (*A, B*) Sagittal and transverse color Doppler images through the distal AAA (*arrows*) show flow in the right limb of the endograft. No flow is seen in the left limb of the graft (*arrow, asterisk*). (*C*) No flow is detected in the left limb. (*D*) Arterial waveforms are present in the right endograft limb. (*E*) Angiogram shows contrast filling the bilateral renal arteries, and endograft within the abdominal aorta and the right endograft limb. No filling is seen in the left limb (*arrows*), consistent with left limb occlusion.

and propagating the dissection. There are usually additional tears in the intimal layer that allow communication between the true and false lumens. Abdominal aortic dissections typically result from extensions of thoracic aortic dissections. Preexisting penetrating ulcers and aneurysms may also increase the risk of aortic dissection. The peak incidence of aortic dissection is in the sixth and seventh decades of life, with a male/female ratio of 2:1.[52] There is high association of aortic dissection with atherosclerosis and hypertension. Other risk factors include Marfan syndrome, Ehlers-Danlos syndrome, aortic coarctation, cocaine use, pregnancy, and trauma. If

dissection is diagnosed within 14 days of initial symptoms, it is considered to be acute. Dissections diagnosed more than 2 weeks after symptom onset are considered chronic.[53]

The false lumen is usually larger in AP diameter and the true lumen may be narrowed, showing increased PSVs on spectral Doppler analysis (**Fig. 19**). The dissection flap is seen on gray scale as an echogenic line within the lumen of the aorta (see **Fig. 19A–C**). An entry point that allows communication between the true and false lumens may also be seen on gray-scale imaging. On occasion the false lumen is thrombosed and in these cases there is no detectable flow in the false lumen

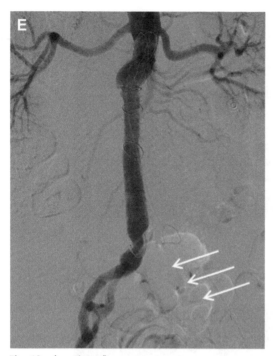

Fig. 18. (continued)

and the echogenic flap is difficult to see. Patent false lumens often display a characteristic to-and-fro pattern on color Doppler, indicating forward flow within the false lumen during systole and reversal of flow during diastole.[54–56]

Assessment of the major aortic branches is necessary in order to diagnose extension of the dissection flap into the SMA, celiac artery, IMA, or renal arteries. Increased PSVs or absent blood flow within the aortic branch should raise concern for extension of the dissection flap into the vessel with subsequent narrowing or occlusion of the involved artery (see **Fig. 19**D, E). In this situation, it is essential to assess perfusion of the end-organ supplied by the affected vessel in order to exclude ischemia or infarction.

ATHEROSCLEROTIC DISEASE OF THE MESENTERIC ARTERIES AND BOWEL ISCHEMIA
Natural History of Bowel Ischemia

Progressive plaque deposition near the ostia of the mesenteric arteries may lead to significant stenosis, thus compromising the blood supply of the bowel and potentially leading to bowel ischemia.

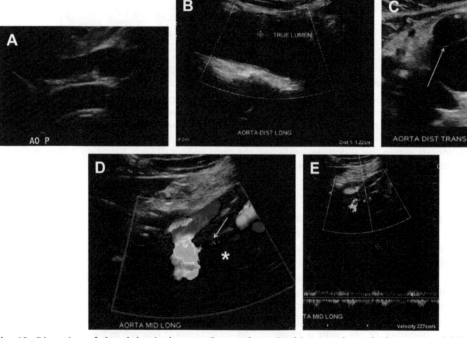

Fig. 19. Dissection of the abdominal aorta. Gray-scale sagittal images through the proximal (*A*) and distal (*B*) abdominal aorta and transverse (*C*) view of the distal aorta show an echogenic line within the lumen of the aorta, consistent with a dissection flap (*arrow* in *C*). (*D*) Color Doppler image through the proximal abdominal aorta at the level of the celiac artery and SMA shows a markedly narrowed true lumen (*arrow*). No flow is present in the false lumen (*asterisk*). (*E*) There is an increased PSV of 227 cm/s in the true lumen of the midaorta on spectral Doppler, confirming significant narrowing.

Because of the presence of a rich supply of collateral vessels, the development of chronic mesenteric ischemia is not usually apparent until 2 or more mesenteric arteries are compromised (celiac artery, SMA, and IMA).[57] Patients with this condition often present with vague postprandial abdominal pain, weight loss related to decreased food ingestion, bloating, and diarrhea. When chronic mesenteric ischemia is suspected, Doppler ultrasonography evaluation of the mesenteric arteries may be considered as the initial noninvasive imaging modality.[58–60] Doppler ultrasonography may not only detect the presence of atherosclerotic plaque and increased velocities in the mesenteric arteries but may also determine the hemodynamic significance of stenotic lesions by showing prestenotic and poststenotic waveform changes. These findings can influence the decision to intervene in the appropriate clinical setting.[61]

Diagnostic Criteria of Mesenteric Artery Stenosis

To date, no absolute consensus has been reached on a set of criteria for the diagnosis of significant mesenteric arterial stenosis. The most commonly accepted criteria are based on PSV measurements, the mesenteric artery/aorta PSV ratio (MAR), and the presence or absence of tardus parvus waveforms (Fig. 20). The established PSV thresholds for the celiac artery, SMA, and IMA are 200 cm/s, 275 cm/s, and 200 cm/s respectively.[61–64] The threshold MARs in the celiac artery, SMA, and IMA are 3.0 to 3.5.[62] The MAR can be calculated by dividing PSV in the mesenteric artery by the PSV at an adjacent site in the abdominal aorta. The presence of tardus parvus waveforms is very specific for the presence of significant proximal stenosis (almost 100%) within the vessel. In

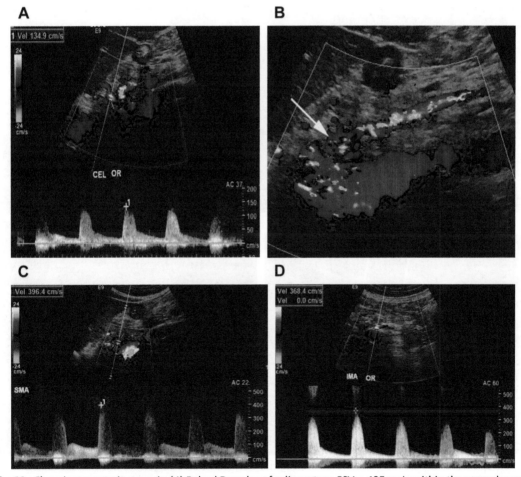

Fig. 20. Chronic mesenteric stenosis. (A) Pulsed Doppler of celiac artery. PSV = 135 cm/s, within the normal range. (B) Color Doppler image of the SMA shows aliasing and color bruit artifact at the site of stenosis (arrow). (C) Pulsed Doppler of SMA at the site of aliasing shows increased PSV (396 cm/s), consistent with significant stenosis. (D) Pulsed Doppler interrogation of the IMA also shows increased PSV (360 cm/s), consistent with significant stenosis.

general, the sensitivity of a tardus parvus waveform is low and specificity is high.

Other secondary signs of stenosis include color bruit artifact, color aliasing, and luminal narrowing (see **Fig. 20**B). Sometimes the presence of collateral vessels is readily apparent. A search for these secondary findings may facilitate the diagnosis of significant mesenteric artery stenosis. It is important to recognize that the presence of multiple abnormal diagnostic criteria improves diagnostic accuracy.

Pitfalls in Diagnosis

There are several pitfalls that can be encountered when performing sonographic evaluation of the mesenteric vessels. One of the most common pitfalls is the presence of increased PSVs in all 3

vessels caused by a high-output state, commonly seen in young or pregnant patients or in patients with metabolic imbalances such as hyperthyroidism. Very low PSVs may be detected in patients with low-output states such as septic shock, blood loss, cardiac dysfunction, and large aneurysms of the aorta, among other causes. In these situations, attention to the MAR helps to detect significant stenosis. A very large or very small ratio should alert the examiner to the presence of a potential pitfall. On occasion, blood flow is increased in 1 mesenteric artery as a result of compensatory flow, when adjacent mesenteric arteries are either occluded or stenotic.[65] In this scenario, increased PSVs are found along the course of the entire vessel, and no secondary signs of stenosis are apparent.

Variant mesenteric arterial anatomy may also affect diagnostic accuracy. The frequently seen

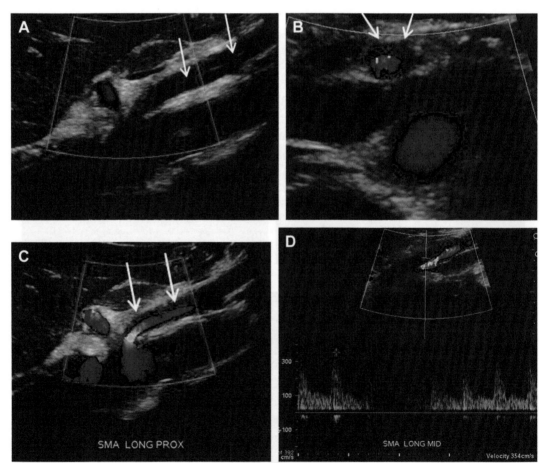

Fig. 21. Spontaneous dissection of the SMA. (*A*) Sagittal view shows an echogenic line within the lumen of the SMA, consistent with a dissection flap (*arrows*). (*B, C*) Transverse and sagittal color Doppler images show flow within the true lumen of the SMA and a thrombosed false lumen (*arrows*). (*D*) Spectral Doppler interrogation of the true lumen reveals increased PSVs (354 cm/s) within the true lumen of the SMA, compatible with significant narrowing. (*E*) Three-dimensional (3D) volume-rendered CT angiography shows small, irregular residual lumen of the SMA (*arrows*).

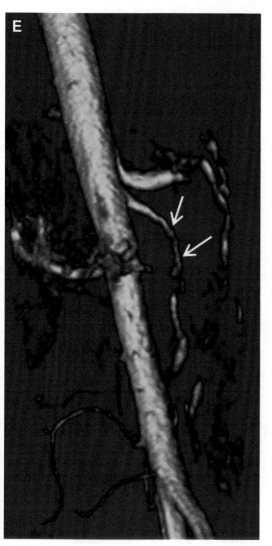

E

Fig. 21. *(continued)*

mesenteric arterial variants include a common origin of the celiac artery and SMA,[58] and variations in the location of the common or right hepatic artery origin. Thorough evaluation of the mesenteric arteries aids in avoiding these pitfalls.

Mesenteric Arterial Occlusion

Occlusion of a mesenteric artery can result from a thromboembolic event or may be caused by progression of an atherosclerotic plaque. It may be acute or chronic in nature. On ultrasonography, there is no detectable flow in the lumen of an occluded mesenteric vessel. With a chronic presentation, there may be reversal of flow with tardus parvus waveforms distal to the occluded segment (as a result of reconstitution by means

of collateral circulation). Increased compensatory flow within an adjacent mesenteric artery may also be seen.

Mesenteric Arterial Dissection

Dissection of the mesenteric arteries usually is a continuation of the aortic dissection. Spontaneous isolated dissection of the mesenteric arteries is very rare. The most frequent artery involved in spontaneous mesenteric dissection is the SMA. Dissections of the hepatic, splenic, left gastric, and celiac arteries are less frequently encountered.[66] Causal factors include atherosclerosis, fibromuscular dysplasia, mycotic infection, trauma, and congenital connective tissue disorders.[67] The location of entry point of isolated SMA dissection is about 1.5 to 3 cm from the orifice. This segment of the SMA is a transition zone of the SMA from a fixed segment under the pancreas to the mobile segment at the mesenteric root. This transition point can be the focus of intimal tear caused by abnormal sheering stress.[68] Although a dissection flap may be difficult to see on imaging because of small vessel size, the chances of identifying a flap may be improved with careful assessment of the arterial lumen on gray-scale imaging (**Fig. 21**A). The false lumen of the dissected artery is commonly thrombosed and can present as asymmetric thickening of the artery (see **Fig. 21**B, C). The true lumen of the dissected artery may be markedly narrowed with associated increased PSVs at this level (see **Fig. 21**D).

Median Arcuate Ligament Syndrome

Median arcuate ligament syndrome (MALS) is an entity that is characterized by a fibrous band that crosses the diaphragmatic crura at the level of the aortic hiatus. This band lies anterior to the celiac artery and can cause significant compression and stenosis of the celiac trunk on expiration. As a result of this compression during expiration, the PSVs within the origin/proximal segments of the celiac artery are markedly increased with posterior displacement of the celiac artery. The typical hooklike appearance of the celiac trunk during expiration is pathognomonic for diagnosis of MALS (**Fig. 22**A, B). Poststenotic dilatation may be present distal to the site of compression. Flow in the celiac trunk normalizes during inspiration, but chronic compression of the celiac artery by the MAL may produce a fixed stenosis with an increased PSV that persists with inspiration (see **Fig. 22**C–F).[69,70]

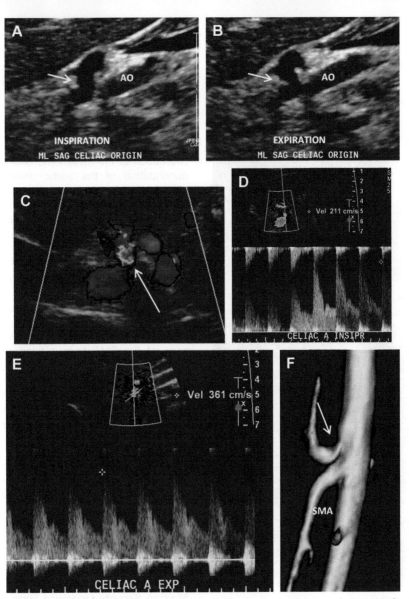

Fig. 22. MALS. A 35-year-old man with postprandial abdominal pain. Sagittal gray-scale images obtained on inspiration (*A*) and expiration (*B*) show a characteristic fish-hook pattern with retraction of the celiac artery on expiration (*arrow*). (*C*) Aliasing is noted in the origin/proximal celiac artery on color Doppler image (*arrow*). (*D, E*) Corresponding spectral Doppler images show increase in the PSV in the proximal celiac artery on expiration (*E*). (*F*) 3D volume-rendered MR angiogram shows narrowing (*arrow*) and compression of the proximal celiac artery.

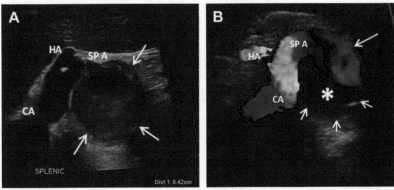

Fig. 23. Splenic artery aneurysm in a 43-year-old man with history of fibromuscular dysplasia. (*A*) Transverse gray-scale image at the level of the celiac artery (CA) shows a large (up to 3.6 cm) partially thrombosed splenic artery aneurysm (SP A). (*B*) Transverse color Doppler image outlining the aneurysmal sac (*short arrows*). Swirling flow (or pseudo–yin-yang sign) is present within the patent part of the aneurysm (*long arrow*). Part of the aneurysm is thrombosed (*asterisk*). HA, common hepatic artery.

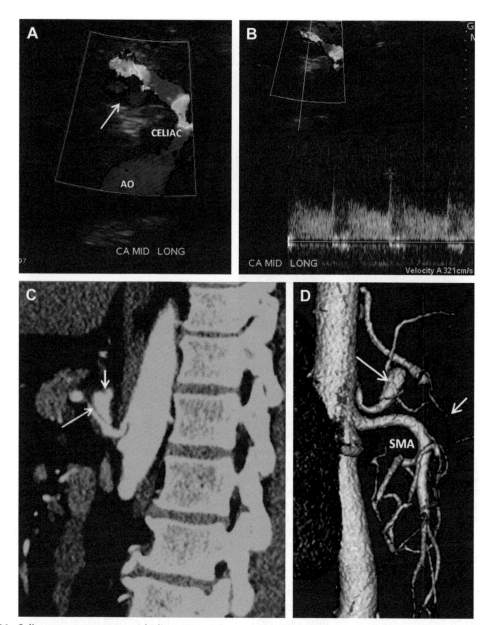

Fig. 24. Celiac artery aneurysm with dissection. Color and pulsed Doppler images show swirling flow within the dissected aneurysm of the celiac artery (*arrow, A*) and increased PSVs in the true lumen of the celiac artery (*B*). The dissection flap is not well seen. (*C*) The dissection flap was not well seen on the Doppler study but was more apparent on the contrast-enhanced CT angiogram (*long arrow, C*). Celiac artery aneurysm (*short arrow*) is association with the dissection flap (*long arrow*). (*D*) 3D volume-rendered CT angiogram reveals an aneurysmal celiac artery (*long arrow*). Note the patent gastroduodenal arcade providing collateral circulation to the celiac artery from the SMA (*short arrow*).

ANEURYSMS AND PSEUDOANEURYSMS OF THE MESENTERIC ARTERIES

Splanchnic artery aneurysms are an uncommon and potentially lethal clinical problem. Therefore it is important to recognize and diagnose these entities in order to facilitate clinical management.

Splanchnic artery aneurysms are most commonly seen in the hepatic, splenic, and celiac arteries. Aneurysms of the pancreatoduodenal, gastroduodenal, SMA and IMA are very rare.[71] Splanchnic artery aneurysms can develop as a result of atherosclerotic disease, a congenital anomaly, or a genetic disease. These aneurysms commonly

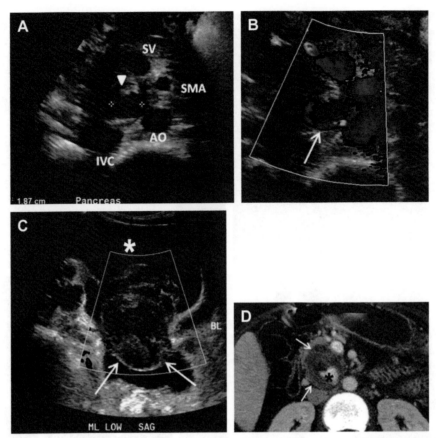

Fig. 25. Ruptured pseudoaneurysm of the inferior pancreatoduodenal artery in a patient with chronic pancreatitis and hematocrit reduction. (*A*) Gray-scale transverse image through the pancreatic area reveals a 1.87-cm complex cystic structure (*arrowhead*) medial to the inferior vena cava (IVC) and lateral to the aorta (AO) and posterior to the splenic vein (SV). (*B*) Yin-yang flow pattern (*arrow*) is present within the structure on color Doppler image. (*C*) Color Doppler image of the lower abdomen shows ascites (*asterisk*) with extensive heterogeneous avascular fluid collection compatible with a retroperitoneal hemorrhage from a ruptured pseudoaneurysm (*arrows*). (*D*) Corresponding contrast-enhanced CT image shows a partially thrombosed pseudoaneurysm (*black arrows*) of the inferior pancreatoduodenal artery with contrast filling the patent part of the pseudoaneurysmal sac (*asterisk*).

present with nonspecific abdominal pain and half of them result in rupture, which for the most part is caused by failure to consider the diagnosis. No established criteria exist to guide their management. The aneurysm can be treated with endovascular embolization or stenting, or it can be surgically resected. Saccular-type and more distal mesenteric aneurysms are more amenable to surgical resection. On ultrasonography, they may be seen as focal dilatation of the vessel lumen and may show a pseudo–yin-yang sign on color Doppler imaging (**Figs. 23** and **24**).

Mesenteric pseudoaneurysms are most commonly seen in the setting of abdominal blunt trauma, infectious/inflammatory processes such as pancreatitis, or they may be iatrogenic (for example, following a biopsy). They are false aneurysms and represent a contained arterial rupture

with injury to 2 or more layers of the arterial wall. On gray-scale imaging, they may be seen as cystic structures with or without mural thrombus. On color Doppler imaging, a yin-yang sign may be seen, but this sign may not be apparent in the case of thrombosis or very slow flow (**Fig. 25**). On rare occasions, the neck of the pseudoaneurysm may also be identified, showing to-and-fro flow on spectral Doppler imaging. Pseudoaneurysms may also present following rupture, with the detection of heterogeneous complex fluid/clot in the peritoneum (see **Fig. 25**). When hemoperitoneum is present, a careful and thorough evaluation of the vascular structures should be performed.

Doppler ultrasonography plays an important role in the evaluation and management of diseases of the aorta and mesenteric arteries. Ultrasonography has proven value in the detection and follow-up of

AAAs. It also can be used in the evaluation of complications following endovascular repair of aortic aneurysms. Ultrasonography is also useful in the detection of mesenteric arterial disease in the setting of chronic mesenteric ischemia and may also detect other abnormalities, including dissection, occlusion, and pseudoaneurysm.

REFERENCES

1. Fisher DF Jr, Fry WJ. Collateral mesenteric circulation [review]. Surg Gynecol Obstet 1987;164(5): 487–92.
2. Bluth EI, LoCascio L. Ultrasonic evaluation of the abdominal aorta. Echocardiography 1996;13: 197–206.
3. Fraser KH, Meagher S, Blake JR, et al. Characterization of an abdominal aortic velocity waveform in patients with abdominal aortic aneurysm. Ultrasound Med Biol 2008;34:73–80.
4. Wilson N, Goldberg SJ, Dickinson DF, et al. Normal intracardiac and great artery blood velocity measurements by pulsed Doppler echocardiography. Br Heart J 1985;53:451–8.
5. Van Bel F, Van Zwieten PH, Guit GL, et al. Superior mesenteric artery blood flow velocity and estimated volume flow: duplex Doppler US study of preterm and term neonates. Radiology 1990;174: 165–9.
6. Lewis BD, James EM. Current applications of duplex and color Doppler ultrasound imaging: abdomen. Mayo Clin Proc 1989;64:1158–69.
7. Jager K, Bollinger A, Valli C, et al. Measurement of mesenteric blood flow by duplex scanning. J Vasc Surg 1986;3:462–9.
8. Cotran RS. Blood vessels. In: Cotran RS, editor. Robbins pathologic basis of disease. Philadelphia: WB Saunders; 1999. p. 493–541, xv.
9. Stary HC. Natural history and histological classification of atherosclerotic lesions: an update. Arterioscler Thromb Vasc Biol 2000;20:1177–8.
10. Holman RL, Mc GH Jr, Strong JP, et al. The natural history of atherosclerosis: the early aortic lesions as seen in New Orleans in the middle of the 20th century. Am J Pathol 1958;34:209–35.
11. Strong JP, Malcom GT, McMahan CA, et al. Prevalence and extent of atherosclerosis in adolescents and young adults: implications for prevention from the Pathobiological Determinants of Atherosclerosis in Youth Study. JAMA 1999;281:727–35.
12. Sensier Y, Bell PR, London NJ. The ability of qualitative assessment of the common femoral Doppler waveform to screen for significant aortoiliac disease. Eur J Vasc Endovasc Surg 1998;15: 357–64.
13. Shaalan WE, French-Sherry E, Castilla M, et al. Reliability of common femoral artery hemodynamics in assessing the severity of aortoiliac inflow disease. J Vasc Surg 2003;37:960–9.
14. Polak JF. Ultrasound assessment of the abdominal aorta. In: Pellerito JS, editor. Introduction to vascular ultrasonography. Philadelphia: Elsevier/Saunders; 2012. p. 450–65. xviii.
15. Audet P, Therasse E, Oliva VL, et al. Infrarenal aortic stenosis: long-term clinical and hemodynamic results of percutaneous transluminal angioplasty. Radiology 1998;209:357–63.
16. Grimshaw GM, Thompson JM. Changes in diameter of the abdominal aorta with age: an epidemiological study. J Clin Ultrasound 1997;25:7–13.
17. Pedersen OM, Aslaksen A, Vik-Mo H. Ultrasound measurement of the luminal diameter of the abdominal aorta and iliac arteries in patients without vascular disease. J Vasc Surg 1993;17: 596–601.
18. Lederle FA, Johnson GR, Wilson SE, et al. Prevalence and associations of abdominal aortic aneurysm detected through screening. Aneurysm Detection and Management (ADAM) Veterans Affairs Cooperative Study Group. Ann Intern Med 1997;126:441–9.
19. Reed D, Reed C, Stemmermann G, et al. Are aortic aneurysms caused by atherosclerosis? Circulation 1992;85:205–11.
20. Bihari P, Shelke A, Nwe TH, et al. Strain measurement of abdominal aortic aneurysm with real-time 3D ultrasound speckle tracking. Eur J Vasc Endovasc Surg 2013;45:315–23.
21. Lederle FA, Wilson SE, Johnson GR, et al. Immediate repair compared with surveillance of small abdominal aortic aneurysms. N Engl J Med 2002; 346:1437–44.
22. Scott RAP, Tisi PV, Ashton HA, et al. Abdominal aortic aneurysm rupture rates: a 7-year follow-up of the entire abdominal aortic aneurysm population detected by screening. J Vasc Surg 1998;28:124–8.
23. Abd Elrazek E, Scott NB, Vohra A. An epidural scoring scale for arm movements (ESSAM) in patients receiving high thoracic epidural analgesia for coronary artery bypass grafting. Anaesthesia 1999;54:1104–9.
24. Brekken R, Bang J, Odegard A, et al. Strain estimation in abdominal aortic aneurysms from 2-D ultrasound. Ultrasound Med Biol 2006;32:33–42.
25. Long A, Rouet L, Bissery A, et al. Compliance of abdominal aortic aneurysms: evaluation of tissue Doppler imaging. Ultrasound Med Biol 2004;30: 1099–108.
26. O'Rourke MF, Staessen JA, Vlachopoulos C, et al. Clinical applications of arterial stiffness; definitions and reference values. Am J Hypertens 2002;15: 426–44.
27. Wilson KA, Lee AJ, Lee AJ, et al. The relationship between aortic wall distensibility and rupture of

infrarenal abdominal aortic aneurysm. J Vasc Surg 2003;37:112–7.

28. Fillinger MF, Marra SP, Raghavan ML, et al. Prediction of rupture risk in abdominal aortic aneurysm during observation: wall stress versus diameter. J Vasc Surg 2003;37:724–32.

29. Brady AR, Thompson SG, Fowkes FG, et al, Participants UKSAT. Abdominal aortic aneurysm expansion: risk factors and time intervals for surveillance. Circulation 2004;110:16–21.

30. Egorova NN, Vouyouka AG, McKinsey JF, et al. Effect of gender on long-term survival after abdominal aortic aneurysm repair based on results from the Medicare national database. J Vasc Surg 2011;54:1–12.e16 [discussion: 11–2].

31. Sweeting MJ, Thompson SG, Brown LC, et al, Collaborators RESCAN. Meta-analysis of individual patient data to examine factors affecting growth and rupture of small abdominal aortic aneurysms. Br J Surg 2012;99:655–65.

32. Thompson SG, Brown LC, Sweeting MJ, et al. Systematic review and meta-analysis of the growth and rupture rates of small abdominal aortic aneurysms: implications for surveillance intervals and their cost-effectiveness. Health Technol Assess 2013; 17:1–118.

33. Lee TY, Korn P, Heller JA, et al. The cost-effectiveness of a "quick-screen" program for abdominal aortic aneurysms. Surgery 2002;132: 399–407.

34. Lederle FA. Ultrasonographic screening for abdominal aortic aneurysms. Ann Intern Med 2003;139:516–22.

35. Collaborators RESCAN, Sweeting MJ, Bown MJ, et al. Surveillance intervals for small abdominal aortic aneurysms. JAMA 2013;309:806–13.

36. Filardo G, Powell JT, Martinez MA, et al. Surgery for small asymptomatic abdominal aortic aneurysms. Cochrane Database Syst Rev 2012;(3):CD001835.

37. Walker DI, Bloor K, Williams G, et al. Inflammatory aneurysms of the abdominal aorta. Br J Surg 1972;59:609–14.

38. Chu P, Howden BP, Jones S, et al. Once bitten, twice shy: an unusual case report of a mycotic aortic aneurysm. ANZ J Surg 2005;75:1024–6.

39. Wanhainen A, Bjorck M, Boman K, et al. Influence of diagnostic criteria on the prevalence of abdominal aortic aneurysm. J Vasc Surg 2001; 34:229–35.

40. Johnston KW, Rutherford RB, Tilson MD, et al. Suggested standards for reporting on arterial aneurysms. Subcommittee on Reporting Standards for Arterial Aneurysms, Ad Hoc Committee on Reporting Standards, Society for Vascular Surgery and North American Chapter, International Society for Cardiovascular Surgery. J Vasc Surg 1991;13: 452–8.

41. McCarthy RJ, Shaw E, Whyman MR, et al. Recommendations for screening intervals for small aortic aneurysms. Br J Surg 2003;90:821–6.

42. Vega de Ceniga M, Gomez R, Estallo L, et al. Analysis of expansion patterns in 4-4.9 cm abdominal aortic aneurysms. Ann Vasc Surg 2008;22:37–44.

43. Vega de Ceniga M, Gomez R, Estallo L, et al. Growth rate and associated factors in small abdominal aortic aneurysms. Eur J Vasc Endovasc Surg 2006;31:231–6.

44. Catalano O, Siani A. Ruptured abdominal aortic aneurysm: categorization of sonographic findings and report of 3 new signs. J Ultrasound Med 2005;24:1077–83.

45. Greenhalgh RM, Brown LC, Kwong GP, et al, EVAR trial participants. Comparison of endovascular aneurysm repair with open repair in patients with abdominal aortic aneurysm (EVAR trial 1), 30-day operative mortality results: randomised controlled trial. Lancet 2004;364:843–8.

46. Thurnher S, Cejna M. Imaging of aortic stent-grafts and endoleaks. Radiol Clin North Am 2002;40:799–833.

47. Wolf YG, Johnson BL, Hill BB, et al. Duplex ultrasound scanning versus computed tomographic angiography for postoperative evaluation of endovascular abdominal aortic aneurysm repair. J Vasc Surg 2000;32:1142–8.

48. Zarins CK, Crabtree T, Bloch DA, et al. Endovascular aneurysm repair at 5 years: does aneurysm diameter predict outcome? J Vasc Surg 2006;44: 920–9 [discussion: 929–31].

49. Zannetti S, De Rango P, Parente B, et al. Role of duplex scan in endoleak detection after endoluminal abdominal aortic aneurysm repair. Eur J Vasc Endovasc Surg 2000;19:531–5.

50. Maldonado TS, Rockman CB, Riles E, et al. Ischemic complications after endovascular abdominal aortic aneurysm repair. J Vasc Surg 2004;40:703–9 [discussion: 709–10].

51. Cochennec F, Becquemin JP, Desgranges P, et al. Limb graft occlusion following EVAR: clinical pattern, outcomes and predictive factors of occurrence. Eur J Vasc Endovasc Surg 2007;34:59–65.

52. Hagan PG, Nienaber CA, Isselbacher EM, et al. The International Registry of Acute Aortic Dissection (IRAD): new insights into an old disease. JAMA 2000;283:897–903.

53. Pretre R, Von Segesser LK. Aortic dissection. Lancet 1997;349:1461–4.

54. Bresnihan ER, Keates PG. Ultrasound and dissection of the abdominal aorta. Clin Radiol 1980;31: 105–8.

55. Clevert DA, Rupp N, Reiser M, et al. Improved diagnosis of vascular dissection by ultrasound B-flow: a comparison with color-coded Doppler

and power Doppler sonography. Eur Radiol 2005; 15:342–7.

56. Risse JH, Vorwerk D, Speckamp F, et al. Color-coded duplex ultrasound in chronic dissecting abdominal aortic aneurysm. Differentiation between true and false aortic lumen with reference to the blood supply to larger abdominal arteries. Radiologe 1995;35:759–66 [in German].

57. Thomas JH, Blake K, Pierce GE, et al. The clinical course of asymptomatic mesenteric arterial stenosis. J Vasc Surg 1998;27:840–4.

58. Zwolak RM. Can duplex ultrasound replace arteriography in screening for mesenteric ischemia? Semin Vasc Surg 1999;12:252–60.

59. Harward TR, Smith S, Seeger JM. Detection of celiac axis and superior mesenteric artery occlusive disease with use of abdominal duplex scanning. J Vasc Surg 1993;17:738–45.

60. Moneta GL. Screening for mesenteric vascular insufficiency and follow-up of mesenteric artery bypass procedures. Semin Vasc Surg 2001;14:186–92.

61. Lim HK, Lee WJ, Kim SH, et al. Splanchnic arterial stenosis or occlusion: diagnosis at Doppler US. Radiology 1999;211:405–10.

62. Moneta GL, Yeager RA, Dalman R, et al. Duplex ultrasound criteria for diagnosis of splanchnic artery stenosis or occlusion. J Vasc Surg 1991;14:511–8 [discussion: 518–20].

63. Perko MJ, Just S, Schroeder TV. Importance of diastolic velocities in the detection of celiac and mesenteric artery disease by duplex ultrasound. J Vasc Surg 1997;26:288–93.

64. Pellerito JS, Revzin MV, Tsang JC, et al. Doppler sonographic criteria for the diagnosis of inferior mesenteric artery stenosis. J Ultrasound Med 2009;28:641–50.

65. Healy DA, Neumyer MM, Atnip RG, et al. Evaluation of celiac and mesenteric vascular disease with duplex ultrasonography. J Ultrasound Med 1992; 11:481–5.

66. Subhas G, Gupta A, Nawalany M, et al. Spontaneous isolated superior mesenteric artery dissection: a case report and literature review with management algorithm. Ann Vasc Surg 2009;23: 788–98.

67. Dushnitsky T, Peer A, Katzenelson L, et al. Dissecting aneurysm of the superior mesenteric artery: flow dynamics by color Doppler sonography. J Ultrasound Med 1998;17:781–3.

68. Yun W, Kim Y, Park K, et al. Clinical and angiographic follow-up of spontaneous isolated superior mesenteric artery dissection. Eur J Vasc Endovasc Surg 2009;37:572–7.

69. Wolfman D, Bluth EI, Sossaman J. Median arcuate ligament syndrome. J Ultrasound Med 2003;22: 1377–80.

70. Lynch K. Celiac artery compression syndrome: a literature review. J Diagn Med Sonogr 2014;30: 143–8.

71. Shanley CJ, Shah NL, Messina LM. Uncommon splanchnic artery aneurysms: pancreaticoduodenal, gastroduodenal, superior mesenteric, inferior mesenteric, and colic. Ann Vasc Surg 1996;10: 506–15.

Sonography of the Bowel

Stephanie R. Wilson, MD[a,b,*], Kerri L. Novak, MD, FRCPC[b]

KEYWORDS

- Ultrasound • Crohn disease • Appendicitis

KEY POINTS

- Ultrasound (US) is a safe, radiation-free, and noninvasive method of imaging the bowel.
- The high-resolution capability of US allows for superior visualization of bowel wall layers and pathology without requirement for contrast injection or other specialized techniques.
- The dynamic real-time capability of US allows for assessment of bowel content, caliber, and motion, improving particularly the prediction of bowel obstruction.
- Meta-analysis shows equivalent accuracy of US to computed tomography and magnetic resonance scan for the detection and diagnosis of inflammatory bowel disease.
- In this era of radiation and cost awareness, US should be a first choice for the evaluation of patients with inflammatory bowel disease and acute abdomen of other causes.

Videos of CD of Neoterminal ileum (NTI), CD of sigmoid colon, incomplete mechanical bowel obstruction, enetero-enteric fistula shown between the thick abnormal terminal ileum in cross-section, perianal fistula shown on transperineal scan, normal and perforated appendix scans accompany this article at http://www.ultrasound.theclinics.com/

INTRODUCTION

The benefits of superb spatial and temporal resolution, which have allowed ultrasound (US) to perform so well in the evaluation of the abdominal and pelvic solid organs, have not been widely shared for the evaluation of the bowel wherein concerns regarding gas artifacts and a fear of unsuccessful examinations have altered its acceptance. These beliefs are inaccurate and today there is keen awareness of radiation risk from computed tomography (CT) scan and cost of imaging tests, both of which have allowed a revival of interest in US of the bowel. This situation is excellent because US has incredible benefits for gut evaluation in multiple different clinical situations, described here.

The Gut Signature

The gut is a continuous hollow tube with *4 concentric layers* (**Fig. 1**). From the lumen outward, they are mucosa, submucosa, muscularis propria, and the serosa or adventitia. These histologic layers correspond with the sonographic appearance, as depicted in **Fig. 2**: the *gut signature*, where up to *5 layers* may be visualized. The sonographic layers appear alternately echogenic and hypoechoic: the first, third, and fifth layers are echogenic; the second and fourth layers are hypoechoic. Only US allows for routine resolution of the gut wall layers without the addition of contrast enhancement. In addition to its location, there are other morphologic features that allow recognition of specific portions of the gut, including the gastric rugae,

Disclosure: None.
[a] Department of Radiology, University of Calgary, 2500 University Drive Northwest, Calgary, AB T2N 1N4, Canada; [b] Division of Gastroenterology, Department of Medicine, University of Calgary, Calgary, AB T2N 1N4, Canada
* Corresponding author. Foothills Medical Centre, 1403 29th Street Northwest, Calgary, AB T2N 2T9, Canada.
E-mail address: stephanie.wilson@albertahealthservices.ca

Ultrasound Clin 9 (2014) 751–773
http://dx.doi.org/10.1016/j.cult.2014.07.008
1556-858X/14/$ – see front matter © 2014 Elsevier Inc. All rights reserved.

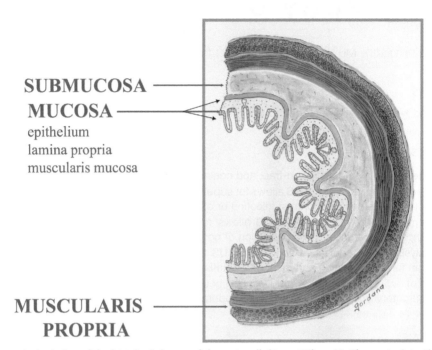

SUBMUCOSA

MUCOSA
epithelium
lamina propria
muscularis mucosa

MUSCULARIS PROPRIA

Fig. 1. Schematic depiction of the histologic layers of the gut wall. (*From* Wilson SR. The gastrointestinal tract. In: Rumack CR, Wilson SR, Charboneau JW, et al, editors. Diagnostic ultrasound. Philadelphia: Elsevier Mosby; 2011. p. 262; with permission.)

the valvulae conniventes, and the colonic haustrations (**Fig. 3**).

A tremendous unique benefit of sonography is its *real-time capability*, allowing for dynamic assessment of the status of the bowel, including its content, its caliber, and its motility, all of which may change with disease.

Gut Wall Pathology

Evaluation of thickened gut on sonography is far superior to the evaluation of normal gut for 2 important reasons. Thick gut, particularly if associated with abnormality of the perienteric soft tissues, creates a *"mass effect,"* which is easily seen on US. In addition, thickened gut is frequently relatively *gasless*, improving its sonographic evaluation. Recognized early was the association of gut pathology with characteristic sonographic appearances, especially the *target pattern*,[1] also described as a *pseudokidney sign*,[2] whereby the hypoechoic external rim corresponds to thickened gut wall, and the echogenic center relates to residual gut lumen or mucosal ulceration (**Fig. 4**), correctly denoting abnormal bowel in more than 90% of cases.

Identification of *thickened gut on sonography* may suggest a benign or malignant process. *Benignancy* is favored by long segment involvement with concentric thickening and wall layer preservation.

The classic benign pathology showing gut wall thickening is Crohn disease (CD). *Malignancy* is favored by short segment involvement with eccentric disease and wall layer destruction. The classic malignant pathology showing gut wall thickening is adenocarcinoma of the stomach or colon.

Gut wall masses, as distinct from thickened gut wall, may be intraluminal, mural, or exophytic, all with or without ulceration (**Fig. 5**). *Intraluminal gut masses* are mucosal and the most difficult because they may be hidden by gas or luminal content. In contrast, gut pathology creating an *exophytic mass* without or with mucosal involvement or ulceration may form masses that are more readily visualized, including most carcinoids and gastrointestinal stromal (GIST) tumors.

Technique

Routine sonograms of the gut are best performed following an *overnight fast*. In urgent or acute situations, the scan may be performed without any prior preparation. A *real-time survey* of the entire abdomen is first performed with a 3.5- to 5-MHz transducer and obvious masses or gut signatures are observed. The pelvis is scanned before and after bladder emptying. Areas of interest then receive detailed analysis, including *compression sonography* (**Fig. 6**),[3] using high-frequency, 5- to 9-MHz, linear or convex linear probes. Normal

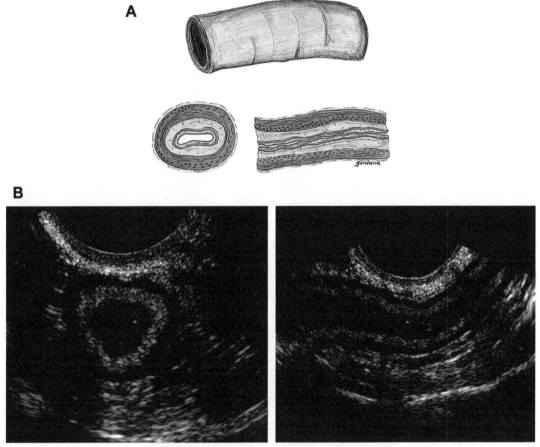

Fig. 2. Gut signature. Top (*A*), schematic, and bottom (*B*), corresponding US in a patient with mild gut thickening from CD. Blue layers, representing the muscle, are black or hypoechoic on the sonogram. Yellow layers, representing the submucosa and the superficial mucosa, are hyperechoic. There is a small amount of fluid and air in the gut lumen on the sonogram. (*From* Wilson SR. The gastrointestinal tract. In: Rumack CR, Wilson SR, Charboneau JW, et al, editors. Diagnostic ultrasound. Philadelphia: Elsevier Mosby; 2011. p. 263; with permission.)

gut will be compressed, and gas pockets displaced away from the region of interest. In contrast, thickened abnormal loops of bowel and/or obstructed noncompressible loops will remain unchanged. In women, *transvaginal sonography* is invaluable for evaluation of the portions of the gut within the true pelvis, most particularly the rectum and sigmoid colon and, in some, the ileum and appendix.

Blood Flow Evaluation of the Gut Wall

Normal gut shows little signal on conventional *color Doppler* because interrogation is difficult in a normal and mobile bowel loop. Both neoplasia and inflammatory disease show increased vascularity when compared with the normal gut wall, whereas ischemic[4] and edematous gut tends to be relatively hypovascular. Historically, these subjective assessments have been made with color Doppler imaging (CDI). Today, however, the use of contrast-enhanced ultrasound (CEUS) improves performance by showing blood flow to the perfusion level.

Gastrointestinal Neoplasms

The role of sonography in the evaluation of gastrointestinal tract neoplasms is similar to that of CT scan. Visualization is rarely obtained in early mucosal lesions or with small intramural nodules, whereas tumors growing to produce an exophytic mass, a thickened segment of gut with or without ulceration, or a sizable intraluminal mass may all be seen. Sonograms are frequently performed early in the diagnostic workup of patients with gastrointestinal tract tumors, often before their initial identification. Vague abdominal symptoms, abdominal pain, a palpable abdominal mass, and anemia are common indications for these scans.

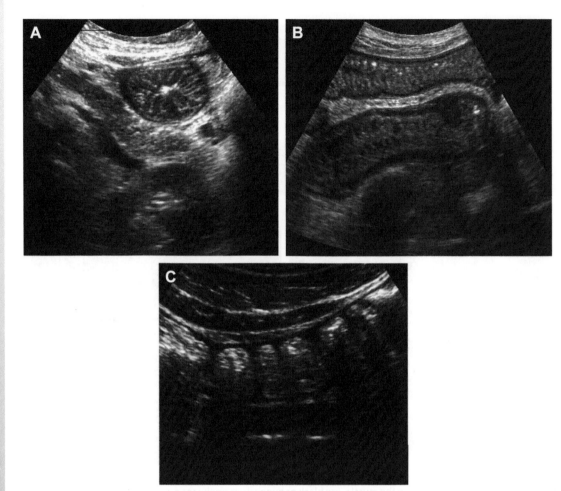

Fig. 3. Gut recognition. (*A*) Cross-sectional views of the stomach show normal gastric rugae. The collapsed stomach shows variable wall thickness. (*B*) Valvulae conniventes of the small bowel, more easily seen when there is fluid in the lumen of the bowel or if the valvulae are edematous. (*C*) Appearance of the colonic haustrations. (*From* Wilson SR. The gastrointestinal tract. In: Rumack CR, Wilson SR, Charboneau JW, et al, editors. Diagnostic ultrasound. Philadelphia: Elsevier Mosby; 2011. p. 264; with permission.)

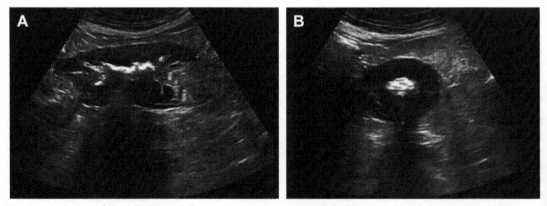

Fig. 4. Lymphoma of the small bowel shows a "target" or "psueudokidney" sign in (*A*), long axis, and (*B*), cross-section. There are no wall layers shown. The black rim is the tumor and the white center is the residual lumen.

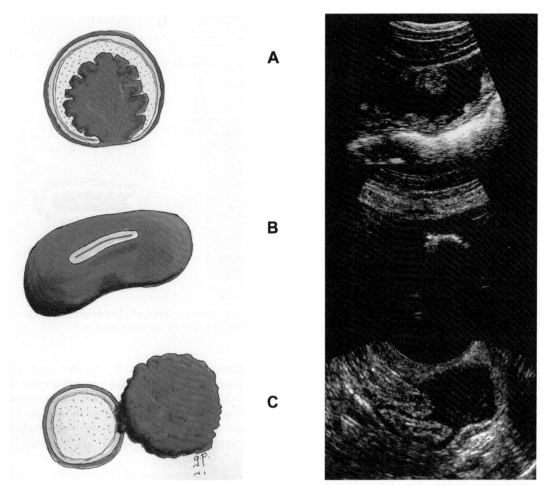

Fig. 5. Gut wall pathology. Schematic of sonographic appearances with sonographic equivalents. (*A*) Intraluminal mass. Inflammatory pseudopolyp on sonogram. (*B*) Pseudokidney sign with symmetric wall thickening and wall layer destruction. Carcinoma of the colon on sonogram. (*C*) Exophytic mass. Serosal seed on visceral peritoneum of the gut on sonogram. (*From* Wilson SR. The bowel wall looks thickened: what does that mean? In: Cooperberg PL, editor. Radiologic Society of North America categorical course syllabus. Chicago: RSNA; 2002. p. 265; with permission.)

Appreciation of the typical morphologies associated with gastrointestinal tract neoplasia may lead to accurate recognition, localization, and diagnosis. While performing careful evaluation of the bowel, incidental masses related to the gut wall are encountered with some regularity. Some of these masses may be small and include GIST and carcinoid tumors, in particular.

INFLAMMATORY BOWEL DISEASE
The Clinical Story

Inflammatory bowel disease (IBD) is a *chronic, idiopathic disease* characterized by a fluctuating course of relapses and periods of remission. Although dysregulation of the immune system is the key to pathogenesis of IBD, the underlying pathophysiology is largely unknown.[5] There are

2 major constituent disorders, *ulcerative colitis (UC)* and *CD*. UC primarily affects the mucosal layer of the colon, whereas CD is an asymmetric, transmural inflammatory disease that can affect any portion of the gastrointestinal tract, characteristically in skip lesion pattern, and showing a predilection for the distal small bowel. Complications of UC are uncommon, while CD is notoriously complex, resulting in a high surgical rate from penetrating or fibrostenotic disease. IBD has a predilection for developed, northern climates and low incidence in the southern hemisphere.[6–8] High rates of disease are present in both Canada and the United States.

The peak *age of onset* of CD is between 20 and 29 years.[9] Before biologic therapy, more than 80% of patients with CD required surgery.[10] *Predictors of severe disease* in addition to young age of onset

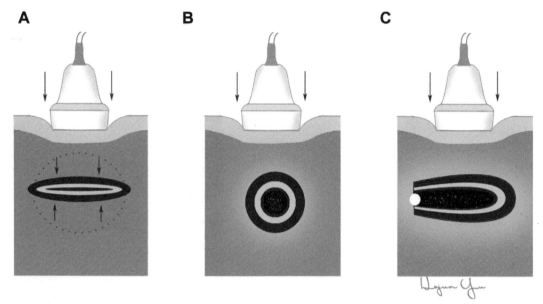

Fig. 6. Compression sonography, schematic depiction. (*A*) Normal gut is compressed. (*B*) Abnormally thickened gut or (*C*) an obstructed loop, such as that seen in acute appendicitis, will be noncompressible.

(less than 40 years) include perianal disease, smoking, extraintestinal manifestations, and the initial requirement of glucocorticoid treatment.[11,12]

Optimizing *medical management* of patients with IBD is paramount given the high likelihood of disease progression and complication without bowel-preserving therapies.[13] The *aim of medical management* is to move beyond symptoms and alter disease course. Complete mucosal healing is the aim of therapy, which is a proven surrogate of improved outcome.[14,15]

Diagnosis and Monitoring of IBD

The demand for methods to safely and effectively diagnose and monitor patients with CD is very high. *Endoscopy* remains the gold standard; however, it is invasive, with consequent risks and need for patient preparation. As neither clinical symptoms or absence of, nor laboratory indicators of, inflammation consistently reflect disease activity,[16,17] the recognition of the necessity for safe and effective imaging to monitor disease activity is paramount today. *Recurrent use of CT* poses possible increased malignancy risk given cumulative ionizing radiation exposure.[18–21] Magnetic resonance (MR) imaging is a very good method for the evaluation of the bowel but is both expensive and relatively inaccessible in many jurisdictions.

US evaluation provides a safe and accurate method of diagnosing and monitoring IBD.[22–25] A large prospective study of patients with inflammatory symptoms by Parente and colleagues[26] showed a positive predictive value for diagnosing CD of 98%. A recent meta-analysis comparing diagnostic modalities showed no significant difference in accuracy with high sensitivity and specificity of US versus CT and MR scan.[27]

Sonography of IBD

The demand for diagnostic imaging in patients with CD is very high, not just for initial diagnosis but for monitoring disease activity, response to therapy, and detection of complications. The challenge of scanning patients with IBD is considerable because symptoms do not correlate with disease activity, and the use of anti-inflammatory drugs may alter presentation. Scanning with IBD presents significant challenge in the total assessment of these patients, as does the complexity of the imaging related to the myriad of possible complications. Therefore, a general heightened search for every possible observation in all patients with IBD is a good "guiding rule."

CD is a chronic, transmural inflammatory process. Thus, in addition to gut wall thickening, changes in the perienteric soft tissue are an expectation. It most commonly affects the terminal ileum and the colon, although any portion of the gut may be involved. Grossly, the gut wall in CD is typically thick and rigid with secondary luminal narrowing. Discrete or continuous ulcers and deep fissures are characteristic, frequently leading to fistula formation. Mesenteric lymph node enlargement and matting of involved loops are common. The mesentery may be markedly thickened and fatty, creeping over the edges of the gut to the antimesenteric border. Perianal disease is also commonly included in the evaluation. From this unique gross pathology, CD provides the major source of patients with IBD referred for an imaging examination. Sonography is an ideal cross-sectional imaging modality because it offers invaluable additional information not only about the gut wall, but also about the adjacent lymph nodes, mesentery, and regional soft tissues.

CLASSIC FEATURES OF IBD
Gut Wall Thickening

Gut wall thickening is the most frequently observed abnormality in patients with CD and its demonstration on sonography is the basis for diagnosis,[28] detection of recurrence, and determining the extent of disease. Observations include the length of thickened bowel and its maximal thickness measured from the luminal surface to the serosa. Involved segments vary from a few millimeters to many centimeters in length. Wall thickness is often considerable, ranging from 5 to 9 mm in most cases, but measuring as much as 1.5 cm in others. The threshold for suggestion of abnormal thickening is variously established at either 3 or 4 mm, with expected variation in sensitivity and specificity.[22–25] The thickened gut should also be evaluated for *gut wall morphology* including *wall layer retention* (**Fig. 7**, Video 1), seen most often in uncomplicated CD, or *wall layer destruction* (**Fig. 8**, Video 2), associated most often with disease of marked acuity. Interobserver agreement in assessing bowel wall thickness can be high ($\kappa = 0.71–1.0$), despite claims US of the bowel lacks standardization.[23] Long-standing and often burnt-out disease may also show subtle wall thickening with fat deposition in the submucosa, which shows an increased echogenicity of this layer (**Fig. 9**). Skip areas are frequent.

The *margination* or definition of the outer bowel wall is also assessed. In most uncomplicated cases, the bowel wall is sharply defined and well differentiated from the surrounding perienteric fat. However, with marked disease acuity, the margin of the gut becomes serrated or appears spiky (**Fig. 10**) as the transmural inflammatory process spreads to involve the perienteric soft tissues. The observation of this *spiculated border* heralds imminent bowel perforation and subsequent perienteric phlegmonous change.

The real-time assessment of the gut for wall thickening should also include assessment of its *compliance*. Normal or mildly abnormal bowel is typically very compliant, showing frequent peristalsis and easy compressibility. Conversely, actively involved gut typically appears rigid and fixed with decreased or absent peristalsis and compressibility.

Inflammatory Fat

Inflammatory fat is a characteristic feature of CD and produces an echogenic halolike "mass effect" that may creep over the border of the abnormal gut or completely engulf it (**Fig. 11**).

Lymphadenopathy

Tender and enlarged *mesenteric* and *perienteric* lymph nodes are common features of active Crohn inflammation. Lymph nodes appear as focal hypoechoic masses circumferentially surrounding the gut and in the expected location of their

A

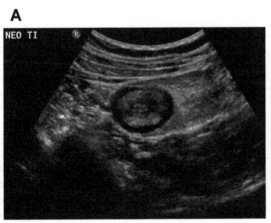

B

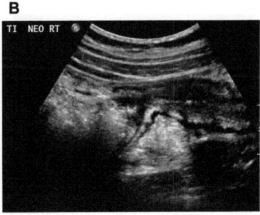

Fig. 7. Thick bowel wall in CD, with wall layer retention. (*A*) Axial and (*B*) long-axis views of the neoterminal ileum show thickening of the bowel wall. The long axis shows luminal apposition on the right side of the image and a gas distended lumen on the left, suggestive of an element of stricture.

A   **B**

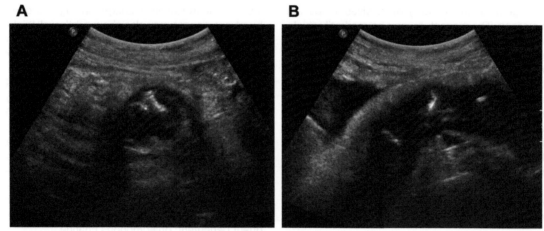

Fig. 8. Thick bowel wall in CD, with complete wall layer destruction, consistent with severe subacute inflammation. (*A*) Axial and (*B*) long-axis views of the terminal ileum show thick black bowel wall with virtually no layers. The bright echogenic foci within the thick wall represent air pockets within deep ulcerations, which extend virtually to the outer margin of the bowel wall.

mesenteric attachment. Nodes are frequently quite round and typically lose their normal linear echogenic streak from the nodal hilum and their reniform shape.

Hyperemia

Neoangiogenesis of the bowel wall is a recognized association of inflammation.[29,30] Therefore, mural blood flow is interpreted as reflective of disease activity, becoming a useful tool to monitor inflammation and response to therapy.

Doppler

Highly sensitive color Doppler allows for evaluation of blood flow involving especially larger blood vessels with relatively rapid blood flow.[31]

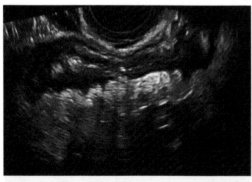

Fig. 9. Spiculation of the border of the bowel wall reflects severe transmural involvement of the serosa and perienteric fat. This long-axis view of the terminal ileum shows spiky projections from the border of the bowel projecting into the inflammatory fat.

Hyperemia, or increased mural blood flow, as detected by color-power Doppler, has been shown to correlate with inflammatory activity (see **Fig. 11**).[32] Larger mesenteric vessel flow is also altered with disease activity, evident with color Doppler.[33]

CEUS

CEUS is performed with the intravenous injection of microbubble contrast agents imaged with specialized US techniques. Evidence suggests US with contrast enhancement is accurate in evaluating blood flow at the perfusion level,[34–37] adding incredible potential for quantification and thus standardization of measures of inflammation.[38] Currently, these agents are not approved for use in evaluation of the bowel in Canada or the United States and are used off-label (**Fig. 12**).[39]

Complications of CD

Sonography is established as an accurate method for the detection of inevitable complications in CD.[40,41] Although these complications may be part of a clinical exacerbation, they may also occur silently in patients who are unaware of their presence.

Strictures

Strictures relate to rigid narrowing of the gut lumen, fixed luminal apposition (**Fig. 13**), and *fixed acute angulations* (**Fig. 14**). Luminal stenoses can be effectively detected by US,[40,41] possibly more accurately with use of color Doppler (**Fig. 15**).[42] In a population of CD from a tertiary referral center, Gasche and colleagues[43]

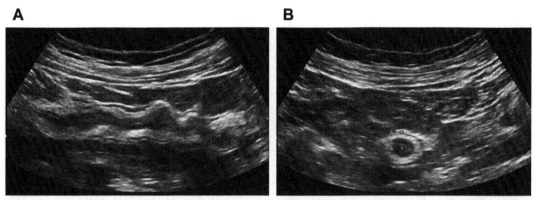

Fig. 10. Inflammatory fat infiltration into the submucosa of the bowel wall increases the echogenicity of the submucosal layer as shown here on (*A*) axial and (*B*) long-axis views of the terminal ileum, occurring most often in chronic long-standing disease.

illustrated 100% sensitivity in detecting strictures, proven intraoperatively. The luminal surfaces of involved segments of the gut most often appear to be in fixed constant apposition, with the lumen appearing as a linear echogenic central linearity within a thickened gut loop. Identification of fixed acute angulations is always of great concern and is a predictor of future obstructive possibilities. Stricture related to segmental active disease shows classic features of gut wall thickening with hyperemia, whereas a fibrotic stricture may show much less blood flow at the obstructive site.[44]

Mechanical Bowel Obstruction

Stricture with the development of incomplete mechanical bowel obstruction is the most frequent indication for surgery in patients with CD.

Occlusion of the gastrointestinal tract lumen in these circumstances is *mechanical*—where an actual physical impediment to the progression of the luminal content exists related in these patients to the intrinsic abnormalities of the gut wall associated with luminal narrowing.

Mechanical bowel obstruction is characterized by:

- Dilation of the intestinal tract proximal to the site of luminal occlusion
- Accumulation of large quantities of fluid and/or gas
- Hyperperistalsis as the gut attempts to pass the luminal content beyond the obstruction (Video 3).

Obstruction in IBD is generally incomplete and may be chronic. At the *transition point* of caliber

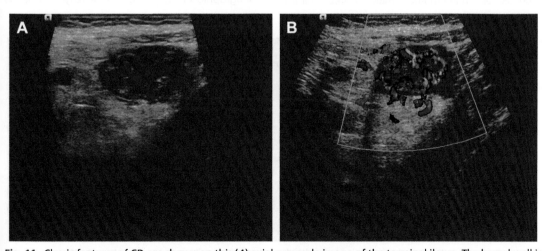

Fig. 11. Classic features of CD are shown on this (*A*) axial grayscale image of the terminal ileum. The bowel wall is thick. There is surrounding echogenic inflammatory fat, and a small perienteric lymph node is shown within the fat. (*B*) The addition of CDI shows vascularity of the bowel wall as a reflection of the active inflammation.

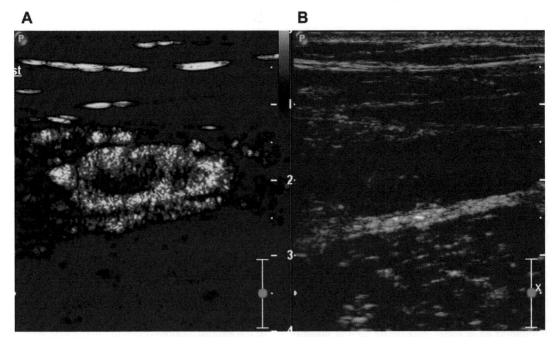

Fig. 12. CEUS of the bowel is shown on this image with the contrast shown on the left (*A*) and the low mechanical index grayscale image, for localization, on the right (*B*). CEUS shows transmural enhancement of the bowel wall.

variation, the observer should assess for segmental wall thickening and stricture, extrinsic masses such as abscesses, and fixed angulations.

Inflammatory Masses

Extraintestinal inflammatory masses are common complications of CD, although actual drainable pus occurs relatively infrequently. They can be very effectively identified on US.[25,43,45] A *phlegmon* is an inflammatory mass noted before

the stage of liquefaction and is evident as an ill-defined hypoechoic zone without fluid content within areas of inflamed fat. Acute angulations between the hypoechoic region and the fat are typical and predictive of a phlegmon as the inflammatory process dissects within the surrounding echogenic inflammatory fat. *Abscess* formation results in a complex or fluid-filled mass. Gas content within an abscess is both helpful in raising suspicion of an abscess and also a potential source of sonographic error, particularly if large quantities

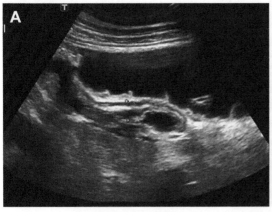
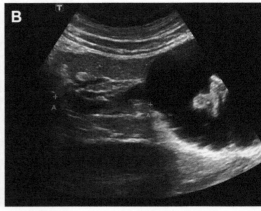

Fig. 13. Crohn complication: incomplete mechanical bowel obstruction is suggested on these 2 different aspects of the same region in a patient with bloating and pain. There is dilated bowel and an obvious transition to a loop with luminal surfaces in apposition and a thickened wall, measured in thickness in (*A*) and in length in (*B*).

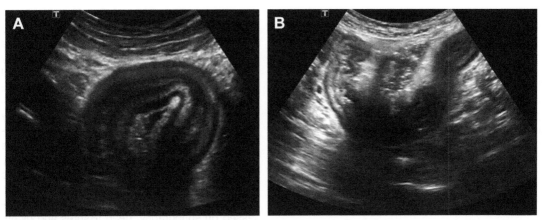

Fig. 14. Acute fixed angulations of the bowel are important observations because they are often identified before the development of mechanical obstruction. (*A*) Tight acute angulation of a thickened loop of terminal ileum and (*B*) in a different patient shows a more gradual and less alarming angulation of the ileum deep in the true pelvis.

are present. Abscesses may be intraperitoneal or extraperitoneal or may be in remote locations, such as the liver, the abdominal wall, or the psoas muscles.

Localized Perforation

Perforation is a frequently encountered complication of CD. Perforations do not occur freely into

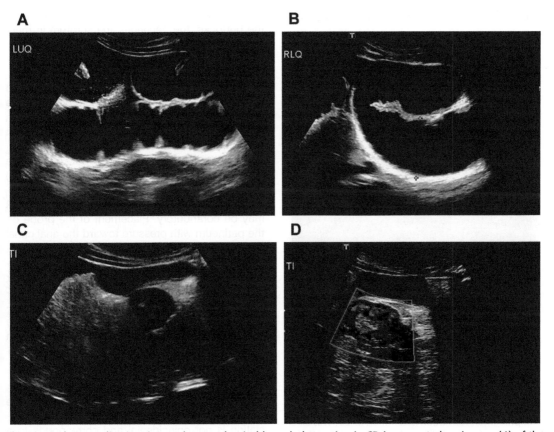

Fig. 15. Crohn complication: incomplete mechanical bowel obstruction in CD is suggested on images (*A*) of the left upper quadrant and (*B*) the right lower quadrant, both showing dilated fluid-filled loops of proximal small bowel. (*C*) Image of the terminal ileum shows thickening of the bowel wall, luminal apposition, and massive surrounding echogenic inflammatory fat. (*D*) Vascularity of the bowel wall on CDI, suggesting obstruction by an inflammatory hyperemic stricture of the terminal ileum.

the peritoneal cavity but have a tendency to be *localized*, seemingly walled off by the frequent inflammatory changes in the surrounding fat and mesentery. These localized perforations are often small and in some circumstances asymptomatic. If *extraluminal gas* is identified, a localized perforation should be suspected (**Fig. 16**). The gas appears as a bright echogenic focus with distal ring-down artifact. Localized perforations may occur anywhere in the abnormal bowel, although they have a predilection for the bowel at the proximal end of a stricture.

Fistula Formation

Fistulas are abnormal communications between epithelial surfaces and are a hallmark of CD. These fistulas often occur between loops of small bowel (enteroenteric) or between the small and large bowel (enterocolonic) (Video 4), as well as the bowel and skin (enterocutaneous). Other organs are less commonly affected, such as the bladder (enterovesical) and vagina (enterovaginal). This process is intrinsically related to transmural inflammation and occurs most commonly at the proximal

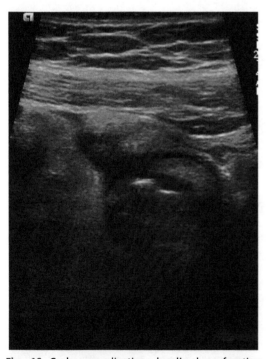

Fig. 16. Crohn complication: localized perforation with phlegmon formation is common in CD. This axial view of the terminal ileum shows disruption of the bowel wall between 10 and 12 o'clock with air projecting beyond the gut lumen. A hook-shaped hypoechoic mass adjacent to the bowel is classic for perienteric phlegmonous change.

end of a thickened and strictured segment of diseased bowel. Tethering of the bowel has a frequent association with fistulization. With fistula formation, linear bands of varying echogenicity can be seen extending from segments of abnormal gut to the skin, bladder, vagina, or other abnormal loops. If there is gas or movement in the fistula during the sonographic study, the fistula will usually appear bright or echogenic, with or without ring-down artifact related to the presence of air in the tract. Conversely, if the tract is empty or partially closed, it may appear as a black or hypoechoic tract.

Although *mucosal ulcerations* are not well assessed on sonography, deep fissures and ulcers in the gut wall appear as echogenic linear areas penetrating deeply into the wall beyond the margin of the gut lumen (see **Fig. 8**).

Perianal Inflammatory Disease

Perianal disease complicating CD is a frequent and debilitating event characterized by the development of highly complex transsphincteric tracts, which may extend to involve the deep tissues of the buttocks, the perineum, the scrotum in men, and the labia and vagina in women. Disease presentation with perianal disease is a poor prognostic indicator.

For appropriate evaluation of the anal canal and the perianal soft tissues, the authors prefer to use a combination of *transvaginal sonography* in conjunction with *transperineal sonography* in women, and transperineal sonography in men. This method of evaluation is not only more comfortable than transrectal ultrasound (TRUS) but also more informative in most patients, allowing for identification of patients on whom MR may be contributory. Placement of the probe on the perineum with pressure toward the anal canal will show the anatomy and identify any inflammatory tracts or collections (**Fig. 17**, Video 5). Furthermore, in women, transvaginal scan is also ideal for showing enterovesical, enterovaginal, and rectovaginal fistulae. Tracts and collections in the perineum, buttocks, scrotum, and labia can also be assessed and followed in a retrograde direction to their connection with the anal canal.[46]

Complicating Neoplasia

Association of CD and adenocarcinoma in the small intestine is uncommon. However, this association is not coincidental and corresponds to a significantly higher relative risk for this population. Affected individuals have generally had a long course of active disease before the development of this unfortunate complication. Preoperative

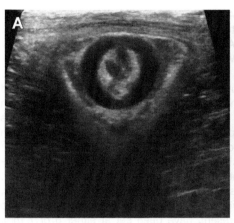
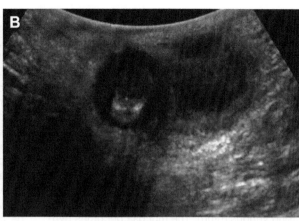

Fig. 17. Crohn complication: transperineal scan to evaluate perianal inflammatory disease in 2 patients. (*A*) An axial image of the anal canal shows a normal appearance. The internal anal sphincter is a complete hypoechoic ring surrounded by a less well-defined echogenic rim, representing the external sphincter. (*B*) The anal canal with an adjacent abscess and a tract at 5 o'clock.

identification of such a neoplasm is unusually difficult as the features of carcinoma may be easily mimicked by the extensive and varied inflammatory changes, which may be shown in these patients. Furthermore, the wall layer destruction associated with severe inflammation is similar to the wall layer destruction of neoplastic infiltration, and abnormal fat and lymph nodes are common to both. Other tumors may also be found in association with CD (**Fig. 18**).

Neoplasia may also complicate long-standing perianal fistulas with development of tumor in the fistulous tracts. Neoplasia is also difficult to recognize and differentiate from chronic inflammatory change.

ACUTE ABDOMEN

Sonography is a valuable imaging tool in patients who may have specific gastrointestinal disease, such as acute appendicitis or acute diverticulitis,[47] although its contribution is far more broad reaching. The real-time aspect of sonographic study allows for direct interaction of the sonographer/physician with the patient with confirmation of palpable masses and/or focal points of tenderness. The doctrine "scan where it hurts" is invaluable and has led sonographers to describe the value of the sonographic equivalent to clinical examination with such descriptors as a sonographic Murphy or sonographic McBurney sign.

Right Lower Quadrant Pain

Acute appendicitis
Acute appendicitis is the most common explanation for the so-called acute abdomen presentation to an emergency department. Patients typically

have right lower quadrant pain, tenderness, and leukocytosis. A mass may also be palpable.

Although presentations may be typical, there is a well-recognized *overlap of symptoms* of appendicitis with a variety of other gastrointestinal and gynecologic conditions, in particular. Therefore, in a patient with *suspected appendicitis*, the objectives of imaging are

- To identify the patient with acute appendicitis
- To identify the patient without acute appendicitis
- In this latter population, to identify an alternate explanation for their right lower quadrant pain.

CT and US both provide sensitive and accurate diagnosis of appendicitis. The choice of imaging

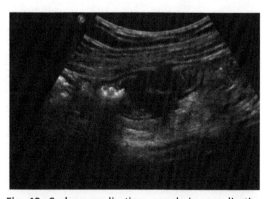

Fig. 18. Crohn complication: neoplasia complicating CD of the small bowel. This long-axis view of the terminal ileum shows thickened bowel disrupted by the presence of a very black lobulated mass. On pathology, this mass is a malignant neuroendoocrine tumor of the bowel.

modality is motivated to some extent on local expertise.[48] Some institutions also screen patients by their weight, sending thin patients for US and reserving CT for larger patients. These considerations aside, the authors recommend sonographic evaluation of all women—with the addition of transvaginal scan in all patients on whom the explanation for the pain is not evident on completion of a traditional suprapubic pelvic sonogram.

The *pathophysiology* in the development of acute appendicitis is thought to be obstruction of the appendiceal lumen, 35% of cases demonstrating a fecalith.[49] Mucosal secretions continue, increasing the intraluminal pressure and compromising venous return. The mucosa becomes hypoxic and ulcerates. Bacterial infection ensues with ultimate gangrene and perforation. Walled-off abscess is more common than free peritoneal contamination.

In 1986, Julien Puylaert described the value of *graded compression sonography* in the evaluation of 60 consecutive patients suspected of having acute appendicitis.[3] The initial reports of the success of Puylaert[3] in diagnosing acute appendicitis with compression sonography depended solely on visualization of *the appendix*:

- A blind-ended, noncompressible, aperistaltic tube
- Arising from the tip of the cecum
- With a gut signature (**Fig. 19**).

However, other investigators have reported seeing *normal appendices* on a sonogram (**Fig. 20**, Video 6).[50,51] The normal appendix is compressible with a wall thickness of less than or equal to 3 mm.[52] Jeffrey and colleagues[53] concluded that the size of an appendix can differentiate the normal from the acutely inflamed. *Threshold levels* for the diameter of the appendix, above which acute appendicitis is highly likely to be present, have been set at either 6 or 7 mm, with resultant change of sensitivity and specificity. Sonographic visualization of an appendix with an *appendicolith*, regardless of appendiceal diameter, should also be regarded as a positive test. Rettenbacher and colleagues[54] have described the additional value of assessment of *appendiceal morphology* in confirming suspicion of appendicitis. A round or partly round appendix had a high correlation with acute appendicitis. Color Doppler is also contributory, showing hyperemia in the appendiceal wall in the acutely inflamed

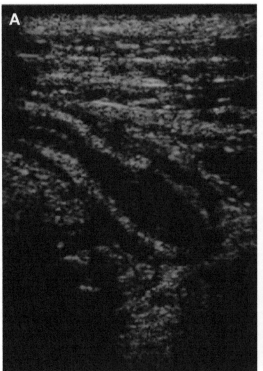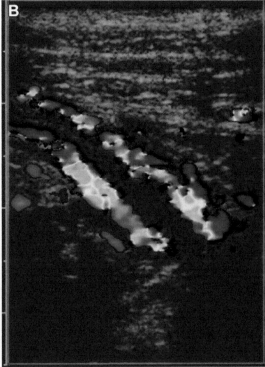

Fig. 19. Acute appendicitis, classic findings. (*A*) A grayscale long-axis view of the appendix show its blind end and fluid distended lumen. It is aperistaltic and noncompressible. (*B*) CDI shows profuse vascularity from the inflamed wall.

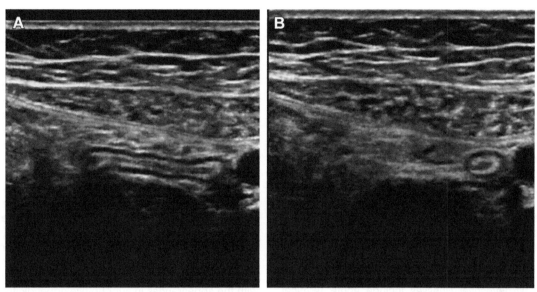

Fig. 20. A normal appendix may be seen, especially in very thin female patients, as here. (*A*) A long-axis and (*B*) axial image of the appendix shows a gut signature, a blind end, and a diameter of 7 mm or less.

appendix. Lee[55] described graded compression sonography with adjuvant use of a posterior manual compression technique for improving the sonographic diagnosis of acute appendicitis.

The appendix is most commonly located caudal to the base of the cecum. It may also be retrocecal and retroileal. In a minority of patients, the appendix may be located in the true pelvis. It is in this situation that confusion in diagnosis occurs, most often in terms of mistaken diagnosis with gynecologic disease. Inflammation of the appendix that is positioned in the true pelvis may be optimally studied with *transvaginal* placement of the US probe because the appendix is often intimately related to either the uterus or the ovaries. The identification of the blind-ended tip of the appendix with

an increased diameter, luminal distention, and inflammation of the surrounding fat is obvious (**Fig. 21**).

Although the sensitivity of sonography for the diagnosis of appendicitis decreases with *perforation*, features statistically associated with its occurrence include

- Loculated pericecal fluid (**Fig. 22**, Video 7).
- Phlegmon or abscess
- Prominent pericecal or periappendiceal fat
- Circumferential loss of the submucosal layer of the appendix[56]

False-positive diagnosis for acute appendicitis may occur if a normal appendix or a thickened

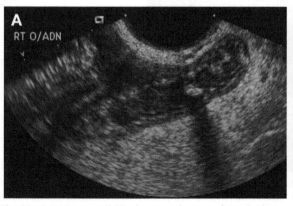
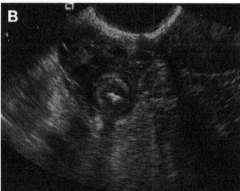

Fig. 21. Acute appendicitis shown only on endovaginal scan, here in (*A*) long-axis and (*B*) axial view. The appendix is blind ended, very large, and shows a shadowing appendicolith and surrounding inflammatory fat.

terminal ileum is mistaken for an inflamed appendix. Awareness of the diagnostic criteria stated previously, particularly related to appendiceal diameter and morphology, should minimize these errors.

Clinical misdiagnosis of appendicitis occurs most frequently in young women with *gynecologic conditions*, especially acute pelvic inflammatory disease, rupture or torsion of ovarian cysts, and postpartum ovarian vein thrombosis. Bendeck and colleagues[57] have recently confirmed that women suspected of having appendicitis benefit the most from preoperative CT or US, with a statistically significant lower negative appendectomy rate than women who undergo no preoperative imaging. They concluded that preoperative imaging should be part of the routine evaluation of women suspected of having acute appendicitis.

Other diseases than those of gynecologic origin may also be misdiagnosed as acute appendicitis. *Gastrointestinal illnesses* include acute terminal ileitis with mesenteric adenitis,[58] acute typhlitis, acute diverticulitis, especially of a cecal tip

diverticulum, and CD in the ileocecal area or involving the appendix itself.[59] *Urologic disease*, especially stone-related and right-sided *segmental omental infarction*, may also mimic acute appendicitis. The value of sonography in establishing an *alternate diagnosis* in patients with suspected acute appendicitis was addressed by Gaensler and colleagues,[60] who found that 70% of patients with another diagnosis had abnormalities visualized on the sonogram.

Crohn appendicitis
Patients with CD may present with acute appendicitis due to inflammatory bowel involvement of the appendix as distinct from acute suppurative appendicitis. The wall of the appendix is typically markedly thickened and hyperemic with wall layer preservation, and the luminal surfaces are often in apposition.[59] This apposition is in sharp contrast with the appearances in suppurative appendicitis, where luminal distention is the expectation and wall thickening is usually moderate at most.

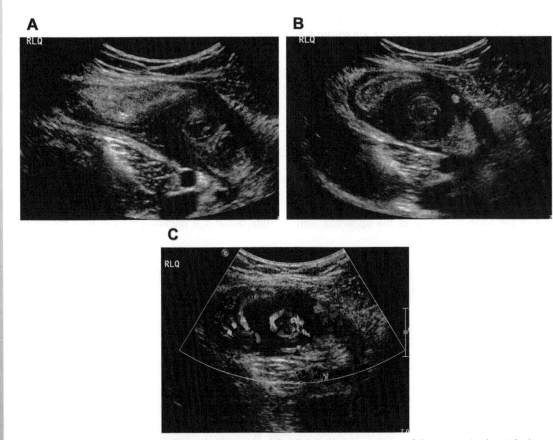

Fig. 22. Appendix rupture is suspected from pericecal fluid. (*A*) A long-axis view of the cecum in the right lower quadrant shows a hetrerogeneous mass caudal to the cecum. (*B*) An axial image shows the cecum displaced to the patient's right side and the distended appendix surrounded by a black rim of inflammatory fluid. (*C*) The addition of CDI confirms hyperemia of the appendiceal wall and also of the adjacent cecum.

Crohn appendicitis is a self-limited process[61,62] and treatment may be conservative if the appropriate diagnosis can be established with noninvasive techniques.

Right-sided diverticulitis

Acute inflammation of a right-sided diverticulum is distinct from the more common diverticulitis that is encountered in the left hemicolon. These diverticula occur more often in women than in men and have a predilection for Asian populations. Most affected patients are young adults. Right-sided diverticula are usually solitary and congenital in origin. Their inflammation is associated with right lower quadrant pain, tenderness, and leukocytosis with a mistaken diagnosis of appendicitis in virtually all cases.

On *sonography*, acute diverticulitis is associated with inflammation of the pericolonic fat. The diverticula may be located in the cecum or the adjacent ascending colon. When inflamed, they may have 1 of 2 appearances.[63] Most commonly, the diverticulum may show as a pouch or saclike structure arising from the colonic wall (**Fig. 23**).[64] Wall layers are continued into the wall of the congenital diverticulum. Hyperemia of the diverticulum and the inflamed fat is typical. If a fecalith is present within the diverticulum, it may show as a bright echogenic focus located within or beyond a segment of thickened colonic wall. On occasion, the culprit diverticulum may not be evident and the only observations may be the inflamed fat and the focal thickening of the colonic wall. In the appropriate clinical milieu, this is highly suspicious for acute diverticulitis.

Treatment of acute diverticulitis is conservative and not surgical, emphasizing the importance of preoperative imaging in patients with right lower quadrant pain attributed to this condition.

Acute typhlitis

Immunocompromised patients are most often affected, with acute myelogeneous leukemia accounting for the overwhelming majority of cases seen today. Previously, AIDS accounted for almost all cases. *Sonography* most commonly shows striking concentric, uniform thickening of the colon wall, usually localized to the cecum and the adjacent ascending colon (**Fig. 24**).[65] The colon wall may be several times larger than normal in thickness, reflecting severe inflammatory infiltration throughout the gut wall.[66,67] *Tuberculous colitis* may similarly affect the right colon and is frequently associated with lymphadenopathy (particularly involving the mesenteric and omental nodes), splenomegaly, intrasplenic masses, ascites, and peritoneal masses, all of which may be assessed using sonography.

Mesenteric adenitis and acute terminal ileitis

Mesenteric adenitis, in association with acute terminal ileitis, is the most frequent gastrointestinal cause of misdiagnosis of acute appendicitis. Patients typically have right lower-quadrant pain

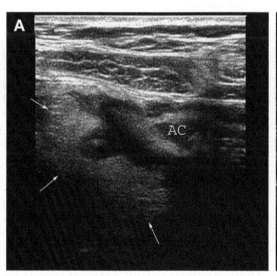 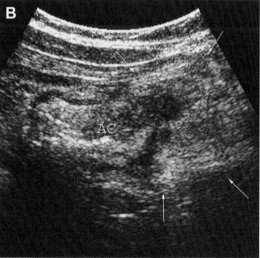

Fig. 23. Right-sided diverticulitis in 2 patients. Transverse sonograms through the ascending colon (AC) show a hypoechoic pouchlike projection, representing the inflamed diverticulum, which arises from the lateral wall of the gut in (*A*) and from the medial border of the gut in (*B*). Both are surrounded by inflamed fat (*arrows*). (*From* Wilson SR. The gastrointestinal tract. In: Rumack CR, Wilson SR, Charboneau JW, et al, editors. Diagnostic ultrasound. Philadelphia: Elsevier Mosby; 2011. p. 261–317; with permission.)

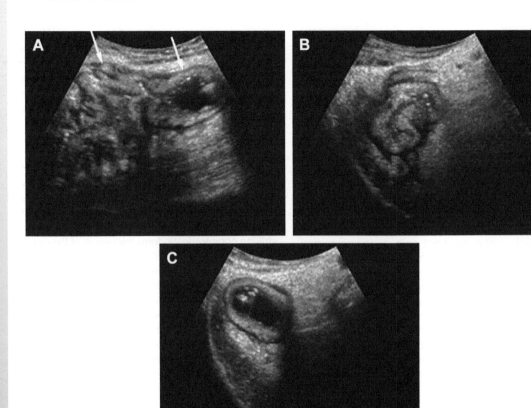

Fig. 24. Acute typhlitis. (*A*) Long-axis view of the ascending colon shows marked mural thickening of the cecum and the wall of the ascending colon. Wall layer preservation is noted. (*B*) At the level of the left arrow in A is a cross-sectional view of the thickened colon, with luminal surfaces in apposition. (*C*) At the level of the right arrow in A is a cross-sectional view of the cecum, which is thick walled and shows a fluid-filled lumen. (*From* Wilson SR. The bowel wall looks thickened: what does that mean? In: Cooperberg PL, editor. Radiologic Society of North America categorical course syllabus. Chicago: RSNA; 2002. p. 219–28; with permission.)

and tenderness. On the *sonographic examination*, enlarged mesenteric lymph nodes and mural thickening of the terminal ileum are noted. *Yersinia enterocolitica* and *Campylobacter jejuni* are the most common causative agents.[58,68]

Right-sided segmental omental infarction
Right-sided segmental infarction of the omentum is a rare condition that is virtually always mistaken clinically for acute appendicitis.[69] Of unknown cause, it is postulated to occur with an anomalous and fragile blood supply to the right lower omentum, making it susceptible to painful infarction. Patients present with right lower-quadrant pain and tenderness and are invariably thought to have acute appendicitis clinically. On *sonography*, a plaque or cakelike area of increased echogenicity suggesting inflamed or infiltrated fat is seen superficially in the right flank with adherence to the peritoneum.[69] No underlying gut abnormality is

shown. As segmental infarction is a self-limited process, its correct diagnosis will prevent unnecessary surgery. CT scan is confirmatory, showing streaky fat in a masslike configuration in the right side of the abdomen without abnormality of the underlying bowel.

Left Lower-Quadrant Pain

Acute diverticulitis
Diverticula of the colon are usually acquired deformities of the left hemicolon and are found most frequently in western urban civilizations.[70] Acute diverticulitis and spastic diverticulosis may both be associated with a *classic triad of presentation*: left lower-quadrant pain, fever, and leukocytosis. Inspissated fecal material is thought to incite the initial inflammation in the apex of the diverticulum, leading to acute diverticulitis.[71] Spread to the peridiverticular tissues and microperforation or macroperforation may follow. Localized abscess

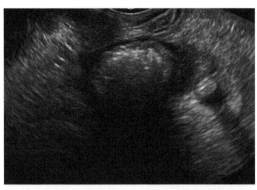

Fig. 25. Acute diverticulitis of the sigmoid colon. The bowel wall is black, reflective of the hypertrophy of the muscular layer. The diverticulum is projecting beyond the bowel wall and appears echogenic with a distal shadow. There is surrounding echogenic inflammatory fat.

formation occurs more commonly than does peritonitis. Surgical specimens demonstrate shortening and thickening of the involved segment of colon, associated with muscular hypertrophy. The peridiverticular inflammatory response may be minimal or very extensive.

Sonography appears to be of value in early assessment of patients thought to have acute diverticulitis.[72] *Classic features* include segmental thickened gut, inflamed diverticula, shown as bright echogenic foci with acoustic shadowing or "ring-down" artifact within or beyond the thickened gut wall, and inflamed perienteric fat (**Fig. 25**). A negative scan combined with a low clinical suspicion is usually a good indication to stop investigation.

Failure to identify gas-containing and interloop abscesses are the major *potential sources of error* when using sonography to evaluate patients thought to have diverticulitis. A meticulous technique of following involved thickened segments of colon in the long-axis and transverse section will help detect even small amounts of extraluminal gas.

The sonographic and clinical features of diverticulitis are more specific than those of acute appendicitis and errors of diagnosis occur less often. However, *torsion of appendices epiploicae* may produce a sonographic appearance so closely resembling acute diverticulitis that differentiation may be difficult.[73] The inflamed/infarcted fat of the appendix shows as a shadowing area of increased

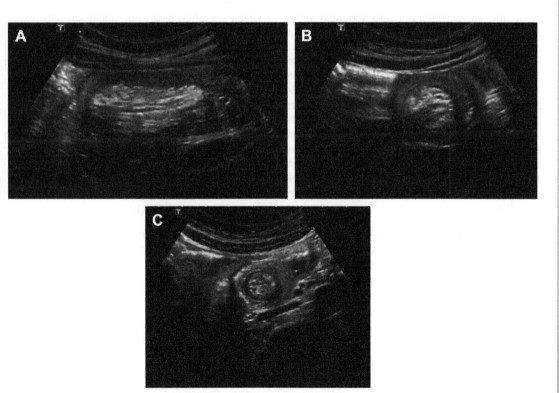

Fig. 26. Intussusception of the proximal small bowel is frequently shown as an incidental observation, as here. (*A*) The long-axis view is likened to the appearance of a hayfork. (*B, C*) Axial views show variable amounts of the fatty component of the mesentery, which appears echogenic. (*C*) Classic description of multiple concentric rings.

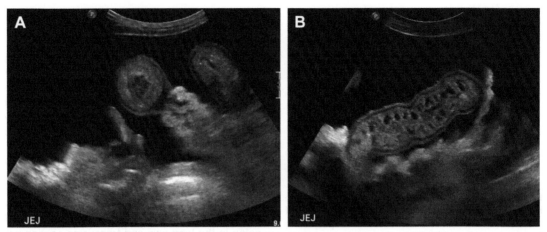

Fig. 27. Edema of the valvulae conniventes of the small bowel shows multiple fluid-filled fingerlike projections projecting from the wall into the bowel lumen, shown here in (A) axial and (B) long-axis views. There is also abundant ascites. This nonspecific observation may be seen in acute vasculitis, shock abdomen, or graft versus host disease.

echogenicity related to the margin of the colon, mimicking an inflamed diverticulum. Regional perienteric inflammatory change, however, is usually minimal and systemic symptoms are fewer.

Unique sonographic features are seen in the following:

Intussusception, invagination of a bowel segment (the intussusceptum) into the next distal segment (the intussuscipiens), may be seen in any patient as a transient observation and is shown with slightly increased frequency in patients with CD. Their observation, therefore, is usually insignificant. A *sonographic appearance* of multiple concentric rings, related to the invaginating layers of the telescoped bowel, seen in cross-section is virtually pathognomonic. The longitudinal appearance suggesting a "hayfork"[74] is not as reliably detected. In both projections, the mesenteric fat, invaginating with the intussusceptum, will show as an eccentric area of increased echogenicity (**Fig. 26**).

Furthermore, intussusception may also be a relatively infrequent cause of mechanical obstruction in the adult in whom it is usually associated with a tumor as a lead point. In the authors' experience, this is frequently a lipoma that appears as a highly echogenic intraluminal mass related to its fat content.

Shock abdomen may show edema of the valvulae conniventes (**Fig. 27**) in association with vasculitis, venous thrombosis, and embolic phenomena.

SUMMARY

US is a valuable modality for the evaluation of patients presenting with the so-called acute abdomen, especially those with specific right or left lower quadrant pain. Furthermore, it is increasingly popular for the routine and emergency evaluation of those with IBD, providing a safe and reliable method for diagnosis of disease, detection of recurrent disease following surgery, monitoring therapy, and identifying those with complications, which are often silent but significant. US is safe and well tolerated and may be repeated as necessary. In this era of radiation and cost awareness, US is surely a valuable modality for the evaluation of the bowel.

ACKNOWLEDGMENTS

Drs S.R. Wilson and K.L. Novak would like to acknowledge Gordana Popovic and Hojun Yu for their artwork that helped to make illustrating this article possible.

SUPPLEMENTARY DATA

Videos related to this article can be found online at http://dx.doi.org/10.1016/j.cult.2014.07.008.

REFERENCES

1. Lutz HT, Petzoldt R. Ultrasonic patterns of space occupying lesions of the stomach and the intestine. Ultrasound Med Biol 1976;2:129–32.
2. Bluth EI, Merritt CR, Sullivan MA. Ultrasonic evaluation of the stomach, small bowel, and colon. Radiology 1979;133:677–80.
3. Puylaert JB. Acute appendicitis: US evaluation using graded compression. Radiology 1986;158:355–60.

4. Teefey SA, et al. Bowel wall thickening: differentiation of inflammation from ischemia with color Doppler and duplex US. Radiology 1996;198:547–51.

5. Xavier RJ, Podolsky DK. Unravelling the pathogenesis of inflammatory bowel disease. Nature 2007;448:427–34.

6. Kyle J. Crohn's disease in the northeastern and northern Isles of Scotland: an epidemiological review. Gastroenterology 1992;103:392–9.

7. Loftus EV, et al. Ulcerative colitis in Olmsted County, Minnesota, 1940–1993: incidence, prevalence, and survival. Gut 2000;46:336–43.

8. Bernstein CN, et al. Epidemiology of Crohn's disease and ulcerative colitis in a central Canadian province: a population-based study. Am J Epidemiol 1999;149:916–24.

9. Bernstein CN, et al. The epidemiology of inflammatory bowel disease in Canada: a population-based study. Am J Gastroenterol 2006;101:1559–68.

10. Michelassi F, Balestracci T, Chappell R. Primary and recurrent Crohn's disease experience with 1379 patients. Ann Surg 1991;214(3):230–40.

11. Beaugerie L, Seksik P, Nion-Larmurier I, et al. Predictors of Crohn's disease. Gastroenterology 2006;130:650–6.

12. Lichtenstein GR, et al. Factors associated with the development of intestinal strictures or obstructions in patients with Crohn's disease. Am J Gastroenterol 2006;101:1030–8.

13. Sandborn WJ, et al. Colectomy rate comparison after treatment of ulcerative colitis with placebo or infliximab. Gastroenterology 2009;137:1250–60 [quiz: 1520].

14. Frøslie KF, Jahnsen J, Moum BA, et al. Mucosal healing in inflammatory bowel disease: results from a Norwegian population-based cohort. Gastroenterology 2007;133:412–22.

15. Schnitzler F, et al. Mucosal healing predicts long-term outcome of maintenance therapy with infliximab in Crohn's disease. Inflamm Bowel Dis 2009;15:1295–301.

16. Regueiro M, et al. Crohn's disease activity index does not correlate with endoscopic recurrence one year after ileocolonic resection. Inflamm Bowel Dis 2011;17:118–26.

17. Rodgers AD, Cummins AG. CRP correlates with clinical score in ulcerative colitis but not in Crohn's disease. Dig Dis Sci 2007;52:2063–8.

18. Brenner DJ, Hall EJ. Computed tomography–an increasing source of radiation exposure. N Engl J Med 2007;357:2277–84.

19. Peloquin JM, et al. Diagnostic ionizing radiation exposure in a population-based cohort of patients with inflammatory bowel disease. Am J Gastroenterol 2008;103:2015–22.

20. Berrington de González A, Darby S. Risk of cancer from diagnostic X-rays: estimates for the UK and 14 other countries. Lancet 2004;363:345–51.

21. Sodickson A, et al. Recurrent CT, cumulative radiation exposure, and associated radiation-induced cancer risks from CT of adults. Radiology 2009;251:175–84.

22. Migaleddu V, et al. Contrast-enhanced ultrasonographic evaluation of inflammatory activity in Crohn's disease. Gastroenterology 2009;137:43–52.

23. Fraquelli M, et al. Reproducibility of bowel ultrasonography in the evaluation of Crohn's disease. Dig Liver Dis 2008;40:860–6.

24. Rigazio C, et al. Abdominal bowel ultrasound can predict the risk of surgery in Crohn's disease: proposal of an ultrasonographic score. Scand J Gastroenterol 2009;44:585–93.

25. Tarján Z, et al. Ultrasound in Crohn's disease of the small bowel. Eur J Radiol 2000;35:176–82.

26. Parente F, et al. Bowel ultrasound and mucosal healing in ulcerative colitis. Dig Dis 2009;27:285–90.

27. Horsthuis K, Bipat S, Bennink RR, et al. Inflammatory bowel disease diagnosed with US, MR, scintigraphy, and CT: meta-analysis of prospective studies. Radiology 2008;247:64–79.

28. Dubbins PA. Ultrasound demonstration of bowel wall thickness in inflammatory bowel disease. Clin Radiol 1984;35:227–31.

29. Danese S, et al. Angiogenesis as a novel component of inflammatory bowel disease pathogenesis. Gastroenterology 2006;130:2060–73.

30. Deban L, Correale C, Vetrano S, et al. Multiple pathogenic roles of microvasculature in inflammatory bowel disease: a Jack of all trades. Am J Pathol 2008;172:1457–66.

31. Spalinger J, et al. Doppler US in patients with Crohn disease: vessel density in the diseased bowel reflects disease activity. Radiology 2000;217:787–91.

32. Esteban J, Maldonado M, Sanchiz V, et al. Activity of Crohn's disease assessed by colour Doppler ultrasound analysis of the affected loops. Eur Radiol 2001;11:1423–8.

33. Britton I, Maguire C, Adams C, et al. Assessment of the role and reliability of sonographic post-prandial flow response in grading Crohn's disease activity. Clin Radiol 1998;53:599–603.

34. Serra C, et al. Ultrasound assessment of vascularization of the thickened terminal ileum wall in Crohn's disease patients using a low-mechanical index real-time scanning technique with a second generation ultrasound contrast agent. Eur J Radiol 2007;62:114–21.

35. Ripollés T, et al. Crohn disease: correlation of findings at contrast-enhanced US with severity at endoscopy. Radiology 2009;253:241–8.

36. De Pascale A, Garofalo G, Perna M, et al. Contrast-enhanced ultrasonography in Crohn's disease. Radiol Med 2006;111:539–50.

37. Robotti D, Cammarota T, Debani P, et al. Activity of Crohn disease: value of Color-Power-Doppler and contrast-enhanced ultrasonography. Abdom Imaging 2004;29:648–52.

38. Medellin-Kowalewski A, Wilkens R, Wilson A. Integration of quantitative contrast-enhanced ultrasound parameters into sonographic evaluation of the bowel in crohn disease. AJR Am J Roentgenol 2014, in press.

39. Wilson SR, Greenbaum LD, Goldberg BB. Contrast-enhanced ultrasound: what is the evidence and what are the obstacles? AJR Am J Roentgenol 2009;193:55–60.

40. Maconi G, et al. Small bowel stenosis in Crohn's disease: clinical, biochemical and ultrasonographic evaluation of histological features. Aliment Pharmacol Ther 2003;18:749–56.

41. Parente F, et al. Bowel ultrasound in assessment of Crohn's disease and detection of related small bowel strictures: a prospective comparative study versus x ray and intraoperative findings. Gut 2002; 50(4):490–5.

42. Kratzer W, et al. Contrast-enhanced power Doppler sonography of the intestinal wall in the differentiation of hypervascularized and hypovascularized intestinal obstructions in patients with Crohn's disease. J Ultrasound Med 2002;21:149–57 [quiz: 158–9].

43. Gasche C, et al. Transabdominal bowel sonography for the detection of intestinal complications in Crohn's disease. Gut 1999;44:112–7.

44. María J, et al. Contrast-enhanced ultrasonography: usefulness in the assessment of postoperative recurrence of Crohn's disease. J Crohns Colitis 2013;7: 192–201.

45. Weissberg DL, Scheible W, Leopold GR. Ultrasonographic appearance of adult intussusception. Radiology 1977;124:791–2.

46. Stewart LK, McGee J, Wilson SR. Sonography of perianal inflammatory disease. AJR Am J Roentgenol 2001;177:627–32.

47. Puylaert JB. Ultrasound of acute GI tract conditions. Eur Radiol 2001;11:1867–77.

48. Birnbaum BA, Wilson SR. Appendicitis at the millennium. Radiology 2000;215(2):337–48.

49. Shaw RE. Appendix calculi and acute appendicitis. Br J Surg 1965;52:451–9.

50. Abu-Yousef MM, et al. High-resolution sonography of acute appendicitis. AJR Am J Roentgenol 1987; 149:53–8.

51. Jeffrey RB, Laing FC, Townsend RR. Acute appendicitis: sonographic criteria based on 250 cases. Radiology 1988;167:327–9.

52. Rioux M. Sonographic detection of the normal and abnormal appendix. AJR Am J Roentgenol 1992; 158:773–8.

53. Jeffrey RB, Laing FC, Lewis FR. Acute appendicitis: high-resolution real-time US findings. Radiology 1987;163:11–4.

54. Rettenbacher T, et al. Ovoid shape of the vermiform appendix: a criterion to exclude acute appendicitis–evaluation with US. Radiology 2003;226: 95–100.

55. Lee J. Graded compression sonography with adjuvant use of a posterior manual compression technique in the sonographic diagnosis of acute appendicitis. AJR Am J Roentgenol 2002;178:863–8.

56. Borushok KF, Jeffrey RB, Laing FC, et al. Sonographic diagnosis of perforation in patients with acute appendicitis. AJR Am J Roentgenol 1990; 154(2):275–8.

57. Bendeck SE, Nino-murcia M, Berry GJ, et al. Imaging for suspected appendicitis: negative appendectomy and perforation rates. Radiology 2002; 225:22–5.

58. Puylaert JB, Lalisang RI, van der Werf SD, et al. Campylobacter ileocolitis mimicking acute appendicitis: differentiation with graded-compression US. Radiology 1988;166:737–40.

59. Agha F, Ghahremani G, Panella JS, et al. Appendicitis as the initial manifestation of Crohn's disease: radiologic features and prognosis. AJR Am J Roentgenol 1987;149(3):515–8.

60. Gaensler EH, Jeffrey RB, Laing FC, et al. Sonography in patients with suspected acute appendicitis: value in establishing alternative diagnosis. AJR Am J Roentgenol 1989;152:49–51.

61. Higgins MJ, et al. Granulomatous appendicitis revisited: report of a case. Dig Surg 2001;18: 245–8.

62. Roth T, Zimmer G, Tschantz P. Crohn's disease of the appendix. Ann Chir 2000;125:665–7 [in French].

63. Chou YH, et al. Sonography of acute right side colonic diverticulitis. Am J Surg 2001;181:122–7.

64. O'Malley M, Wilson SR. US of gastrointestinal tract abnormalities with CT correlation. Radiographics 2003;23:59–72.

65. Teefey A, Goldfogel GA. Sonographic neutropenic diagnosis typhlitis of neutropenic typhlitis. AJR Am J Roentgenol 1987;149(4):731–3.

66. Balthazar EJ, Megibow AJ, Fazzini E, et al. Cytomegalovirus colitis in AIDS: radiographic findings in 11 patients. Radiology 1985;155:585–9.

67. Frager DH, et al. Gastrointestinal complications of AIDS: radiologic features. Radiology 1986;158: 597–603.

68. Puylaert JB. Mesenteric adenitis and acute terminal ileitis: US evaluation using graded compression. Radiology 1986;161:691–5.

69. Puylaert JB. Right-sided segmental infarction of the omentum: clinical, US, and CT findings. Radiology 1992;185:169–72.

70. Painter NS, Burkitt DP. Diverticular disease of the colon, a 20th century problem. Clin Gastroenterol 1975;4:3–21.

71. Fleischner FG, Ming SC. Revised concepts on diverticular disease of the colon. II. So-called diverticulitis: diverticular sigmoiditis and perisigmoiditis; diverticular abscess, fistula, and frank peritonitis. Radiology 1965;84:599–609.

72. Wilson SR, Toi A. The value of sonography in the diagnosis of acute diverticulitis of the colon. AJR Am J Roentgenol 1990;154:1199–202.

73. Derchi LE, Reggiani L, Rebaudi F, et al. Appendices epiploicae of the large bowel. Sonographic appearance and differentiation from peritoneal seeding. J Ultrasound Med 1988;7:11–4.

74. Meiser G, Meissner K. Sonographic differential diagnosis of intestinal obstruction–results of a prospective study of 48 patients. Ultraschall Med 1985;6:39–45 [in German].

Ultrasound of the Abdominal Wall

Jason M. Wagner, MD*, Justin C. North, MD

KEYWORDS

• Sonography • Abdominal wall • Superficial • Subcutaneous • Mass • Hernia

KEY POINTS

- The use of dynamic ultrasound techniques, including Valsalva maneuver and upright imaging, is recommended when evaluating for hernias.
- Ultrasound is highly accurate for the diagnosis of hernia in the setting of a palpable mass, but may have reduced accuracy in the setting of possible occult hernia.
- Inguinal hernias can be characterized based on their location. Indirect hernias arise superior and lateral to the inferior epigastric artery and direct hernias are inferior and medial.
- Dynamic compression imaging is useful to evaluate reducibility of hernias and to identify abscesses with hyperechoic contents.
- Lipomas are the most common neoplasm of the abdominal wall, but must be distinguished from fat-containing hernias.

 Videos of an inguinal fat-containing hernia enlarging with Valsalva maneuver, transverse sonography of an indirect inguinal hernia containing fluid, and transverse sonography of a direct inguinal hernia containing bowel accompany this article at http://www.ultrasound.theclinics.com/

INTRODUCTION

Ultrasound is a highly valuable imaging modality for evaluation of the abdominal wall because of its high spatial resolution, lower cost, and lack of ionizing radiation. Ultrasound has the major advantage of allowing dynamic imaging, including imaging in the upright position, imaging during Valsalva maneuver, and imaging during dynamic compression. Doppler technology is useful in evaluation of vascular abnormalities of the abdominal wall.

The abdominal wall is affected by a wide variety of pathology, including hernias, fluid collections, tumors, and tumor-like conditions. Ultrasound is effective in the evaluation of a large number of these conditions and may also be used to guide drainage of fluid collections and biopsy of tumors when appropriate. This article reviews the anatomy of the abdominal wall, sonographic technique, and common pathologies involving the abdominal wall.

ANATOMY

Knowledge of a few key ultrasound-visible structures and adjacent structures of the abdominal wall is crucial to making accurate diagnoses. The abdominal wall is divided into the anterior, lateral, and posterior portions with the anterior and lateral portions being the most important for ultrasound evaluation.

The anterior abdominal wall consists primarily of the rectus abdominis, a paired midline muscle connected centrally by the linea alba (**Fig. 1**). It is divided into individual muscle bellies at tendinous intersections (**Fig. 2**). The rectus is contained by the rectus sheath, a continuation of the

Department of Radiological Sciences, University of Oklahoma Health Sciences Center, 940 Northeast 13th Street, Suite 4G4250, Oklahoma City, OK 73104-5008, USA
* Corresponding author.
E-mail address: jason-wagner@ouhsc.edu

Ultrasound Clin 9 (2014) 775–791
http://dx.doi.org/10.1016/j.cult.2014.07.005
1556-858X/14/$ – see front matter © 2014 Elsevier Inc. All rights reserved.

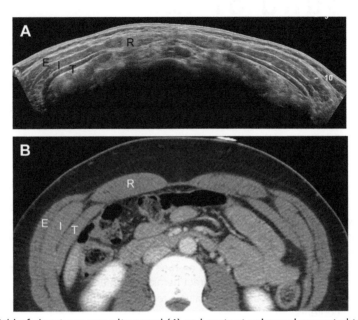

Fig. 1. Extended field of view transverse ultrasound (*A*) and contrast-enhanced computed tomography (CT) (*B*) of the abdominal wall demonstrate the paired rectus centrally, the layered muscles of the lateral abdominal wall, and their tendinous junctions. E, external oblique muscle; I, internal oblique muscle; R, rectus abdominus muscle; T, transversus abdominus muscle.

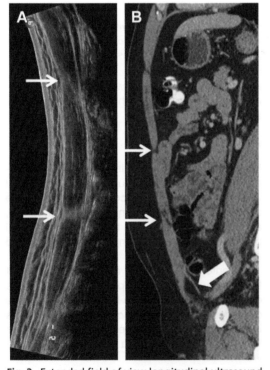

Fig. 2. Extended field of view longitudinal ultrasound (*A*) and sagittal reformatted CT image (*B*) through the paramidline rectus shows the tendinous intersections dividing individual muscle bellies (*thin arrows*). On the CT image, the inferior epigastric vessel (*thick arrow*) can be seen entering the muscle at the level of the arcuate line.

aponeurosis of the lateral abdominal wall musculature.[1] The deep aspect of the rectus sheath folds anterior to the rectus at the arcuate line, just below the level of the navel. Although the arcuate line is not visible by ultrasound, the superior epigastric vessels anastomose with inferior epigastric vessels at this level. This level can be identified as the superior epigastric vessels exit their course in the rectus and rectus sheath, and the inferior epigastric vessels run posterior to the rectus.

The lateral abdominal wall musculature consists of three layers. From superficial to deep these are the external oblique, internal oblique, and transverse abdominis (see **Fig. 1**). These attach medially to the rectus through the aponeurosis of the tendons of these muscles. They attach similarly to the iliac crest and inguinal ligament inferiorly.

Although the anatomy in the inguinal region is complex, most groin hernias can be correctly diagnosed according to their relation to the inguinal triangle (Hesselbach triangle). This triangle is formed by the intersection of the rectus muscle medially, the inferior epigastric vessels superolaterally, and the inguinal ligament inferiorly.

The superficial layers of the abdominal wall are also important because differential diagnosis is derived from the layer where the lesion arises. The layers from superficial to deep are epidermis, dermis, subcutaneous fat, fascia of the muscles of the abdominal wall, and the muscles themselves (**Fig. 3**).

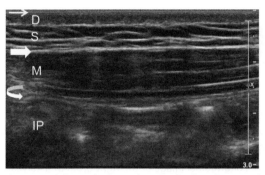

Fig. 3. High-resolution longitudinal ultrasound through the rectus abdominis muscle showing the superficial layers of the abdominal wall. From superficial to deep: epidermis (*thin arrow*), dermis (D), subcutaneous fat (S), echogenic fascia (*thick arrow*), and the muscle (M). Subjacent to the muscle are the transversalis fascia, parietal peritoneum (*curved arrow*), and intraperitoneal contents (IP).

SONOGRAPHIC TECHNIQUE

Sonographic evaluation of the abdominal wall should be optimized for each patient based on the clinical question being addressed. A high-frequency ($\geq$12 MHz) linear transducer is used for most applications in the anterior abdominal wall. Lower-frequency curved transducers are also commonly used, particularly in larger patients. If a mass or fluid collection is encountered, it is highly important that an appropriate imaging depth is used to allow complete visualization of the entire structure and the adjacent deeper structures. Extended field of view imaging is helpful to fully visualize larger structures (**Fig. 4**). We advocate comparison views of the contralateral side, particularly when a patient presents with focal symptoms and no sonographic abnormality is discovered. By convention, most examinations of

the abdominal wall are performed primarily in the longitudinal and transverse planes. When evaluating for inguinal hernias, we consider the longitudinal plane to be parallel with the inguinal ligament and the transverse plane to be perpendicular to the inguinal ligament.

The major advantage of ultrasound with regard to imaging of the abdominal wall is the ability to perform dynamic maneuvers.[2] Imaging during Valsalva maneuver (**Fig. 5**, Video 1) and with upright positioning (**Fig. 6**) is highly useful for the evaluation of suspected hernia. Many hernias may spontaneously resolve with the patient resting in the supine position, making them undetectable without dynamic maneuvers.[2,3] Additionally, some hernias may only contain bowel during Valsalva or other dynamic maneuvers (**Fig. 7**). Dynamic compression imaging is helpful to determine reducibility of hernias. Dynamic compression is also helpful in the detection of abscess.[4,5]

HERNIAS

A hernia is the protrusion of a structure through the tissues normally containing it, either through a focal defect in the tissue or stretching of the tissue.[3] Hernias are a common problem and the annual rate of inguinal hernia repair is 200 per 100,000 population.[6] Many hernias are diagnosed clinically with no additional benefit from imaging. In the setting of a clinically apparent mass suspected to be hernia, ultrasound has been shown to be highly accurate, with one study showing a sensitivity and specificity of 100%.[7] A meta-analysis of sonography in the diagnosis of inguinal hernias found an overall sensitivity of 96.6%, specificity of 84.8%, and a positive predictive value of 92.6%.[8] The diagnostic accuracy of ultrasound, however, is reduced in the absence of a

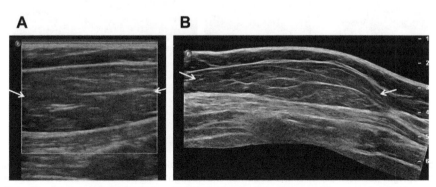

Fig. 4. The benefit of extended field of view imaging. Transverse ultrasound image of a right upper quadrant mass in a 54-year-old woman (*A*) demonstrates apparently thickened subcutaneous tissues (*arrows*) shown to be a large lipoma on a subsequent extended field of view image (*B*).

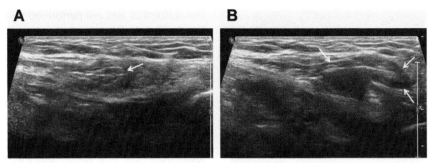

Fig. 5. The benefit of imaging during Valsalva maneuver. (*A*) Longitudinal image of the right groin of a 46-year-old woman with bilateral groin pain performed at rest demonstrates a possible small hernia (*arrow*). (*B*) With Valsalva maneuver, the fat-containing hernia becomes significantly larger (*arrows*). Also see Video 1.

clinically palpable hernia.[8] Although one study found ultrasound to have a 98.3% positive predictive value in the setting of clinically suspected occult hernia, a recent meta-analysis found ultrasound to have only a sensitivity of 86% and a specificity of 77% in this clinical setting.[9,10] Sonography has been reported to be effective in the postsurgical evaluation of hernias repaired with mesh.[11]

Groin hernias consist of indirect inguinal hernias, direct inguinal hernias, and femoral hernias (**Fig. 8**). Indirect inguinal hernias are the most common groin hernia, involve the internal inguinal ring, are more common in men, and are considered congenital.[2] Indirect inguinal hernias enter the inguinal canal superior and lateral to inferior epigastric artery and then extend inferior and medial, superficial to the artery (**Fig. 9**, Video 2). Indirect inguinal hernias are more likely than direct inguinal hernias to extend down into the scrotum or labia majus (**Fig. 10**). The contents of an indirect inguinal hernia tend to be located superficial to the spermatic cord.[2]

Direct inguinal hernias directly enter the inguinal canal through the conjoined tendon, which is composed of the aponeuroses of the internal oblique and transverse abdominis muscles and the underlying transversalis fascia. Direct inguinal hernias arise inferior and medial to the inferior epigastric artery and, therefore, do not cross superficial to the artery (see **Fig. 9**, Video 3). The contents of a direct inguinal hernia tend to be located deep to the spermatic cord within the inguinal canal.[2] Direct inguinal hernias are acquired and frequently bilateral.

Femoral hernias are the least common groin hernia detected by ultrasound. However, they are the most likely type of groin hernia to incarcerate. Femoral hernias are more common in women, possibly because of pregnancy. Femoral hernias arise within the femoral canal inferior to the inguinal ligament and are most commonly located medial to the common femoral vein.[2]

Midline anterior abdominal wall hernias are characterized as epigastric (superior to the umbilicus), umbilical, and hypogastric (inferior to the

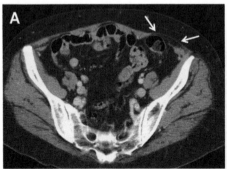
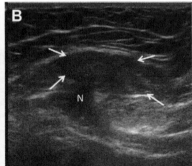

Fig. 6. The benefit of imaging in the upright position. A 73-year-old woman with a chronic tender lump, mostly noticed in the upright position. (*A*) CT of the abdomen shows slight bulge of the left anterior abdominal wall at the lateral border of the rectus abdominis muscle (*arrows*). (*B*) Subsequent transverse ultrasound image of the left mid abdomen performed in the upright position demonstrates a fat-containing spigelian hernia (*arrows*). N, neck of the hernia.

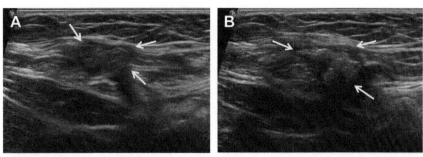

Fig. 7. Inguinal hernia (*arrows*) in a 69-year-old woman that only contains fat at rest (*A*), but contains bowel with Valsalva maneuver (*B*).

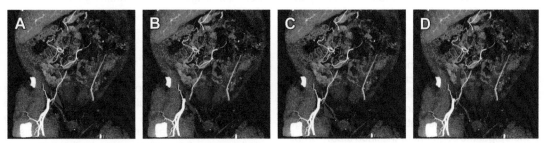

Fig. 8. The common groin hernias depicted with relation to the inguinal triangle (*A, red triangle*). Direct inguinal hernias pooch directly through the inguinal triangle. The inguinal triangle is bordered by the rectus medially, the inferior epigastric artery superolaterally, and the inguinal ligament inferomedially. (*B*) Indirect hernias extend through the inguinal canal just lateral to the inferior epigastric vessels. (*C*) Femoral hernias extend under the inguinal ligament. (*D*) Spigelian hernias arise in the oblique and rectus aponeurosis at or superior to the inferior epigastric vessels.

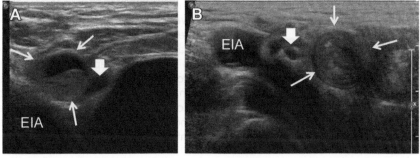

Fig. 9. (*A*) Right indirect inguinal hernia containing fluid and fat in a 13-year-old girl with ascites caused by immature teratoma. Note that the hernia (*thin arrows*) is lateral to the inferior epigastric artery (*thick arrow*). Also see Video 2. (*B*) Right direct inguinal hernia containing bowel in a 50-year-old man. Note that the hernia (*thin arrows*) is medial to the inferior epigastric artery (*thick arrow*). EIA, external iliac artery. Also see Video 3.

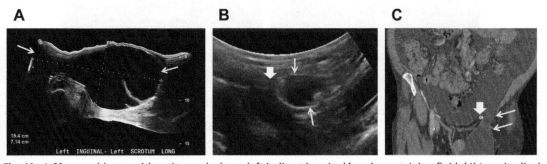

Fig. 10. A 60-year-old man with ascites and a large left indirect inguinal hernia containing fluid. (*A*) Longitudinal extended field of view sonographic image shows the large hernia extending inferiorly into the superior scrotum (*arrows*). Transverse ultrasound of the neck of the hernia (*B*) and coronal reformatted contrast-enhanced CT (*C*) demonstrates the neck of the hernia (*thin arrows*) to be lateral to the inferior epigastric vessels (*thick arrows*).

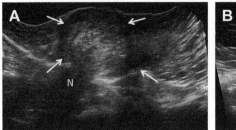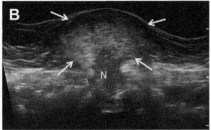

Fig. 11. Extended field of view longitudinal (*A*) and transverse (*B*) images of a fat-containing umbilical hernia (*arrows*) in a 65-year-old man. N, neck of the hernia.

umbilicus). Epigastric and hypogastric hernias occur through focal defects in the linea alba. Diastasis of the rectus muscles is a related condition with thinning and stretching of the linea alba that generally extends the entire craniocaudal length of the epigastric segment of the linea alba.[2] Umbilical hernias protrude through a widened umbilical ring and may be congenital or occur later in life (**Fig. 11**).

Spigelian hernias occur through a defect in the spigelian fascia, which is located at the lateral border of the rectus muscle at the semilunar line (see **Fig. 6**).[12] Most spigelian hernias occur near the inferior aspect of the semilunar line where the spigelian fascia is penetrated by the inferior epigastric vessels.[2] Incisional hernias occur through prior surgical sites, such as laparoscopic port and ostomy sites, and are the only type of hernia that penetrates through muscle. There are several, less common types of hernias that are generally not evaluated with ultrasound, including obturator hernias, lumbar hernias, and various types of internal hernias.[12]

FLUID COLLECTIONS

Fluid collections are commonly observed in the abdominal wall, particularly in patients who have recently had surgery. A common clinical scenario is a new bulge near a recent abdominal incision and, in our opinion, ultrasound with dynamic imaging techniques is an ideal modality to distinguish incisional hernia from postoperative fluid collections. Abdominal wall fluid collections include seroma, hematoma, and abscess. At ultrasound, a hematoma should be an avascular collection, which may be hyperechoic acutely, but most commonly is hypoechoic (**Fig. 12**).[13,14] Hematomas should have a clinical explanation, such as recent surgery. Unexplained hematomas, particularly intramuscular, should be approached with caution because the sonographic appearance of hematoma and sarcoma overlap and sarcoma can present with internal hemorrhage.[15,16] When delayed diagnosis of a soft tissue sarcoma is the result of an incorrect sonographic diagnosis, hematoma is the most common errant diagnosis.[17–19]

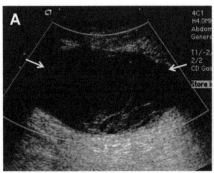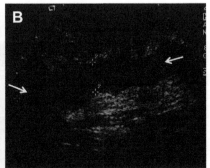

Fig. 12. A 53-year-old woman who presented with a tender mass in the anterior abdominal wall following abdominoplasty after successful weight loss associated with gastric bypass. (*A*) Ultrasound with color Doppler shows an avascular heterogenous large collection (*arrows*). Surgical drainage confirmed a sterile hematoma. (*B*) Post-drainage imaging demonstrates near complete evacuation of the hematoma (*arrows*).

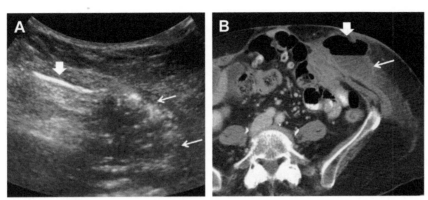

Fig. 13. A 73-year-old woman with an abscess in the left mid abdominal wall after a colostomy takedown. Transverse ultrasound (*A*) and axial CT (*B*) both demonstrate a large air and fluid collection. The *thin arrows* indicate the abscess fluid, which contains nonshadowing echogenic reflectors. The *thick arrows* indicate gas within the collection, which produces an echogenic reflector with "dirty" deep acoustic shadowing.

Ultrasound is an effective modality to evaluate for superficial abscess.[5] Abscess generally presents as an avascular collection of variable echogenicity with surrounding hyperemic, edematous tissue. Dynamic compression is very helpful to identify the mobile contents of an abscess, particularly when the contents are hyperechoic. Gas may be seen within an abscess (**Fig. 13**). Ultrasound is also effective in guiding aspiration and drainage of abdominal wall abscesses. A common differential diagnosis with regard to abdominal wall collections is sterile hematoma versus abscess. Although the two conditions may certainly have similar ultrasound features, in our experience, the contents of an abscess tend to be more mobile with dynamic compression.

When an abdominal wall fluid collection is discovered, the deep aspect should be carefully evaluated to exclude a hernia containing fluid (**Fig. 14**). When fluid is present in a hernia, motion of the fluid with respiration may be observed in the hernia neck, which can mimic a pseudoanerysm at Doppler interrogation.[20]

MASS LESIONS

We are frequently asked to perform an ultrasound examination to evaluate a mass or lump of the abdominal wall. The differential diagnosis in this situation includes entities that occur throughout the body, such as lipoma, other mesenchymal tumors, fat necrosis, and epidermal inclusion cysts. The differential diagnosis for the abdominal wall also includes hernia presenting as a mass, endometriosis, desmoid, and metastatic disease. Evaluation of a focal mass should include focused

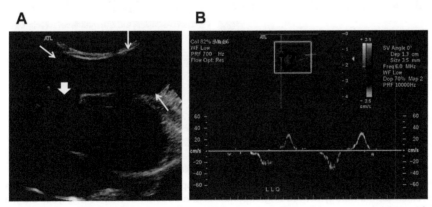

Fig. 14. (*A*) Abdominal wall hernia (*thin arrows*) containing ascites. There is a communication with intraperitoneal ascites at the neck of the hernia (*thick arrow*). (*B*) Color and spectral Doppler interrogation of the neck of the hernia shows a to-and-fro pattern of fluid motion.

history and physical examination, correlation of sonographic findings with palpation, and Doppler evaluation with settings optimized for slow flow. Ultrasound has good accuracy in the characterization of small, superficial masses.[21,22] Masses that are larger than 5 cm or deep to the fascia generally require computed tomography or MR imaging for further characterization.

Lipomas are the most common benign soft tissue tumor, most commonly present in middle-aged adults, are rare in children, and are multiple in 5% of patients.[23,24] Lipomas are usually soft or rubbery and mobile to palpation. Lipomas are generally nontender, although angiolipomas may present with tenderness.[25] By sonography, lipomas are most commonly subcutaneous, solid masses with smooth well-defined borders, variable echogenicity, minimal or no internal blood flow by color Doppler, wider than tall shape, and no acoustic shadowing.[21,26] Unlike conventional lipomas which range from hyperechoic to hypoechoic, angiolipomas tend to be hyperechoic.[27] Lipomas that are isoechoic or hypoechoic as compared with the adjacent subcutaneous fat generally have internal gently curved echogenic linear structures (**Fig. 15**).

In the abdominal wall, lipomas can be subtle and appear to be prominent fat lobules. The distinction of prominent adipose tissue from lipoma is aided by correlation with palpation and comparison views of the contralateral side (**Fig. 16**). In the abdominal wall, fat-containing hernias and lipomas can have a similar appearance and the deep border of any potential lipoma should be carefully interrogated for any shadowing that may indicate the neck of a nonreducible hernia (**Fig. 17**). Additionally, lipomas generally have little or no refractive edge shadowing and the presence of edge shadowing may indicate a hernia (**Fig. 18**). All potential lipomas occurring in a location where hernia is possible should be evaluated with dynamic imaging including Valsalva maneuver and upright imaging.

Fat necrosis is occasionally discovered involving the abdominal wall (**Fig. 19**). Fat necrosis is a benign aseptic saponification of adipose tissue, usually encountered in the breast or subcutaneous tissue, which presents as a palpable, possibly painful nodule.[28,29] Fat necrosis has a variable sonographic appearance, including a well-defined isoechoic mass with a hypoechoic halo and a poorly defined area of hyperechogenicity. Acoustic shadowing may be present. Because of the variable sonographic appearance and symptomatic presentation, fat necrosis may require further characterization with computed tomography or MR imaging and/or biopsy.

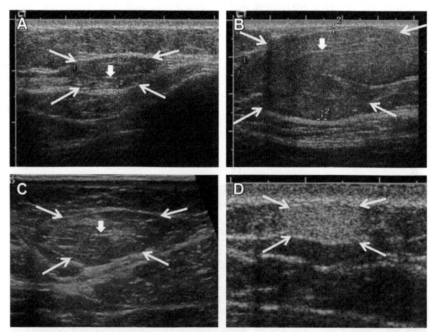

Fig. 15. Pathology-proved lipomas (*thin arrows*) of the left upper quadrants of a 43-year-old woman (*A*) and a 41-year-old woman (*B*). Pathology-proved angiolipomas of the abdominal wall of a 49-year-old man (*C*) and a 25-year-old man (*D*). Lipomas may demonstrate a range of echogenicity, from slightly hypoechoic to hyperechoic. Note that the more hypoechoic lipomas (*A–C*) have internal gently curved echogenic linear structures (*thick arrows*).

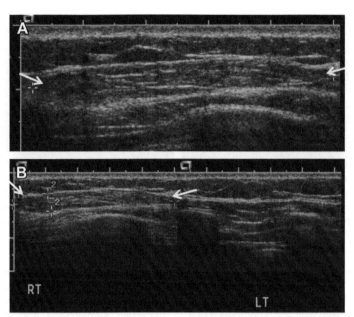

Fig. 16. Pathology-proved lipoma (*arrows*) in the deep subcutaneous tissues of the right upper quadrant of a 43-year-old man. (*A*) Transverse view of the right upper quadrant demonstrates a well-defined mass that is essentially isoechoic with the adjacent subcutaneous fat and has internal linear echogenic structures. (*B*) A split screen transverse image provides comparison with the contralateral tissues, indicating this is an asymmetric mass.

Although lipoma is by far the most common neoplasm of the body wall, other benign and malignant mesenchymal neoplasms can involve the abdominal wall. Benign neoplasms of the superficial tissues other than lipoma are often solid

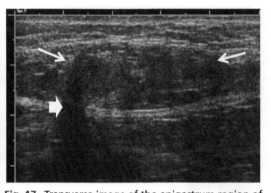

Fig. 17. Transverse image of the epigastrum region of a 41-year-old man demonstrates a slightly hypoechoic mass (*thin arrows*) that contains linear echogenicities and mostly has a well-defined deep margin. The appearance would be compatible with a lipoma, except there is focal loss of the deep margin at the right lateral aspect of the mass with associated shadowing (*thick arrow*). This shadowing corresponds to the neck of this fat-containing epigastric hernia. This hernia did not change with Valsalva maneuver or upright positioning.

hypoechoic masses without specific ultrasound features (**Fig. 20**). Although most soft tissue tumors are benign, primary sarcomas do rarely occur in the abdominal wall.[30]

Nonneoplastic conditions that present as masses, such as epidermal inclusion cysts, also involve the body wall (**Fig. 21**). Epidermal inclusion cysts have been described as having a pseudotestis pattern of echogenicity, should be adjacent to the dermis, have no internal blood flow by Doppler imaging, often have increased acoustic transmission, and may have refractive edge shadowing.[31,32]

Desmoid tumors, or aggressive fibromatosis, are uncommon mesenchymal neoplasms that have locally aggressive behavior without potential for distant metastasis (**Fig. 22**). The abdominal wall and within the abdominal cavity are the most common locations for desmoids to occur.[33] There is a distinct form of desmoid tumor that tends to involve the anterior abdominal muscles in women and be associated with pregnancy, postpartum state, or oral contraceptive use.[34]

Endometriosis may occur in the anterior abdominal wall associated with surgical scars, such as incisions for caesarean section and laparoscopic port sites (**Fig. 23**). The reported incidence of abdominal wall endometriosis following caesarean section varies from 0.03% to 1.7%.[35] Classically, a woman presents with a fixed tender mass near a

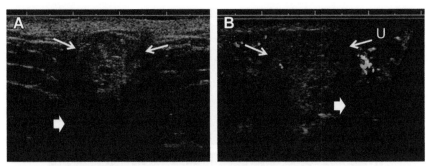

Fig. 18. Transverse (*A*) and longitudinal (*B*) images of a fat-containing hernia (*thin arrows*) at the superior aspect of the umbilicus (U) of a 27-year-old man with a tender lump. This hernia did not change appearance with Valsalva maneuver or upright position. Although the hyperechoic echotexture and subcutaneous location would be compatible with a lipoma, the location near the umbilicus, ill-defined posterior border, refractive edge shadowing (*thick arrows*), and tenderness are all suggestive of a hernia.

scar and complains of cyclical pain. Cyclical pain was observed in 11 of 18 patients with abdominal wall endometriosis in a series reported by Ozel and colleagues.[36] Abdominal wall endometriosis has a small chance of malignant transformation into endometrioid or clear cell carcinoma.[35,37]

In our experience, the most common malignant tumor encountered in the abdominal wall is metastatic disease. Metastatic deposits are generally hypoechoic solid masses (**Fig. 24**), although we have observed hyperechoic metastatic ovarian cancer (**Fig. 25**). Metastatic deposits involving the parietal peritoneum at the deep aspect of the abdominal wall can usually be visualized by

ultrasound and may be the most easily accessible site for biopsy (**Fig. 26**). Ultrasound is an excellent tool for evaluating abdominal wall abnormalities of uncertain significance encountered in patients with cancer undergoing surveillance imaging by other modalities (**Fig. 27**). In these cases, if a suspicious abnormality is found, it can be immediately biopsied with ultrasound guidance.

VASCULAR ABNORMALITIES

Vascular abnormalities of the abdominal wall are occasionally encountered, particularly in patients with portal hypertension. In the setting of portal

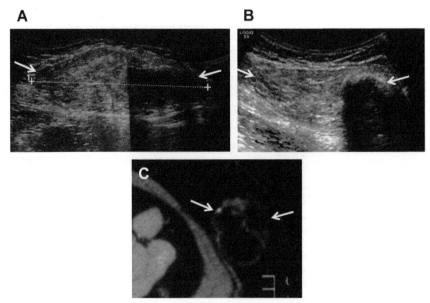

Fig. 19. Longitudinal (*A*) and transverse (*B*) ultrasound images of a partially shadowing solid subcutaneous abdominal wall mass (*arrows*) in a 71-year-old man. (*C*) The corresponding CT image demonstrates predominantly fatty consistency with small areas of soft tissue density and calcification (*arrows*). Needle biopsy confirmed fat necrosis.

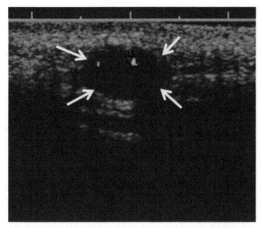

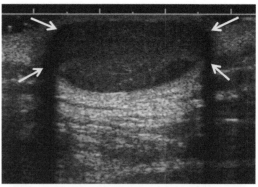

Fig. 21. Epidermal inclusion cyst involving the abdominal wall of a 56-year-old man. This cyst has a "pseudotestis" echo pattern, well-defined borders, deep acoustic enhancement, and refractive edge shadowing (*arrows*). The cyst broadly abuts the dermis. Color Doppler (not shown) revealed no internal flow.

Fig. 20. Neurofibroma involving the posterolateral body wall of a 21-year-old woman. This small hypoechoic mass (*arrows*) has a nonspecific sonographic appearance with a broad differential diagnosis. The presence of more than minimal color Doppler signal and the lack of internal linear echogenic structures argue against lipoma.

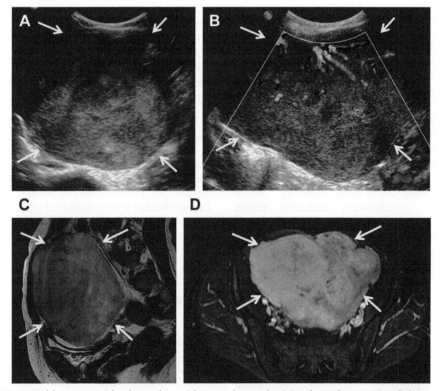

Fig. 22. A 38-year-old woman with a large desmoid tumor (*arrows*) arising from the anterior abdominal wall near the medial aspect of the left rectus muscle. Longitudinal (*A*) and transverse (*B*) ultrasound images demonstrate a large solid mass involving the anterior abdominal wall and filling much of the pelvis. Transvaginal sonography (not shown) demonstrated the mass to be separate from the uterus. Sagittal T2 (*C*) and axial postcontrast T1 with fat saturation (*D*) MR images demonstrate homogeneous T2 signal and diffuse enhancement.

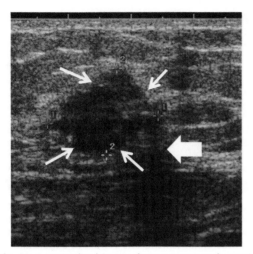

Fig. 23. Longitudinal image demonstrates endometriosis (*thin arrows*) in the abdominal wall of a 33-year-old woman. The mass has a nonspecific sonographic appearance of an aggressive/invasive lesion with ill-defined borders, but the location adjacent to a surgical scar from caesarean section (shadowing from the surgical scar indicated by the *thick arrow*) is characteristic. Additionally, this patient reported cyclical pain, worsened during menstrual flow.

hypertension, dilated paraumbilical veins can be observed taking blood from the left portal vein to the systemic venous circulation via collateralization with the epigastric veins near the umbilicus (**Fig. 28**).[38] The presence of enlarged paraumbilical veins and abdominal wall varices is helpful in confirming the diagnosis of portal hypertension. Rarely, umbilical varices cause major hemorrhage.[39,40]

Evaluation of the vasculature of the abdominal wall is of particular importance in patients requiring paracentesis. Hemorrhagic complications occur in 0.2% to 3% of paracentesis procedures, with most being minor bleeding.[41] Major hemorrhagic complications, including death, have been reported following paracentesis.[41–43] The patient's coagulation status has not been

consistently found to determine the risk of hemorrhage and we are convinced that the most important determinate of bleeding from paracentesis is whether or not a major vascular structure is traversed. The inferior epigastric artery is the most dangerous structure because its deep position allows hemorrhage into the peritoneal cavity and prevents effective manual compression. The course of the inferior epigastric artery can be somewhat difficult to predict clinically because of obesity, stretching of the abdominal wall by ascites, hernias, and distortion from prior surgery. Although not proved in the literature, we believe that large venous varices, which occasionally occur along the deep aspect of the abdominal wall, pose a similar threat of major bleeding if disrupted during paracentesis (**Fig. 29**). Our protocol is to always evaluate the abdominal wall with color Doppler optimized to detect low flow before choosing a puncture site for paracentesis. Routine use of ultrasound before paracentesis has been proposed and may reduce cost by decreasing complications.[41,44]

Vascular abnormalities of the abdominal wall can also occur because of disease of the major systemic arteries and veins. Patients with occlusion of major pelvic veins can develop collateral venous vessels along the abdominal wall (**Fig. 30**). In the setting of chronic arterial disease, collateral flow to the lower extremities can develop involving the superior circumflex iliac artery and the superior and inferior epigastric arteries (**Fig. 31**).

MISCELLANEOUS CONDITIONS

Foreign bodies are occasionally encountered in the abdominal wall. Ultrasound is sensitive and specific for the detection of foreign bodies.[45,46] Foreign bodies are generally echogenic structures that may produce deep acoustic shadowing or comet tail artifact (**Fig. 32**).

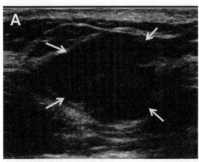
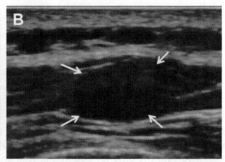

Fig. 24. (*A*) Metastatic melanoma (*arrows*) involving the flank of a 46-year-old woman. (*B*) A 52-year-old woman with neck squamous cell carcinoma (*arrows*) metastatic to the muscle of the posterolateral body wall.

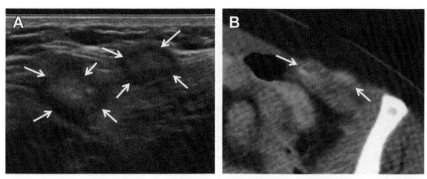

Fig. 25. Metastatic papillary ovarian cancer involving the anterior abdominal wall of a 46-year-old woman. The superior spatial resolution of ultrasound (*A*) allows the two adjacent tumors (*arrows*) to be more clearly visualized as compared with CT (*B*).

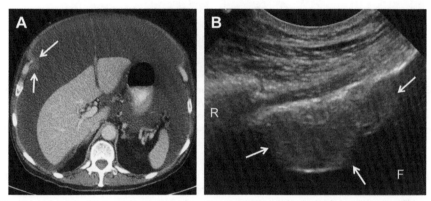

Fig. 26. A 78-year-old man with no previous history of cancer who presented with abdominal distention. (*A*) CT demonstrated large volume ascites and peritoneal nodularity (*arrows*) concerning for peritoneal carcinomatosis. (*B*) Targeted ultrasound demonstrated a solid nodule (*arrows*) involving the parietal peritoneum adjacent to a rib (R) with surrounding ascites (F). This nodule was biopsied, revealing metastatic colon cancer.

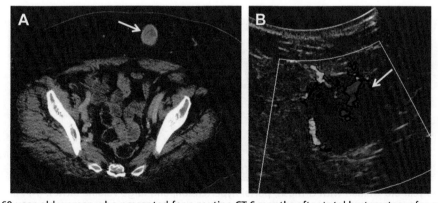

Fig. 27. A 69-year-old woman who presented for a routine CT 6 months after total hysterectomy for endometrial cancer. (*A*) A single-phase postcontrast CT demonstrated a mass or high-attenuation collection in the umbilicus (*arrow*). (*B*) Subsequent targeted ultrasound demonstrated a solid mass (*arrow*) with internal blood flow. An ultrasound-guided biopsy was performed at the same time and confirmed metastatic disease.

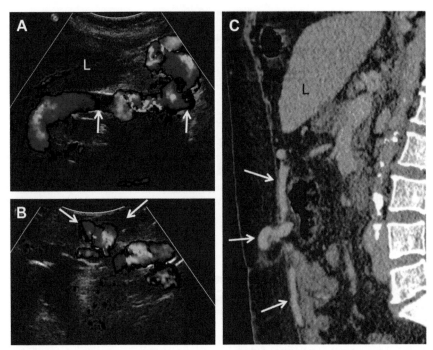

Fig. 28. A 53-year-old woman with cirrhosis and portal hypertension. (*A*) Longitudinal image of the left lobe of the liver (L) demonstrates a large paraumbilical vein (*arrows*) extending inferiorly along the abdominal wall. (*B*) Transverse view through the umbilicus shows an umbilical hernia containing a dilated vein and a small amount of fluid (*arrows*). (*C*) Sagittal reformatted image of a contrast-enhanced CT also demonstrates the varix (*arrows*).

During the evaluation of upper abdominal pain, fracture of a lower rib should be considered in the differential diagnosis, particularly if the patient has focal pain made worse with intercostal scanning. Potential rib abnormalities should be evaluated with a high-resolution linear transducer, focused on the area of patient discomfort (**Fig. 33**). Ultrasound may be more sensitive for rib fractures than radiography.[47]

The sonographer and radiologist should remember to visually examine the skin, particularly in older patients with acute, lateral abdominal pain and no observed sonographic abnormality. We have made the diagnosis of herpes zoster (shingles) in several patients presenting for ultrasound to evaluate acute abdominal pain. The pain associated with herpes zoster may begin 2 to 3 days before the rash appears, leading to initial

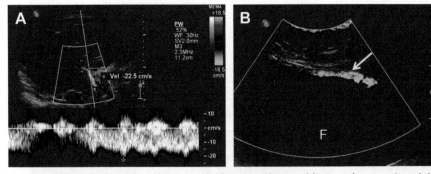

Fig. 29. A 55-year-old woman with cirrhosis, portal hypertension, and large-volume ascites. (*A*) Pulsed Doppler interrogation of the main portal vein demonstrates reversed flow. (*B*) Sonographic survey of the abdomen wall before therapeutic paracentesis revealed large-volume ascites (F) and a dilated vein along the deep aspect of the abdominal wall (*arrow*). Similar dilated veins were found in all four quadrants of the abdomen, necessitating careful real-time ultrasound guidance during paracentesis.

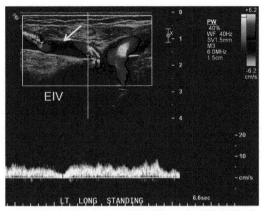

Fig. 30. Dilated venous collateral taking flow from the left common femoral vein superiorly along the abdominal wall (*arrow*), despite imaging in the upright position. Essentially no flow was visualized in the external iliac vein (EIV). Subsequent CT demonstrated chronic occlusion of the left common iliac vein.

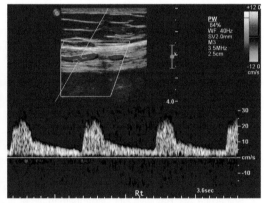

Fig. 31. Large superior epigastric artery with vigorous low resistance flow in a 57-year-old man, providing collateral flow to the lower extremities. A CT showed extensive atherosclerotic disease of the distal aorta.

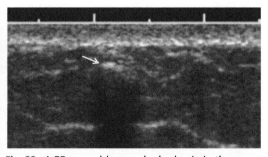

Fig. 32. A 55-year-old man who had pain in the superficial right upper quadrant during lumbar spine MR imaging. A radiograph indicated a metallic foreign body and ultrasound was used to localize the foreign body (*arrow, with deep shadowing*) before surgical removal.

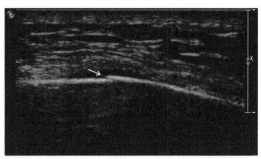

Fig. 33. A 66-year old who presented with right upper quadrant pain who was found to have a right lower rib fracture (*arrow*) that was well demonstrated on high-resolution ultrasound imaging. This minimally displaced fracture was poorly visualized on a CT performed before the ultrasound.

diagnostic confusion.[48] It is therefore possible for a patient to be evaluated clinically before the rash appears, but to present with skin findings at the time of outpatient sonography.

SUMMARY

Ultrasound is a highly valuable imaging modality for evaluating the abdominal wall because of its high spatial resolution and dynamic imaging capability. Imaging during Valsalva maneuver and in the upright position is critical for full evaluation of many abnormalities of the abdominal wall, particularly hernias. Lipomas are the most common neoplasm of the abdominal wall and can be distinguished from fat-containing hernias with careful interrogation.

SUPPLEMENTARY DATA

Videos related to this article can be found online at http://dx.doi.org/10.1016/j.cult.2014.07.005.

REFERENCES

1. Netter FH. Atlas of human anatomy. Summit, (NJ): Ciba-Geigy; 1989.
2. Stavros AT, Rapp C. Dynamic ultrasound of hernias of the groin and anterior abdominal wall. Ultrasound Q 2010;26(3):135–69.
3. Jamadar DA, Jacobson JA, Morag Y, et al. Sonography of inguinal region hernias. AJR Am J Roentgenol 2006;187(1):185–90.
4. Bureau NJ, Chhem RK, Cardinal E. Musculoskeletal infections: US manifestations. Radiographics 1999; 19:1585–92.
5. Adhikari S, Blavias M. Sonography first for subcutaneous abscess and cellulitis evaluation. J Ultrasound Med 2012;31:1509–12.

6. Kingsnorth AN. Hunterian Lecture. Hernia surgery: from guidelines to clinical practice. Ann R Coll Surg Engl 2009;91(4):273–9.

7. Bradley M, Morgan D, Pentlow B, et al. The groin hernia: an ultrasound diagnosis? Ann R Coll Surg Engl 2003;85(3):178–80.

8. Robinson A, Light D, Nice C. Meta-analysis of sonography in the diagnosis of inguinal hernias. J Ultrasound Med 2013;32:339–46.

9. Bradley M, Morgan J, Pentlow B, et al. The positive predictive value of diagnostic ultrasound for occult herniae. Ann R Coll Surg Engl 2006;88(2):165–7.

10. Robinson A, Light D, Kasim A, et al. A systematic review and meta-analysis of the role of radiology in the diagnosis of occult inguinal hernia. Surg Endosc 2013;27(1):11–8.

11. Jamadar DA, Jacobson JA, Girish G, et al. Abdominal wall hernia mesh repair: sonography of mesh and common complications. J Ultrasound Med 2008;27:907–17.

12. Sinha R, Rajiah P, Tiwary P. Abdominal hernias: imaging review and historical perspectives. Curr Probl Diagn Radiol 2007;36(1):30–42.

13. vanSonnenberg E, Simeone JF, Mueller PR, et al. Sonographic appearance of hematoma in liver, spleen and kidney: a clinical, pathologic, and animal study. Radiology 1983;147:507–10.

14. Jain N, Goyal N, Mukherjee K, et al. Ultrasound of the abdominal wall: what lies beneath? Clin Radiol 2013;68:85–93.

15. Ward WG Sr, Rougraff B, Quinn R, et al. Tumors masquerading as hematomas. Clin Orthop Relat Res 2007;465:232–40.

16. Kontogeorgakos VA, Martinez S, Dodd L, et al. Extremity soft tissue sarcomas presented as hematomas. Arch Orthop Trauma Surg 2010;130(10): 1209–14.

17. Doyle AJ, Miller MV, French JG. Ultrasound of soft-tissue masses: pitfalls in interpretation. Australas Radiol 2000;44:275–80.

18. Brouns F, Stas M, De Wever I. Delay in diagnosis of soft tissue sarcomas. Eur J Surg Oncol 2003;29(5): 440–5.

19. Coates M. Ultrasound and soft-tissue mass lesions: a note of caution. N Z Med J 2003;116(1187):1–2.

20. Middleton MA, Middleton WD. Femoral hernia simulating a pseudoaneurysm on color Doppler sonography. AJR Am J Roentgenol 1993;160:1291–2.

21. Wagner JM, Lee KS, Rosas H, et al. Accuracy of sonographic diagnosis of superficial masses. J Ultrasound Med 2013;32(8):1443–50.

22. Lakkaraju A, Sinha R, Garikipati R, et al. Ultrasound for initial evaluation and triage of clinically suspicious soft-tissue masses. Clin Radiol 2009;64(6): 615–21.

23. Widmann G, Riedl A, Schoepf D, et al. State-of-the-art HR-US imaging findings of the most frequent musculoskeletal soft-tissue tumors. Skeletal Radiol 2009;38(7):637–49.

24. Nielsen GP, Mandahl N. Lipoma. In: Fletcher CD, Unni KK, Mertens F, editors. World Health Organization classification of tumours: pathology and genetics of tumours of soft tissue and bone. Lyon (France): International Agency for Research on Cancer; 2002. p. 20–2.

25. Choong K. Sonographic appearance of subcutaneous angiolipomas. J Ultrasound Med 2004;23:715–7.

26. Chiou HJ, Chou YH, Chiu SY, et al. Differentiation of benign and malignant superficial soft-tissue masses using grayscale and color Doppler ultrasonography. J Chin Med Assoc 2009;72(6):307–15.

27. Bang M, Kang BS, Hwang JC, et al. Ultrasonographic analysis of subcutaneous angiolipoma. Skeletal Radiol 2012;41(9):1055–9.

28. Robinson P, Farrant JM, Bourke G, et al. Ultrasound and MRI findings in appendicular and truncal fat necrosis. Skeletal Radiol 2008;37(3):217–24.

29. Walsh M, Jacobson JA, Kim SM, et al. Sonography of fat necrosis involving the extremity and torso with magnetic resonance imaging and histologic correlation. J Ultrasound Med 2008;27:1751–7.

30. Pencavel T, Strauss DC, Thomas JM, et al. The surgical management of soft tissue tumours arising in the abdominal wall. Eur J Surg Oncol 2010;36(5): 489–95.

31. Huang CC, Ko SF, Huang HY, et al. Epidermal cysts in the superficial soft tissue: sonographic features with an emphasis on the pseudotestis pattern. J Ultrasound Med 2011;30:11–7.

32. Kim HK, Kim SM, Lee SH, et al. Subcutaneous epidermal inclusion cysts: ultrasound (US) and MR imaging findings. Skeletal Radiol 2011;40(11):1415–9.

33. Shinagare AB, Ramaiya NH, Jagannathan JP, et al. A to Z of desmoid tumors. AJR Am J Roentgenol 2011;197(6):W1008–14.

34. Dinauer PA, Brixey CJ, Moncur JT, et al. Pathologic and MR imaging features of benign fibrous soft-tissue tumors in adults. Radiographics 2007;27(1): 173–87.

35. Uysal A, Mun S, Taner CE. Endometrioma in abdominal scars: case reports of four cases and review of the literature. Arch Gynecol Obstet 2012;286(3):805–8.

36. Ozel L, Sagiroglu J, Unal A, et al. Abdominal wall endometriosis in the cesarean section surgical scar: a potential diagnostic pitfall. J Obstet Gynaecol Res 2012;38(3):526–30.

37. Li X, Yang J, Cao D, et al. Clear-cell carcinoma of the abdominal wall after cesarean delivery. Obstet Gynecol 2012;120(2 Pt 2):445–8.

38. Lafortune M, Constantin A, Breton G, et al. The recanalized umbilical vein in portal hypertension: a myth. AJR Am J Roentgenol 1985;144:549–53.

39. Assis DN, Pollak J, Schilsky ML, et al. Successful treatment of a bleeding umbilical varix by

percutaneous umbilical vein embolization with sclerotherapy. J Clin Gastroenterol 2012;46(2): 115–8.

40. Lewis CP, Murthy S, Webber SM, et al. Hemorrhage from recanalized umbilical vein in a patient with cirrhosis. Am J Gastroenterol 1999;94(1):280.

41. Sekiguchi H, Suzuki J, Daniels CE. Making paracentesis safer: a proposal for the use of bedside abdominal and vascular ultrasonography to prevent a fatal complication. Chest 2013;143(4):1136–9.

42. Seidler M, Sayegh K, Roy A, et al. A fatal complication of ultrasound-guided abdominal paracentesis. J Clin Ultrasound 2013;41(7):457–60.

43. Webster ST, Brown KL, Lucey MR, et al. Hemorrhagic complications of large volume abdominal paracentesis. Am J Gastroenterol 1996;91(2):366–8.

44. Mercaldi CJ, Lanes SF. Ultrasound guidance decreases complications and improves the cost of care among patients undergoing thoracentesis and paracentesis. Chest 2013;143(2):532–8.

45. Jacobson JA, Powell A, Craig JG, et al. Wooden foreign bodies in soft tissues: detection at US. Radiology 1998;206:45–8.

46. Bray PW, Mahoney JL, Campbell JP. Sensitivity and specificity of ultrasound in the diagnosis of foreign bodies in the hand. J Hand Surg Am 1995;20(4): 661–6.

47. Turk F, Kurt AB, Saglam S. Evaluation by ultrasound of traumatic rib fractures missed by radiography. Emerg Radiol 2010;17(6):473–7.

48. Cohen JI. Clinical practice: herpes zoster. N Engl J Med 2013;369(3):255–63.

Ultrasound-Guided Intervention in the Abdomen and Pelvis
Review from A to Z

Corinne Deurdulian, MD*, Nicole French, MD

KEYWORDS

• Ultrasound • Biopsy • Drainage • Procedure • Fusion • Complication • Lesion • Collection

KEY POINTS

- Ultrasound (US) guidance for invasive procedures is a necessary tool and should be considered the first-line modality for most procedures in the abdomen and pelvis.
- There are many steps in ensuring patient safety and optimal procedure environment, including setup of room and equipment, sonographer and nursing support, and comprehensive review of the patient history and imaging.
- US with fusion further increases the utility of US in the setting of invasive procedures.

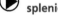

Videos of Hydrodissection, liver biopsy-related hemorrhage, renal biopsy-related hemorrhage, and splenic biopsy accompany this article at http://www.ultrasound.theclinics.com/

INTRODUCTION

Image-guided percutaneous biopsy and fluid collection drainage are commonly performed radiologic interventions in the abdomen. Both US and computed tomography (CT) guidance are used for image-guided procedures. Advantages of the sonographic approach include decreased procedure time, absence of radiation, low cost, portability, real-time visualization of needle placement, and real-time Doppler imaging to avoid vessel puncture or to rapidly confirm complications such as bleeding.[1,2] US also allows for rapid, real-time guidance for aspirations and drainages, precluding the need for CT scanning and radiation to confirm needle or catheter placement in many patients.[3]

When deciding whether to use US or CT guidance, a good general rule is to consider US first.

If the lesion cannot be seen under US guidance or if a safe pathway is not identified, then CT may be considered. Occasionally, both modalities may need to be used. For example, the initial access may be easier under US guidance, with confirmation of the needle or catheter placement under CT. However, US alone is more than sufficient for most types of abdominal intervention.[4,5]

Newer applications in procedures such as the use of US contrast, volume navigation, and fusion further expand the capabilities of US. US contrast helps visualize lesions that may be suboptimally seen by conventional sonography and also helps identify foci of residual or recurrent tumor after ablation.[6] Volume navigation assists in selecting trajectories from various entry points based on the location of the target. Fusion technology allows for overlay of CT, magnetic resonance imaging (MRI), and positron emission tomography

The authors have no disclosures.
Department of Radiology, USC Keck School of Medicine, 1500 San Pablo Street, Los Angeles, CA 90033, USA
* Corresponding author.
E-mail address: Corinne.Deurdulian@med.usc.edu

Ultrasound Clin 9 (2014) 793–820
http://dx.doi.org/10.1016/j.cult.2014.07.012

(PET)/PET-CT images, with the sonographic images to target biopsies and ablations.

IMAGING REVIEW

Before scheduling a procedure, it is important to review other imaging modalities such as CT, MRI, or PET to help localize or characterize the target lesion or fluid collection. Cross-sectional imaging may help identify other lesions that are more amenable to biopsy, such as supraclavicular lymph nodes or soft-tissue nodules. Additional lesions may upstage the diagnosis, which can affect which lesion is most appropriate to biopsy.

The radiologist can then review the patient's history, laboratory values, and allergy information. Interventional or surgical backup may be sought for high-risk cases. Patients who are at a higher risk of bleeding than the general population should be informed of their risk and consented accordingly.

SONOGRAPHER

The sonographer plays an important role both before and during the procedure. The sonographer should have all the appropriate supplies ready so there is no need to leave the room after the procedure has started. This preparation includes having doubles of most supplies in case one is dropped or inadvertently contaminated. The sonographer should also coordinate with the imaging nurse for patient monitoring and review of preprocedure laboratory results.

The prescan is important to localize the respective lesion or fluid collection. Before the radiologist enters the room, the sonographer can identify the region of interest and help assess possible trajectories for needle entry. In cases in which changes in patient positioning may be necessary, the sonographer can also provide information of which position allows for optimal visualization of the target. Once the target is identified and patient position optimized, the distance from the skin to the target and/or from the top of the needle guide to the target can be estimated. The sonographer can look for impediments in the possible trajectories, such as bowel, lung, or large vessels. It is imperative that color Doppler imaging be performed, as large vessels should be avoided. The radiologist can then more expeditiously confirm the appropriate trajectory.

During the procedure, the sonographer should capture images demonstrating adequate placement of the needle within the target (**Fig. 1**). The sonographer can capture cine loops of the procedure when there is a question of whether the target was reached, especially in hard-to-visualize targets.

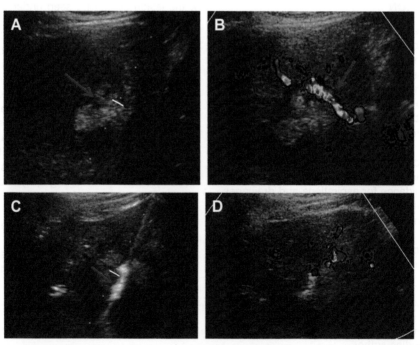

Fig. 1. Necessary steps during a biopsy. (*A*) Assess trajectory to lesion (echogenic liver mass, *arrow*). (*B*) Apply color Doppler and look for vessels in the path (*arrow*). (*C*) Record each pass showing needle location (*arrow*). (*D*) Postscan with and without color Doppler to look for bleeding (none detected).

ROOM SETUP

A movable, height-adjustable stretcher allows for a comfortable working level for the radiologist to minimize unnecessary strain. A functioning oxygen source with the appropriate tubing or masks should be readily available. A sharps container is a requirement for in-room disposal of needles, scalpels, and other sharp objects. In addition, the crash cart should be easily accessible for emergent situations.

The US unit should ideally be opposite the radiologist with respect to the patient (**Fig. 2**). This setup allows for the radiologist to see the needle entering the patient and the US monitor simultaneously and gives the sonographer room on the opposite side to record the necessary images. When the US machine is on the same side as the radiologist, the radiologist cannot look at the monitor and the needle at the same time and may not be able to correlate the needle placement with the US images effectively or efficiently. This setup also promotes neck strain during the procedure. Newer monitor configurations with adjustable articulating arms help alleviate part of this problem. However, if the sonographer needs to document images during the procedure, the same space occupied by the radiologist, US machine, and sonographer quickly gets crowded.

IMAGING NURSE

Moderate- to higher-risk procedures usually necessitate the presence of an imaging nurse to assess and monitor the patients. The nurse should review pertinent history and laboratory results and review the allergy profile, including prior reactions to procedure-related medications. The nurse plays a vital role in raising any potential red flags that may become an issue during the procedure or recovery. The nurse also delivers conscious sedation medication to provide some level of pain control and anxiolysis.

PATHOLOGY SUPPORT

Communication with the pathology department is important to help guide whether fine needle aspiration (FNA), core specimens, or both types of samples are needed. Review of the FNA or touch preparation of the core specimens by the cytopathology personnel during the procedure decreases the chance of inadequate or insufficient sampling. If lymphoma is suspected, FNA specimens may need to be sent for flow cytometry. The pathology department may also provide different solutions for specific biopsies such as renal biopsies.[7]

NEEDLE SELECTION

FNAs for abdominal biopsies are typically performed with 18- to 22-gauge needles and can be used independently or through a coaxial introducer. Most abdominal core biopsies are obtained with 18-gauge needles. In patients with mild coagulopathy or with deep lesions where prominent blood vessels may be traversed, downsizing to a 20-gauge needle or performing FNA instead of core biopsy may be considered, as larger needle size has been linked to bleeding complications.[8,9] However, many studies report no change in bleeding risk with respect to needle size.[10,11] Lesions that are small or adjacent to vital structures may necessitate using needles with a smaller throw distance, such as 1 cm instead of the usual 2 cm.

Needles that are too short do not reach the target, and needles that are too long may bend, making it difficult to efficiently reach the target. The actual length of the core needle is typically shorter than stated on the label (**Fig. 3**). Many 10-cm-long core biopsy needles have an effective length of 8 cm when cocked. That means a

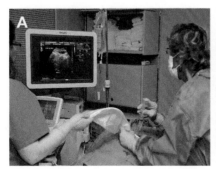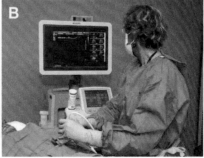

Fig. 2. Room setup. (*A*) Ideal juxtapostion of radiologist facing the patient, needle and transducer position, and ultrasound monitor in a straight line. Sonographer has room to obtain images and assist with the procedure. (*B*) Nonideal position where radiologist turns away from the patient, unable to see the needle and transducer position while looking at the ultrasound monitor. There is no room for the sonographer to obtain images of the procedure.

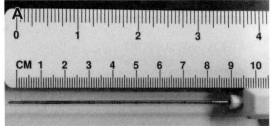
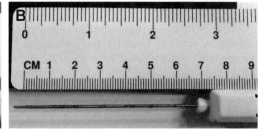

Fig. 3. Differences in needle size. (*A*) A 9-cm core biopsy needle is just less than 9 cm in length. (*B*) However, when cocked, actual needle length is less than 7 cm. Therefore, target must be less than 6.5 cm from skin entry point.

15-cm-long needle may be necessary to reach a target depth beyond 7 or 8 cm. In addition, when subcutaneous anesthesia such as lidocaine is administered, it slightly increases the distance to the target. Similar problems exist with the coaxial needles, which are typically shorter than the length on the label and also shorter than the biopsy needle. For example, the coaxial needle on an 18-gauge 10-cm-long system may be only about 6 to 7 cm long. If lesion depth exceeds the length of the biopsy needle in a coaxial system, a longer system is required. Sometimes, the stated length includes the hub, so this has to be taken into account.

CATHETER SELECTION

When selecting drainage catheters, it is important to select a caliber appropriate for the fluid to be drained. Simple collections usually drain with 8F and 10F catheters. More viscous collections such as pus and complex fluid may necessitate larger catheters such as 12F and 14F. A 10F catheter from 2 different vendors may have different-sized pigtails and side holes (**Fig. 4**). Catheters with smaller pigtails may be easier to place in smaller collections, and larger side holes promote faster drainage, especially of more viscous fluid.

Whether to use a modified Seldinger technique or single-stick trocar technique depends on the circumstances. The Seldinger technique is helpful when the collection is small and deep or the optimal access window is narrow or in a sensitive location. If the collection is large and there is a broad access window in a nonsensitive location, the trocar technique provides a simple and rapid method of catheter placement.[12] Many drainage catheters today have a default trocar configuration that obviates the Seldinger technique when applicable.

TRANSDUCER SELECTION

The curved-phased array transducer (eg, 4–6 MHz with range down to 1 or 2 MHz) is used for most types of abdominal intervention because of its depth of penetration, wide field of view, and excellent spatial resolution. However, a larger window and subcostal approach are often necessary. A vector transducer has a smaller footprint and is easier to use in smaller spaces, especially intercostal. Although traditionally the smaller field of view is a disadvantage, newer high-resolution transducers with virtual convex capability compensate for this deficiency and allow for targeting of deeper lesions.[13] If the target is

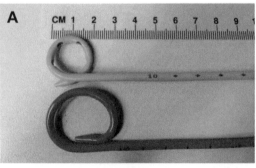
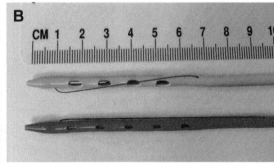

Fig. 4. Two different 10F catheters. (*A*) Two different-size pigtails of 10F catheters. Note the top catheter pigtail is less than 2 cm in diameter and the bottom catheter pigtail exceeds 3 cm in diameter. The smaller pigtail is advantageous for smaller collections, as a shorter length of the catheter needs to be inserted into the collection. (*B*) Differences in size of side holes of different catheters. Note the top catheter has larger side holes, which drain more viscous collections better than smaller side holes.

superficial or in a thin patient, a higher-frequency transducer (eg, 9 MHz linear transducer) may sometimes visualize the lesion better. These transducers have needle guides that can be used to aid in accessing the target.

Appropriate scanning should be performed before the start of the procedure to select the transducer that best images the target and optimal trajectory. If a needle guide is being used with a curved transducer, the air gap between the transducer edge and skin entry point should be minimized to improve needle visibility at the entry point, which can be achieved by slightly tilting the transducer so that the curved edge maintains contact with the skin.

COAGULATION AND BLEEDING RISK

Prothrombin time (PT)/international normalized ratio (INR) and platelet count are the most important laboratory values used to assess bleeding risk before procedures. Normal PT ranges about 11 to 14 seconds, and normal INR typically ranges from 0.9 to 1.1. An INR of 1.5 has been used as a traditional cutoff for most procedures.[14] Many studies have shown that the bleeding risk with an INR up to 1.7 is not significantly increased compared with a normal INR.[15,16]

The activated partial thromboplastin time (aPTT) is generally not considered as important as the INR or platelet count. Studies have shown that elevated aPTT is the most common abnormal coagulation test, it does not predict blood lost in the operating room, and abnormal aPTT values are often transient.[17,18]

The normal platelet count ranges from 150,000 to 450,000, with a traditional threshold of 50,000 for invasive procedures.[14] Although many radiologists are hesitant to perform procedures in patients with platelet counts less than 50,000, there are studies showing lower counts are safe in patients undergoing many types of procedures.[19] Platelet counts less than 10,000 or 20,000 are associated with spontaneous hemorrhage.[20]

ANTICOAGULANTS

Clopidogrel (Plavix) and similar agents may not be able to be discontinued depending on the clinical indication. Neither clopidogrel nor aspirin can be stopped if a patient has had a drug-eluting cardiac stent placed in the last 12 to 24 months or a bare metal stent in the last month.[21,22] If a patient administered clopidogrel needs an invasive procedure, the comparative risks of continuing or stopping the use of clopidogrel for the procedure should be discussed with the patient's cardiologist and clinical team. Patient consent should be obtained for increased risk of excessive hemorrhage or cardiovascular event.

For patients recently administered Clopidogrel, the procedure may be modified so that FNA can be performed instead of core or a smaller-gauge core device can be used (eg, 20 gauge instead of 18 gauge). The postprocedure observation period may be increased beyond the usual recovery time, and vital signs can be obtained more frequently. The patient can also be scheduled for a follow-up appointment soon after the procedure if needed.

Hemostatic Agents

Platelets
Platelets may be administered in a 5- to 6-unit dose pack or 1 pheresis pack. There is a general increase of 5,000 to 10,000 platelets per individual unit or 25,000 to 50,000 per pack or unit dose. Optimally, the last unit of platelets should be given at the start of the procedure. When a procedure nurse is not available to monitor for potential transfusion reaction, the procedure should be performed within 1 to 2 hours of platelet administration. After platelet administration, it is generally recommended not to recheck the platelet count before the procedure. Many times this delays the procedure, which, in turn, decreases the platelets' effectiveness.

Fresh frozen plasma
Fresh frozen plasma (FFP) is administered to patients to decrease an elevated INR. The higher the INR, the greater the correction per unit of FFP (**Table 1**). Typically, two units of FFP may theoretically decrease coagulopathy when the INR is about 2.5 or greater. However, there are little data to either support or refute the benefits of

Table 1
Estimate of INR correction per unit of FFP

Pretransfusion INR	Correction per FFP Unit Mean & Range
1.3–1.7	0.1 (0.1–0.2)
1.7–2.3	0.2 (0.1–0.3)
2.4–2.9	0.4 (0.1–0.7)
3.0–4.3	0.7 (0.2–1.5)
4.4–20.0	3.5 (1.1–8.4)

The higher the INR, the greater the estimated correction per unit FFP.

Adapted from Plapp FV. Essentials of transfusion medicine. ClinLab Navigator, 2008. Available at: http://www.clinlabnavigator.com. Accessed April 28, 2014.

FFP.[23] Plasma transfusion has a minimal effect on normalizing a mildly elevated INR, and FFP is inappropriately ordered in 10% to 83% of patients.[15] Mild to moderate clotting abnormalities do not typically pose a significantly increased bleeding risk, and FFP transfusion may not actually decrease postprocedure bleeding.[16]

The risk of transfusion reactions should also be considered when platelets or FFP may be given. Transfusion reactions include but are not limited to allergy, fever, shortness of breath, volume overload, and transfusion-associated lung injury.[24]

The 2009 consensus statement from the Society of Interventional Radiology is a useful guide for performing procedures in patients with abnormal coagulation parameters or known coagulopathy.[25] It was updated in 2012 and addended in 2013.[26,27] Procedures were divided into low, moderate, and high bleeding risk, with recommendations for laboratory analysis and management.[14,27] A modification of these tables is given in **Tables 2–4**.

Much of the data currently used for imaging-guided procedures have been extrapolated from older surgical data. Therefore, there may be variable clinical practice due to lack of randomized controlled trials. Patient management ultimately depends on comprehensive assessment, procedure type, and experience. Newer studies suggest one may be able to be more liberal with some procedures than the traditional 1.5 INR and 50,000 platelet thresholds. In an interinstitutional and multidisciplinary paper, O'Connor and colleagues[19] proposed more liberal guidelines with an evidence-based summary (**Table 5**).

Using these recommendations, Kitchin and colleagues[28] demonstrated that when the coagulation threshold criteria for their imaging-guided liver biopsies were loosened from an INR of 1.5 to 2 and from platelet count of 50,000 to 25,000, they observed an overall decrease in the hemorrhagic complication rate in 1846 patients. Preprocedure platelet and FFP transfusions decreased 5-fold. Although the individual risk of bleeding was higher in those patients with suboptimal INR and platelet values, they noted that transfusions did not decrease the additional bleeding risk when the laboratory test values were abnormal.

Patients with liver failure may be more prone to bleeding and need laboratory tests more often due to changes in clinical status. However, these patients undergo more procedures more frequently than many other patients, which may account for higher numbers of bleeding-related complications. Patients on the liver transplant list who receive platelets and FFP may show improved coagulation parameters on follow-up laboratory tests, which downgrades them on the transplant list and delays potentially life-saving transplant surgery.

Contraindications

Although there are no absolute contraindications to image-guided procedures, relative contraindications include severe uncorrectable coagulopathy, severely compromised cardiopulmonary function or hemodynamic instability, lack of a safe pathway to the lesion or target (eg, large blood vessels, lung, or bowel), the patient's inability to tolerate the

---

Table 2
Low bleeding risk

Procedure	Preprocedure Laboratory Tests	Management

Vascular
• Dialysis access/intervention
• Venography
• CVC removal
• IVC filter or PICC placement
	INR
	• Warfarin/liver disease
	  (recommended[a])
	aPTT
	• IV heparin (recommended[a])
		INR—correct if >2.0 (FFP or
		  vitamin K)
		aPTT—no consensus
		PLT—transfusion if <50 K
		Clopidogrel (Plavix)—withhold
		  0–5 d[a]

Nonvascular
• Drainage catheter exchange
• Thoracentesis/paracentesis
• Superficial aspiration/biopsy
  (eg, thyroid, superficial lymph
  node or mass)
	PLT—not routinely
	  recommended
		ASA—do not withhold
		LMWH (therapeutic dose)
		• Withhold 1 dose before
		  procedure
		• No need to withhold prophy-
		  lactic dose

Please refer to official guidelines for comprehensive review.
Abbreviations: ASA, aspirin; CVC, central venous catheter; IV, intravenous; IVC, inferior vena cava; LMWH, low molecular weight heparin; PICC, peripherally inserted central catheter; PLT, platelet count.
  [a] New recommendations. Indicates changes with 2013 addendum.
Data from Refs.[14,25,26], *Modified and simplified from* SIR Consensus Guidelines.

Table 3
Moderate bleeding risk

Procedure	Preprocedure Laboratory Tests	Management
Vascular • Arterial angiography (7F)/venous intervention • Chemoembolization/UAE • Transjugular liver biopsy • Tunneled CVC/subcutaneous port	INR aPTT[a] PLT[a]	INR correct if >1.5 aPTT—no consensus, may correct if >1.5× normal PLT—transfusion if <50 K Clopidogrel (Plavix)—withhold 5 d
Nonvascular • Intra-abdominal, lung, chest wall, or retroperitoneal biopsy or abscess drainage • Percutaneous cholecystostomy or gastrostomy • RFA • Spine procedures (LP, vertebroplasty/kyphoplasty)		ASA—do not withhold LMWH (therapeutic dose) • Withhold 1 dose before procedure • Do not need to withhold prophylactic dose

Please refer to official guidelines for comprehensive review.
Abbreviations: ASA, aspirin; CVC, central venous catheter; LMWH, low molecular weight heparin; LP, lumbar puncture; PLT, platelet count; RFA, radiofrequency ablation; UAE, uterine artery embolization.
[a] New recommendations. Indicates changes with 2013 addendum.
Data from Refs.[14,25,26], *Modified and simplified from SIR Consensus Guidelines.*

procedure (eg, breath hold, positioning, or uncooperative), and patient refusal. Other organ-specific relative contraindications are listed in each section where applicable.

INTERVENTIONAL TECHNIQUES

When performing interventions, it is important to always visualize the needle tip with the optimal field of view, focus, and gain settings using the highest-frequency transducer that penetrates the target. The needle is best seen in-plane (longitudinal) whereby needle is parallel to the long axis of the transducer and angled with respect to the US beam, so that the full length of the needle shaft and tip are visualized.

After local anesthesia is instilled into the dermis, it should then be administered to the capsule of the target organ or target lesion if outside an organ. Using the needle guide, anesthesia can be administered using a spinal needle to reach the desired location. The authors prefer the use of

Table 4
High bleeding risk

Procedure	Preprocedure Laboratory Tests	Management
Vascular • TIPS	INR aPTT[a] PLT	INR—correct if >1.5 aPTT—stop or reverse heparin if >1.5× normal PLT—transfusion if <50 K Clopidogrel (Plavix)—withhold 5 d
Nonvascular • Renal biopsy • Biliary intervention (new tract) • Nephrostomy placement • RFA (complex)		ASA—withhold 5 d LMWH—withhold for 24 h or up to 2 doses

Please refer to official guidelines for comprehensive review.
Abbreviations: ASA, aspirin; LMWH, low molecular weight heparin; PLT, platelet count; RFA, radiofrequency ablation; TIPS, transjugular intrahepatic portosystemic shunt.
[a] New recommendations. Indicates changes with 2013 addendum.
Data from Refs.[14,25,26], *Modified and simplified from SIR Consensus Guidelines.*

Table 5
Recommendation summary

Intervention	INR	PLT
FNA ≤20 g	Any	Any
Paracentesis	≤3.0	≥25 K
Thoracentesis, liver biopsy, or other	≤2.0	≥25 K

FNA ≤20 g refers to fluid aspiration anywhere in the body.
Recommendations proposed by O'Connor and colleagues. If laboratory tests are normal within 4–6 months of the procedure and there is no significant clinical change, they recommended not repeating laboratory tests unless warranted by clinical history.
Adapted from O'Connor SD, Taylor AJ, Williams EC, et al. Coagulation concepts update. AJR Am J Roentgenol 2009;193(6):1658.

20-gauge needles for this purpose, as smaller needles tend to bend in the abdomen or retroperitoneum. If moderate sedation is also being administered, the patient should remain awake enough to be able to breath hold when needed.

Several techniques can be used when there is difficulty in accessing a target for biopsy or drainage. Changing patient positioning and respiration are simple maneuvers that can improve access. Hydrodissection is a useful technique that uses injection of saline or sterile water to displace intervening structures away from a target (**Fig. 5**, Videos 1–4). This technique may be especially helpful in accessing retroperitoneal structures such as the adrenal gland (by displacing the pleura laterally and expanding the posterior paravertebral space, allowing a posterior extrapleural approach).[29] In addition, continuously applied pressure with the US transducer over the access site can help displace bowel loops out of the way.

BIOPSY TECHNIQUES

The 2 techniques used for US-guided biopsies are freehand and guided techniques. Each technique has its advantages and limitations.[30] The guided technique provides a predicted needle trajectory but is limited by the fixed angle. The number of fixed angles depends on the needle guide, ranging from 1 to 4. The trajectory can be changed using the same incision point by changing the angle on the guide. The freehand technique requires more technical skill and may be challenging for

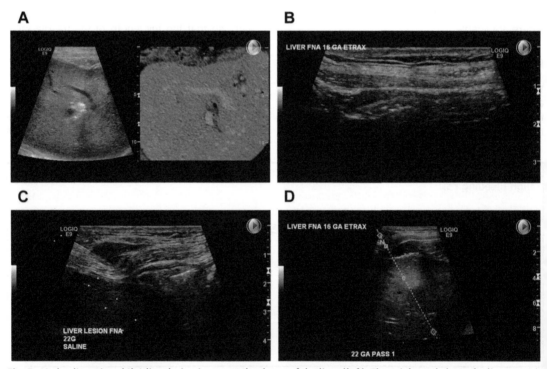

Fig. 5. Hydrodissection. (*A*) A liver lesion is seen at the dome of the liver (*left*). There is bowel along the liver margin in the trajectory of the needle seen better on the CT fusion image (*right*). (*B*) Bowel along the anterior margin of the liver on US imaging. (*C*) Hydrodissection performed with 100 to 150 mL saline separates the bowel from the liver surface to provide a safe entry point. (*D*) Biopsy can then be safely performed. (*Courtesy of* Tchelepi H, MD, Los Angeles, CA.)

beginning or inexperienced interventionalists, as readjustment and tract correction are more often needed. However, the absence of the fixed angle limitation can allow more flexibility in changing the angle without making the change on a guide apparatus or creating a new entry site incision. In a study using phantoms, the guided technique was superior to free hand by allowing faster, more efficient, and reproducible technique; this was especially true for less experienced interventionalists. There was a significant reduction in the number of attempts to insert the needle, overall reduction in the time required to perform the biopsy, and decreased number of passes.[31]

An additional consideration in percutaneous biopsy is using a coaxial system. The advantage of the coaxial technique is that the coaxial needle is usually placed only once into the organ or lesion, obviating multiple entries. This technique may decrease the risk of complications such as hemorrhage, pneumothorax, and tumor seeding along the needle tract. In addition, multiple samples can be obtained from a lesion by slightly changing the needle's trajectory without completely extracting the needle. If a coaxial needle is placed with a biopsy guide, the guide apparatus may need to be detached from the coaxial needle to keep the needle from moving during the procedure unless a second pair of hands can hold the transducer apparatus and needle in place.

Generally, there are the 2 types of samples that can be obtained: FNA and core needle biopsy (CNB). FNA biopsy specimens in the abdomen are typically acquired using 18- to 22-gauge needles and are analyzed cytologically, whereas CNB specimens are obtained using larger 14- to 20-gauge needles, usually 18 gauge, and are analyzed histologically. The main advantage of FNA includes decreased risk of bleeding, given smaller needle size. Advantages of CNB include preservation of tissue architecture, which may be required to diagnose well-differentiated hepatomas and lymphoma, and the ability to use special stains and immunohistochemical techniques. In a comparison study of FNA cytology and needle core biopsy in the sampling of abdominal masses by Stewart and colleagues,[32] FNA cytology was more sensitive and accurate than CNB (FNA cytology was diagnostic in 122 of 141 [86.5%] cases, and CNB was diagnostic in 113 of 141 [80.1%] cases). However, one advantage of CNB was the ability to perform specific tumor subtyping (identifying tumor origin or characterizing tumor). The combination of the 2 techniques yielded the highest accuracy.

Touch preparation is a useful adjunct tool with CNB in that it allows on-site evaluation to provide real-time assessment of material quality and may supply additional diagnostic material if the core tissue does not survive processing. In a retrospective review comparing FNA with CNB with or without touch preparation of 154 renal lesions using US- or CT-guided imaging, CNB with touch preparation yielded a greater specimen adequacy than FNA.[33] In this study, FNAs were obtained with multiple passes of a 21-gauge or smaller needle, and core biopsies were obtained with needles of 20 gauge or larger. The specimen adequacy was satisfactory in 86% of FNAs, 94% of CNBs, and 95% of CNBs with touch preparation. CNB with or without touch preparation had a higher specimen adequacy and diagnostic yield than FNA. Another advantage of CNB is that it provided more diagnostic information (subtype and nuclear grade) in the diagnosis of renal cell carcinoma.

For biopsies of necrotic lesions, the needle should be aimed toward the periphery of the lesion to yield adequate cellular material. Obtaining FNA or touch preparation in these cases also minimizes the chance of inadequate sampling as the trajectory or target lesion can be changed if the original sampling is nondiagnostic.

The number of biopsy passes may be aided by an on-site cytotechnologist or pathologist who performs rapid touch preparation smears of the core biopsy samples or analyzes the FNA samples. This rapid evaluation helps avoid nondiagnostic biopsy results. However, on-site cytology for every biopsy procedure may not be possible because of limited resources. In a study by Appelbaum and colleagues,[34] although lesion size and location did not influence the number of passes needed for diagnosis, metastatic lesions required fewer passes. Without the presence of a cytologist, a predetermined number of 3 passes would be diagnostic in almost 90% of all US-guided focal liver biopsies using an 18-gauge CNB. At the authors' institution, two to three 18-gauge core passes are obtained for most solid-organ biopsies.

DRAIN PLACEMENT TECHNIQUES

Two methods are used for percutaneous US-guided drainage of fluid collections. These include the Seldinger and trocar methods. In the Seldinger method, after localizing the fluid collection under US guidance, a 5F 19-gauge Yueh (Cook Medical, Bloomington, IN) catheter needle is advanced into the fluid collection. On aspiration of the fluid, the outer sheath is advanced from the needle and the needle is then removed. A 0.035- or 0.038-in guidewire is inserted through the sheath and coiled in the collection. The outer sheath is removed over the guidewire, and serial dilation is performed. Typically, dilators can be used in increments of 2F up to the final catheter size. The catheter of choice is then advanced over the guidewire, making sure all side holes are located within the cavity, and the guidewire is removed. The pigtail of the catheter is formed and a drainage bag is connected to the catheter. Advantages of this technique include the ability to manipulate the wire in the exact location before final catheter positioning. Disadvantages of this technique include increased procedure time compared with the trocar method, problems with wire kinking, and leakage of fluid contents around the wire during removal of the needle or dilators.[35]

In the trocar method, the catheter is directly mounted onto a stylet or trocar and no serial dilatation is performed. After the collection is localized and local anesthesia is given, the selected catheter is advanced into the fluid collection. After ensuring adequate placement with aspiration of fluid and direct US visualization, the pigtail is deployed and a drainage bag is connected to the catheter. Advantages of this technique include faster placement from reduced number of steps compared with the Seldinger method and reduced leakage of fluid along the tract.[34]

A needle guide is used for catheter drainage to assist in prompt access into the collection. Via the trocar method, an 8.5F catheter is placed through the largest guide clip. Alternatively, the guide can be used to direct the Yueh access needle via the Seldinger technique. After the guidewire has been placed and the access needle removed, the guide apparatus is detached and the catheter can then be placed over the guidewire.

Drainages are performed with direct access into the collection or through a respective organ, such as liver, kidney, and spleen. Posttransplant hematomas and seromas usually do not require drainage. Lymphoceles, abscesses, and urinomas are usually amenable to drainage.[13]

PATIENT POSITIONING

Generally, patients are most comfortable in the supine position with a comfortable pillow and a wedge or foam roller underneath their knees to reduce lower back pressure. Although some patients may need to be placed in oblique or prone positions for procedures, ensuring patient comfort with adequate use of pillows, towels, or foam wedges decreases patient movement during the procedure.

HEPATIC INTERVENTIONS
Indications

Liver biopsy is one of the most commonly performed procedures in the abdomen, both targeted and nontargeted. Many indications for liver biopsy include diagnosis of acute and chronic hepatitis, iron and copper metabolism abnormalities, glycogen storage disorders, infection, primary biliary cirrhosis, diagnosis of malignancy, and differentiating benign from malignant neoplasms. Liver biopsy in the post–liver transplant patient is commonly performed in the case of suspected rejection. Percutaneous aspiration and catheter drainage is performed for the treatment of both pyogenic and amebic liver abscesses and symptomatic hepatic cysts and hydatid cysts.

Potential Contraindications

Encephalopathy, hepatic failure with severe jaundice, and serious systemic disease may preclude liver intervention. Extrahepatic obstruction and bacterial cholangitis are also contraindications, which may both lead to peritonitis and septicemia. Large volume of ascites may complicate access to the liver, but it can be ameliorated with paracentesis before the procedure and should not be considered a contraindication. According to Little and colleagues,[36] perihepatic ascites does not affect the complication rates of liver biopsies.

Procedure

A transparenchymal approach, in which there is interposing normal liver tissue in between the site of proposed biopsy, may decrease the risk of intraperitoneal hemorrhage; this is especially important in preventing peritoneal spillage in suspected echinococcal disease. Intercostal, subcostal, and epigastric approaches can all be used. The epigastric or subcostal approach is often used to access the left hepatic lobe and can avoid pleural transgression (**Fig. 6**). Intercostal and subcostal approaches are used for the right hepatic lobe (**Fig. 7**). When using the intercostal approach, the needle should be placed immediately above the rib to avoid the intercostal vessels. If an intercostal approach is used, it should be borne in mind that the pleura extends to approximately the 12th rib posteriorly, the 10th rib laterally, and the 8th rib anteriorly. Pneumothorax is rare even if some pleura is traversed if aerated lung is avoided. Childs and Tchelepi[13] recommend looking for the sliding echogenic lung sign during inspiration to help select a trajectory without lung parenchyma in the way. Every effort should be made to avoid vascular structures, especially hepatic arteries and central vessels.[37]

Manual pressure is held over the biopsy site after each pass by the radiologist or the sonographer if possible. After the procedure, pressure

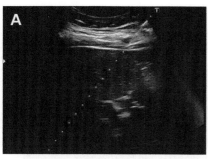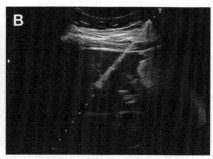

Fig. 6. US-guided biopsy of transplant liver with needle guide using 18-gauge core biopsy needle. (*A*) Prefire and (*B*) postfire.

may be held over the biopsy site for at least 2 minutes. Postprocedure scan can then be performed if desired to assess for bleeding. If the patient is coagulopathic, gelfoam embolization of the biopsy tract through the coaxial needle may be considered to help prevent bleeding. However, transjugular liver biopsies should be considered in patients with severe coagulopathy.[38]

Image-guided percutaneous needle aspiration or catheter drainage in combination with antibiotic therapy has become the treatment of choice for pyogenic and amebic liver abscesses. Percutaneous needle aspiration is performed under real-time sonographic imaging to localize the abscess and guide insertion of the needle. Needle sizes range from 18 to 22 gauge depending on the size of the collection. The change in cavity size should be monitored under real-time sonographic imaging during aspiration. Percutaneous catheter drainage is performed with either the trocar or the Seldinger technique. Catheter sizes typically range from 8F to 12F depending on the size of the collection. After placement of the catheter, aspiration should be performed immediately. The catheter should be secured to the skin for continuous external drainage and left in place until drainage has stopped. Perihepatic abscesses sometimes are difficult to discern from hepatic or subcapsular abscesses (**Fig. 8**). Large

symptomatic cysts are also amenable to drainage (**Fig. 9**).

In a retrospective study by Giorgio and colleagues,[39] 87 percutaneous needle aspirations were performed under US guidance in patients with pyogenic liver abscesses. This treatment in combination with antibiotic therapy was effective in all patients, and there were no recurrences. For most patients, one session of percutaneous needle aspiration was sufficient, and only 7.7% of patients required a second session. However, several studies advocate the use of catheter drainage over percutaneous aspiration. In a randomized prospective study of 60 patients with pyogenic liver abscesses, percutaneous needle aspiration was only successful in 67% of patients, whereas percutaneous catheter drainage was curative in 100% of patients.[40] Similarly, in a randomized study of 50 patients with liver abscesses undergoing percutaneous needle aspiration versus catheter drainage, percutaneous catheter drainage was more effective. Percutaneous needle aspiration was successful in only 60% of patients, whereas catheter drainage was curative in all patients.[41] Although most hepatic abscesses less than 4 or 5 cm usually respond to antibiotic therapy alone, abscesses in the left lobe close to the pericardium are usually drained because of risk of rupture into the pericardium.[13]

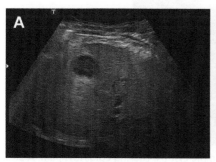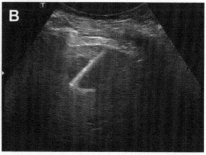

Fig. 7. US-guided biopsy 2.3 cm right hepatic lobe mass (*A*) using coaxial technique freehand (*B*) with 18-gauge core biopsy needle. Pathology demonstrated hepatocellular carcinoma.

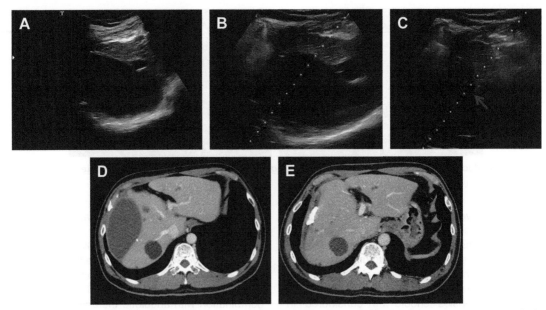

Fig. 8. US-guided drainage of perihepatic abscess (*A*) with placement of 10F catheter, transhepatic approach. (*B, C*) A total of 230 mL pus was aspirated with drain left in place (*arrow*). CT images before (*D*) and after (*E*) drain placement demonstrate interval resolution of abscess.

Percutaneous treatment of hydatid cysts was first introduced in 1985 by Mueller and colleagues[42] (**Figs. 10** and **11**). Before this, percutaneous needle puncture or aspiration for hydatid cysts was always contraindicated because of potential complication of anaphylatic shock or spread of cysts to the peritoneum. In the percutaneous treatment of hydatid cysts, prophylatic

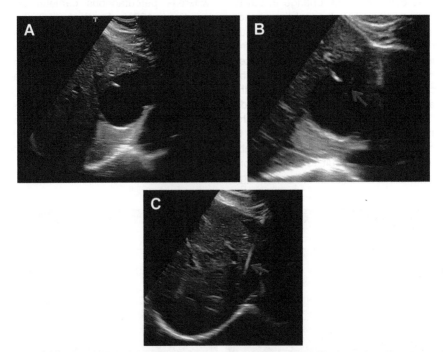

Fig. 9. US-guided aspiration of left hepatic lobe 6 cm simple cyst (*A*) causing epigastric pain. A 5F Yueh catheter (*B, arrow*) was used for aspiration. Postaspiration US (*C*) demonstrated complete resolution of cyst (*arrow*). Patient's epigastric pain resolved.

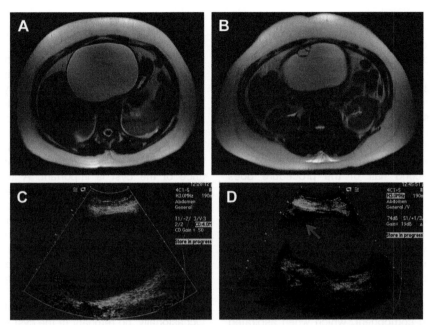

Fig. 10. US-guided drain placement for left hepatic lobe echinococcal cyst seen on MRI. T2-weighted MRI images (*A, B*) demonstrate a large cyst (*C*) replacing the left hepatic lobe. A smaller cystic structure more inferiorly within the cyst is suspicious for daughter cysts. A 12F pigtail catheter (*D, arrow*) was placed within the fluid collection with aspiration of 60 mL of dark green fluid. Postprocedure US imaging demonstrated decreased size of cyst with drain left in place.

albendazole, 15 to 20 mg/kg, is given twice a day by mouth starting 1 week before the procedure and continuing for a total of 4 weeks. Two different scolicidal agents can be injected into the cyst, including absolute alcohol or 20% to 30% hypertonic saline. These agents work on the principle that alcohol causes protein denaturation, cell death, and fibrosis of the cyst wall. Several methods have been reported for the management of hydatid cysts. One method for cysts less than 6 cm uses the puncture, aspiration, injection, and reaspiration technique described by Ben Amor and colleagues.[43] Puncture of the cyst is performed with a 19-gauge needle under sonographic guidance, followed by aspiration of half the volume of the cyst, injection of 20% hypertonic saline solution amounting to one-third the initial estimated cyst volume, a 20-minute wait, and reaspiration of the cyst fluid. Catheterization is used for cysts larger than 6 cm. After injection of the hypertonic saline solution, a 6F to 9F pigtail catheter is placed into the cavity for 24 hours of gravity drainage. If a cystographic study through the pigtail catheter shows no communication between the cyst cavity and the biliary tract, a volume of absolute alcohol half the initially estimated

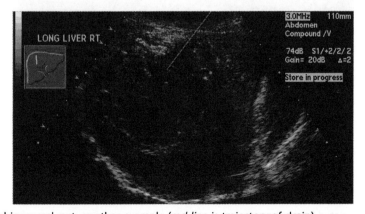

Fig. 11. Hepatic echinococcal cyst, another example (*red line* is trajectory of drain).

volume of the cyst is injected for 20 minutes to pro-duce protoscolecidal and sclerosing effects. If, however, a communication is seen, alcohol should not be used because secondary sclerosing chol-angitis may result.

The double puncture-aspiration-injection (D-PAI)[44] method involves fine needle puncture of the liver cyst, removal of the cyst fluid, and injec-tion of 95% sterile alcohol into the cyst to replace 50% to 60% of the drained fluid. The procedure is then repeated 3 days after the initial aspiration, and the second half of the procedure does not include reaspiration of the scolicidal agent (95% sterile alcohol) or catheter drainage. In a re-view of more than 225 cysts treated by D-PAI by Giorgio and colleagues,[45] success from this technique was equal to that of surgical interven-tion. In long-term follow-up on average of 48 months postprocedure, 48.4% of cysts disap-peared, 46.2% showed a solid pattern on US im-aging, and the remaining 5.3% presented with a minimal fluid component, which when aspirated under US guidance showed no viable scolices. No new intrahepatic or extrahepatic cysts were found. Local recurrences occurred in 5% of cases.

Additional benefits of US-guided hepatic inter-vention include placement of needles and probes for ablation, sclerotherapy of symptomatic hepatic cysts, and placement of localization coils into metastatic lesions before chemotherapy and metastasectomy.[13,46]

Postprocedure Management

Postprocedure monitoring regimens vary by prac-tice, typically ranging from 2 to 6 hours. At the authors' institution, the patient is monitored for 2 to 4 hours depending on the patient, with close monitoring of vital signs. If a right intercostal approach is used, the patient lays on the right side. Postprocedure imaging is usually not per-formed unless the patient is severely symptomatic and a procedure-related complication is sus-pected. A chest radiograph is obtained if pneumo-thorax is suspected.

In the management of hydatid cysts, US follow-up to evaluate the size and sonographic appear-ance of the cyst is important. A large volume reduction should be noted immediately after the procedure, and a gradual change in sonographic appearance from cystic to solid should occur over months to years. Persistence of a round shape and anechoic appearance, smooth (nonirre-gular) and thin cyst wall, and absence of a ruptured endocyst during the routine follow-up examina-tions are worrisome for recurrence. At complete cure, only a solid cyst remnant should be seen. Occasionally, no remnant of the cyst is detected.

Complications

Complications include hemorrhage (**Figs. 12** and **13**, Video 5), pneumothorax, and needle-tract seeding. The complication rate for biopsy of liver lesions and liver abscess drainage is low. In an analysis of complications from a center in which 2320 liver biopsies were performed, there were no major complications after FNA or CNB.[47] Minor complications included self-limited hemoperito-neum (0.3%), vasovagal reaction (0.04%), and transient hypotension (0.08%). No cases of tu-moral seeding along the needle tract were observed. Similarly, in the same study, no major

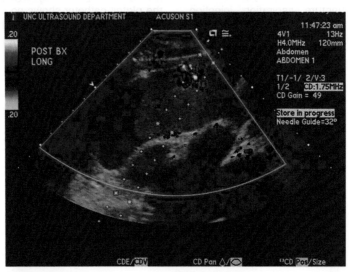

Fig. 12. Liver biopsy-related hemorrhage.

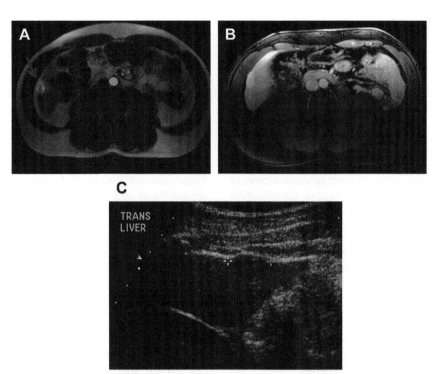

Fig. 13. Complications. The liver lesion seen on MRI (*A, B, arrow*) and US (*C, calipers*) may have bled as it was directly biopsied without going through normal intervening parenchyma. Biopsy demonstrated hepatocellular carcinoma (HCC). Now most biopsies of presumed HCC can be avoided due to diagnostic MRI. (*Courtesy of* W. Chong, MD, Chapel Hill, NC.)

complications were observed after liver abscess drainage. Minor complications included transient hyperthermia and mild pain, which resolved within 24 hours. Imaging follow-up is not typically obtained during or after the recovery period unless the patient is severely symptomatic and clinically a procedure-related complication is suspected.

For hydatid cysts, long-term results from one institution that treated a total of 72 patients with 106 hepatic hydatid cysts reported an 11.1% rate of minor complications, including urticaria and fever. Major complications included infection of the cyst cavity (2.8%), development of biliary fistula (5.6%), and recurrence (2 patients at follow-up 6-month US imaging).[48]

ADRENAL GLAND

Indications of adrenal biopsy include differentiating a benign versus malignant adrenal mass, characterizing an adrenal lesion in a patient with multiple malignancies, determining the source for unknown primary malignancy, and staging a known malignancy with an adrenal lesion.

Contraindications

Adrenal biopsy should be avoided if pheochromocytoma is suspected.

Procedure

It is often advantageous to use both CT and US with or without fusion to biopsy adrenal lesions, with CT providing the best spatial resolution and US providing the best temporal resolution. With US, freehand, guided, or fusion guidance techniques can be used. Conscious sedation may be used; however, the patient must be able to cooperate with breath holding, given the close location of the adrenal gland to the diaphragm. A posterior approach can be used for adrenal biopsy; however, placing the patient in an ipsilateral decubitus position may be more optimal to avoid pneumothorax. Alternative approaches also include anterior, transpancreatic, transhepatic, and transsplenic approaches. A caudal-to-cephalad approach is useful to avoid the kidney and diaphragm. If the mass to be biopsied is highly vascular or bleeding is identified during real-time US evaluation, gelfoam tract embolization should be considered before withdrawing the needle.

Postprocedure Management

At the authors' institution, the patient is monitored for 2 to 4 hours, with close monitoring of vital signs. Postprocedure imaging is not performed unless the patient is symptomatic.

Complications

The most common complications include hemorrhage and pneumothorax. Less common complications include pancreatitis if an anterior approach is used. Needle-tract seeding is extremely rare, with a higher reported incidence in primary adrenocortical carcinoma. Coaxial technique is useful in reducing the incidence of needle-tract seeding. In a study by Mody and colleagues,[49] which examined the immediate and delayed complications of percutaneous biopsy of adrenal masses in 79 cases, the complication rate for adrenal biopsy was higher for the transhepatic approach (12%) than for the posterior approach (8%). Reported complications included pneumothorax, pain, perinephric hemorrhage, subcapsular and intrahepatic hematoma, and one case of hepatic needle-tract metastasis.

RENAL INTERVENTIONS
Indications

In the past, biopsy of renal masses was performed for diagnosis of lymphoma, metastases, infection, or tumors in patients with surgical risk. However, the indications for renal biopsy have expanded to include patients with a renal mass and known extrarenal primary malignancy, patients with a renal mass and imaging features that suggest unresectable renal cancer, patients with a renal mass and surgical comorbidity, and patients with a renal mass that may have been caused by infection. Emerging indications include patients with a small (≤3 cm), hyperattenuating, homogeneously enhancing renal mass; patients with a renal mass considered for percutaneous ablation; and patients with an indeterminate cystic renal mass.[50]

Nontargeted cortical biopsies of native kidneys are performed in patients with diffuse parenchymal disease and laboratory test values indicating proteinuria, hematuria, or unexplained acute renal failure, in which case definitive diagnosis is important for guiding management (ie, determining if the process is active and potentially reversible vs chronic and potentially irreversible).

Nontargeted cortical biopsies are performed in renal transplants in the setting of renal transplant dysfunction. The most common indication for biopsy of a transplant kidney is for diagnosis of allograft rejection.

Contraindications

Contraindications include uncontrolled hypertension (systolic blood pressure >180 mm Hg) and renal or perirenal infection for nontargeted biopsies.

Procedure

Transplant kidneys only require local anesthesia as they are no longer innervated. For a native renal biopsy, the patient should be lying prone or possibly in an oblique decubitus position. A pillow or bolster should be placed under the patient's lower abdomen to straighten the natural lordosis of the spine and help level the entry point over the respective kidney. A subcostal approach is often used to avoid pleural transgression. The lower pole cortex is usually targeted, with the needle aiming as far peripherally as possible to avoid the renal hilum and vessels. Percutaneous biopsy of a renal transplant may be technically easier to perform than biopsy of the native kidneys, given the superficial location of the allograft kidney within the pelvis (**Figs. 14** and **15**). The patient is able to lie supine in most cases.

For biopsy of renal masses, an 18-gauge core biopsy needle, as well as FNA, is used (**Fig. 16**). Renal cortical biopsies are performed using an 18-gauge or larger core biopsy gun, as a smaller sample may provide too thin a core that does not provide adequate material. The appropriate needle gauge is usually determined by the pathology department requirements. Some pathology departments request a cytotechnologist be present during biopsy to ensure appropriate sample size and number. About 2 or 3 samples, each 2 cm in length, are often sufficient for diagnosis. Generally, at least one specimen is placed in 10% formalin for light microscopy and another is placed in 2.5% glutaraldehyde for electron microscopy. The specimen used for immunofluorescence is typically placed in Zeus (Michel) solution.[51]

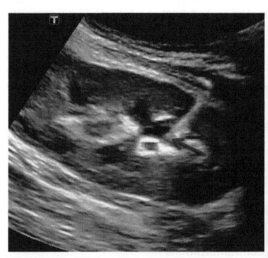

Fig. 14. US-guided biopsy of renal transplant (performed by a nephrologist) with inappropriate placement of needle tip (*arrow*) in the renal collecting system.

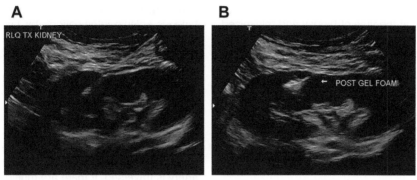

Fig. 15. US-guided biopsy of renal transplant performed by a radiologist with appropriate placement of needle tip in the superior pole of the right lower quadrant renal transplant (*A*). Gel foam embolization (*B*) was also performed.

If there is concern for posttransplant lymphoproliferative disorder, an additional core specimen or flow cytometry analysis is suggested. For renal mass biopsies, a cytotechnologist may need to be present during biopsy to ensure appropriate samples are taken. As the needle is withdrawn, color Doppler may be used to evaluate for bleeding along the biopsy site. Bleeding can usually be controlled with 5 to 10 minutes of compression. Gelfoam tract ablation can also be considered.

Postprocedure Management

After the procedure, patients should rest in bed for 4 to 6 hours depending on department policy, with close monitoring of vital signs.

Complications

Complications include bleeding, hematuria, pseudoaneurysm, arteriovenous fistula, pneumothorax, and needle-tract seeding. Minor bleeding is the most common complication and is generally

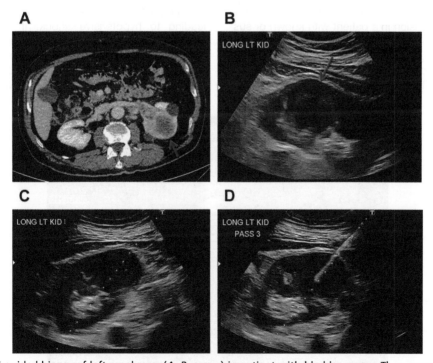

Fig. 16. US-guided biopsy of left renal mass (*A, B, arrow*) in patient with bladder cancer. Three passes were obtained using 18-gauge coaxial technique with needle guide (*C, D*). Pathology demonstrated high-grade invasive urothelial carcinoma.

self-limited (**Fig. 17**, Video 6). This bleeding is usually detected at the time of biopsy and minimized by applying US-guided compression after the biopsy. Hematuria is usually self-limited, but it is important to have patients be aware of postprocedure. In one case series, hematuria occurred in 5% to 7% of patients.[52] Less common complications include pseudoaneurysm and arteriovenous fistula formation, which are often asymptomatic and resolve spontaneously but can cause persistent pain and bleeding. If spontaneous resolution does not occur, transcatheter embolization is performed. Pneumothorax is uncommon but can occur if an intercostal approach is used. Needle-tract seeding is a rare complication estimated to be less than 0.01% of cases.[53] Therefore, this should not be considered a deterrent to biopsy.

SPLENIC INTERVENTIONS
Indications

Percutaneous splenic interventions are not as commonly performed as in other organs, most likely due to concern for increased risk of hemorrhage. However, there are data showing that percutaneous splenic interventions are safe in adults and children and do not pose a significantly higher risk of postprocedure complications.[54] The main indications for splenic biopsy include an indeterminate solid or cystic lesion in a patient with known extrasplenic neoplasm and characterization of a splenic lesion in a patient with known or suspected lymphoma. Other indications include catheter drainage and aspiration of infected fluid collections or abscesses and alcohol ablation in patients with symptomatic splenic cysts and

splenic hydatid cysts. In a 10-year review of percutaneous splenic interventions by Lucey and colleagues,[55] the success rate was 91% for splenic biopsy, 100% for fluid aspiration, and 86% for fluid drainage.

Procedure

Both subcostal and intercostal approaches can be used depending on the location of the spleen. The intercostal approach, however, has risk for pneumothorax and bleeding if pleura or an intercostal artery is traversed. If there are multiple splenic lesions, it is preferred to biopsy the one located more peripherally to avoid the splenic hilum. The needle sizes used for core biopsy range from 18 to 20 gauge and 18 to 22 gauge for FNA (**Fig. 18**, Videos 7 and 8). Gelatin sponge injection along the needle tract may be performed if desired. For catheter placement of infected splenic collections and abscesses, an 8F to 12F catheter can be used, depending on how viscous the fluid initially aspirated is. The trocar method is more commonly used than the Seldinger technique. Good catheter care, including 10-mL flushes of normal saline, is essential for adequate drainage. For splenic cysts and hydatid cysts, please see procedure used for management of hepatic cysts.

Complications

The greatest risk for splenic biopsy is hemorrhage leading to hypotensive shock. If this occurs, aggressive fluid resuscitation and blood transfusion are performed, and if needed, splenic embolization or splenectomy. Other complications include pneumothorax if intercostal approach is

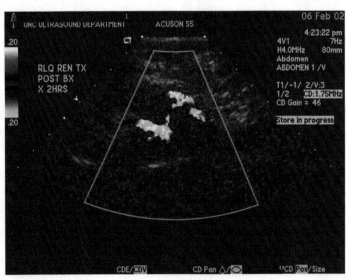

Fig. 17. Renal biopsy-related hemorrhage. (*Courtesy of* W. Chong, MD, Chapel Hill, NC.)

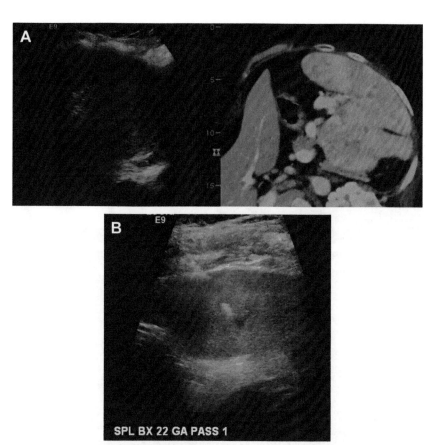

Fig. 18. Splenic biopsy. (*A*) Multiple small splenic lesions. Fusion with CT helps localize lesions on US imaging. (*B*) FNA of splenic lesion demonstrated lymphoma. (*C*) Setup of small splenic lesion biopsy with CT image fusion. (*D*) Fusion with CT helped target an extremely small lesion for biopsy. (*Courtesy of* H. Tchelepi, MD, Los Angeles, CA.)

used and colonic injury. It is suggested that the complication rate for splenic interventions is not much greater than that for biopsy of other abdominal organs. However, this may be because splenic biopsies are much less commonly performed than biopsies of other organs. In a study in which 147 biopsies were performed, the major complication rate was 1.9% requiring splenectomy and the minor complication rate was 14.7%.[56] However, in the study by Lucey and colleagues,[55] 24 biopsies were performed in which 1 patient had a small amount of bleeding requiring no further intervention, whereas 1 patient had significant bleeding requiring splenectomy. Both of these biopsies were performed as FNAs. The risk of complications increased in another study when using larger-caliber 14-gauge CNB needles; however, no significant complications were observed when using core biopsy needles 18 gauge or smaller.[57] In a study by Venkataramu and colleagues,[58] when FNA of splenic lesions was performed in 35 patients using a 22-gauge spinal needle, there was only 1 case of intra-abdominal bleeding,

which did not require intervention. The risk of significant bleeding requiring splenectomy is higher for splenic catheter drainage. This complication occurred in 1 of 7 patients in the study by Lucey and colleagues and 1 of 9 patients in a study by Tasar and colleagues.[59] Hemorrhage-related complications from splenic biopsy are reported in the literature from 0% to 2%, similar to biopsy of other abdominal and pelvic organs.

PELVIC INTERVENTIONS
Indications

Indications include drainage of fluid collections such as seromas, lymphoceles, and abscesses most commonly arising in the setting of diverticulitis, appendicitis, and pelvic inflammatory disease and drainage of lymphoceles. Biopsies of pelvic masses may also be performed under US guidance.

Procedure

Several approaches are used for the drainage of pelvic fluid collections depending on the location

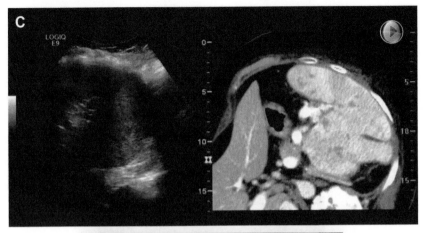

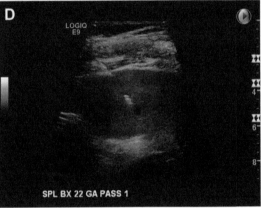

Fig. 18. (*continued*)

of the collection. These approaches include percutaneous (transabdominal [**Fig. 19**] and transgluteal) and endocavitary (transvaginal [**Fig. 20**] and transrectal) techniques. A transgluteal approach allows access to the deeper portions of the pelvis, including posterior to the rectum and sigmoid colon. Conscious sedation is often given in addition to local sedation, as this approach is considered more painful. With the patient in prone position, a curved 3- to 5-MHz transducer is used to localize the fluid collection using the greater sciatic foramen as a window. For this approach, the puncture site needs to be caudal and as close to the sacrum or coccyx as possible to avoid damage to the major neurovascular structures (sciatic nerve and gluteal vessels) that course laterally through the greater sciatic foramen anterior and superior to the piriformis muscle. Bony landmarks are used, and the entry point should be as close and caudal to the coccyx as possible. The drainage catheter should pass inferiorly in the foramen and at or below the level of the sacrospinous ligament.[60]

Transrectal and transvaginal approaches require the use of an endocavitary probe. Compared with the transgluteal approach, these approaches are considered safe in that they avoid damage to the major neurovascular structures.[61] Transvaginal drainage is excellent for drainage of collections in the pouch of Douglas (see **Fig. 20**). For collections deep in the pelvis and palpable through the rectum, a transrectal approach is useful. Conscious sedation and/or local sedation can be used but are not as important as for the transgluteal approach, as these approaches are considered much less painful. Typically, 7-MHz endocavitary probes are used and a drainage guide is attached with a peel-away sheath. The trocar technique is typically used to advance the catheter into the fluid collection under direct US guidance.

Postprocedure Management

Catheter clogging can be minimized by rigorous catheter care after placement. Daily irrigation of

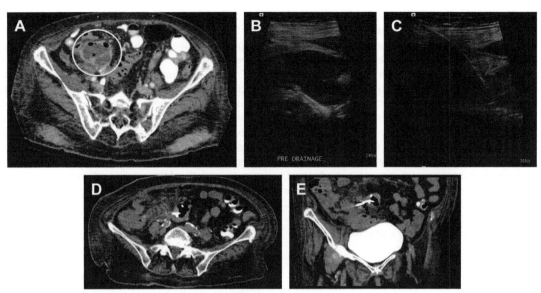

Fig. 19. US-guided drainage of transabdominal approach of periappendiceal abscess (*A, B*) secondary to perforated appendicitis. After placement of an 8.5F pigtail catheter (*C, arrow*) into abscess (*A, circle*) using the Seldinger technique, CT was performed to confirm appropriate placement. CT (*D, E*) demonstrated inadvertent placement of pigtail catheter (*arrow*) beyond abscess cavity into adjacent sigmoid colon. Pigtail catheter was left in place to allow for fistulization.

the catheter is recommended with 10-mL aliquots of saline. Monitoring catheter output allows appropriate removal after ensuring effective catheter drainage. For complex abscesses or hematomas, thrombolytic administration through the catheter can also be performed.

Complications

Immediate postprocedure complications include mainly pain and hemorrhage. Pain radiating to the leg is secondary to placing the catheter too far laterally and proximal to the sciatic nerve, which can occur with the transgluteal approach.

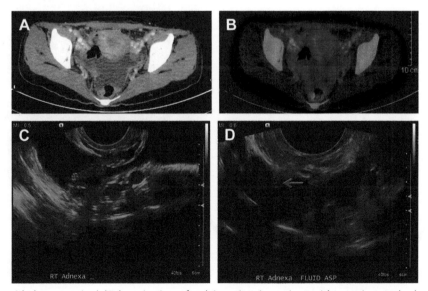

Fig. 20. US-guided transvaginal (TV) aspiration of pelvic ascites in patient with gastric antral adenocarcinoma with new intrapelvic ascites (*C*) seen on prior PET-CT (*A, B*) with diffuse slightly increased fluorodeoxyglucose activity (max standard uptake value [SUV] 1.7) suspicious for carcinomatosis. A 20-gauge Chiba needle (*D, arrow*) was placed into the intrapelvic free fluid under real-time TV US guidance. Cytology demonstrated metastatic adenocarcinoma.

Postprocedure pain is most often due to the transpiriformis approach and violation of the sacral plexus, which lies just anterior to the piriformis muscle. This situation is best avoided by placing the catheter inferior to the piriformis muscle. Hemorrhage occurs secondary to injury to the superior and inferior gluteal vessels, which lie anterior to the piriformis muscle. An infrapiriformis approach can avoid this complication.[62]

In a review of transvaginal drainage of pelvic fluid collections in which 45 aspirations and 40 catheter drainage procedures were performed, there was clinical success in 75% of cases. Minor complications included inadvertent bladder transgression, infection, catheter-related pain, and premature dislodgement of the catheter.[63]

PARACENTESIS
Indications

Paracentesis is one of the most commonly performed abdominal interventions. It can have both a diagnostic role, including evaluation for infection or malignancy, and a therapeutic role in relieving increased intra-abdominal pressure from a large volume of ascites.

Procedure

The patient is positioned with the head of the bed elevated so that fluid can accumulate in the lower abdomen. The optimal puncture site should be in the largest pocket of fluid that avoids the inferior epigastric vessels (**Fig. 21**), usually one of the lower quadrants. A midline approach between the pubis and umbilicus can also be used as long as the bladder is avoided. Many patients requiring paracentesis have cirrhosis with portal hypertension, so prescanning with color Doppler to evaluate for portosystemic collaterals and other vessels before needle puncture is imperative. Most paracentesis kits include a 5F needle with a plastic sheath. At the authors' institution, a 5F Yueh catheter needle is used. US guidance during needle placement is especially important if the collection of fluid is small and to detect moving bowel. After the needle is removed, the sheath is left in place to allow gravity or vacuum drainage of fluid. If a large volume of ascites (>5 L) is removed, intravenous serum albumin (8 g/L) or terlopressin may be given to prevent hypotension.[4,64]

Complications

Complications include bleeding, infection, bowel perforation, and hypotension.

MISCELLANEOUS

Retroperitoneal intervention such as lymph node biopsy performed with US guidance has advantages over CT, including real-time needle visualization,

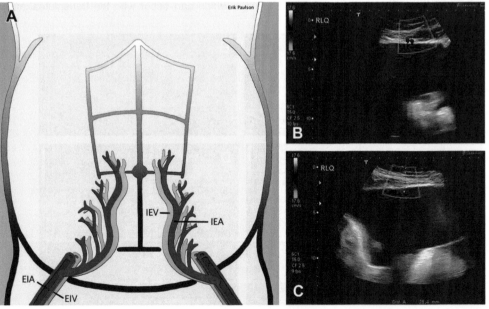

Fig. 21. Diagram of inferior epigastric vessels. (*A*) The inferior epigastric arteries and veins and their perforators (*exaggerated in red and blue*) should be avoided during paracentesis and can be visualized by color Doppler imaging. (*B*) Color Doppler imaging over right lower quadrant (RLQ) showing inferior epigastric artery and vein. (*C*) More lateral positioning along RLQ where no vessels are seen. EIA, external iliac artery; EIV, external iliac vein; IEA, inferior epigastric artery; IEV, inferior epigastric vein. (*Courtesy of* Erik Paulson, DO, California, USA.)

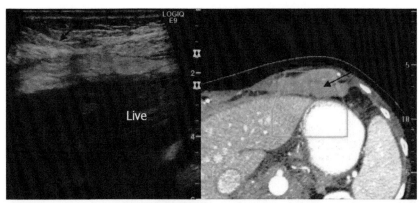

Fig. 22. Biopsy of omental cake. US-guided biopsy of omental cake. Fusion technology helps identify the thickest point of soft tissue (*arrow, CT*) to direct biopsy approach (*arrow, US*) and avoid puncture of liver. Pathology demonstrated lymphoma. (*Courtesy of* H. Tchelepi, MD, Los Angeles, CA.)

multiplanar capability, and decreased distance to the target.[65,66] If visualization with US is difficult, a transhepatic approach can also be considered.

Subcutaneous fluid collections are common in the postoperative setting and are easily amenable to drainage with US guidance given their superficial location. These fluid collections typically include postoperative seromas, hematomas, or infected fluid collections. Simple aspiration or catheter drainage can be used. Subcutaneous masses are easily accessible sonographically. If sarcoma is in the differential, the needle entry and trajectory should be in keeping with a surgical approach.

The omentum is easily visible on US guidance when it is thickened. Given its superficial location and the ability to differentiate the omentum from bowel on real-time US imaging, omental biopsy

with US guidance is useful (**Fig. 22**). Firm transducer pressure can help decrease the distance to the target and can help fixate mobile lesions, if needed.

Serosal lesions can be approached similar to omental lesions but tend to be more fixed, as they are located along the organ (**Fig. 23**). Care should be taken not to puncture the subjacent organ, if possible.

Pancreatic interventions such as pseudocyst or abscess drainage and pancreatic biopsy can be performed using a variety of techniques, including endoscopic US guidance, surgery, and percutaneous US or CT guidance. Endoscopic US guidance is more commonly used, as it avoids the need for an open incision or an external drainage catheter. Percutaneous drainage of pancreatic or

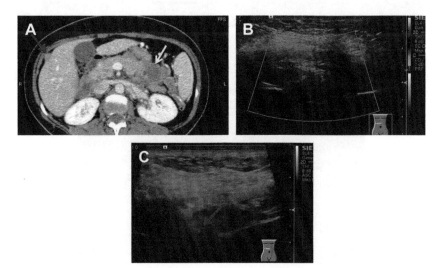

Fig. 23. Serosal implant along the liver in a patient with a hypoenhancing pancreatic tail mass. (*A*) CT image demonstrating pancreatic tail mass (*yellow arrow*) and serosal implant along liver (*red arrow*). (*B*) US image showing serosal lesion with possible flow. (*C*) Biopsy of serosal lesion with FNA (*red arrow*). CNB was also performed; this was proven to represent pancreatic adenocarcinoma and not a metastasis from a second primary.

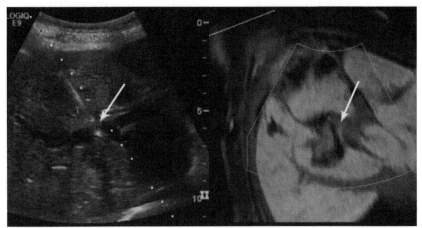

Fig. 24. Biopsy using ultrasound fusion with MRI. Small central hepatic lesion biopsy targeted at the area of bile duct wall thickening (*arrows*), which is better seen with MRI. US images are synched with MRI images, and the lesion can be targeted under US guidance. Biopsy showed cholangiocarcinoma. (*Courtesy of* Tchelepi H, MD, Los Angeles, CA.)

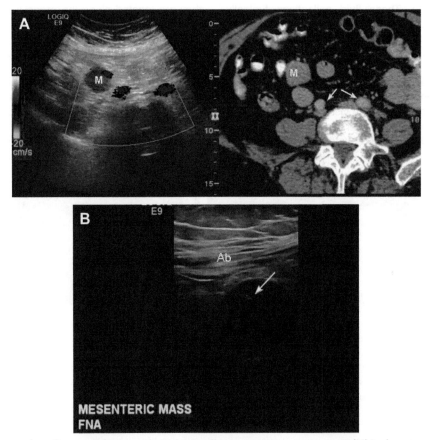

Fig. 25. Biopsy using ultrasound fusion with CT. (*A*) Small mesenteric mass seen on CT (M) is also seen on US image when images are linked. Color Doppler shows blood flow in iliac vessels (*arrows* on CT). Compression helps displace bowel out of the way so biopsy can be performed. (*B*) FNA was safely performed (*arrow*) avoiding bowel and blood vessels. (*Courtesy of* H. Tchelepi, MD, Los Angeles, CA.)

peripancreatic collections can be performed under US guidance; however, the pancreatic duct must be patent, and direct communication with the pancreatic duct results in increased time for drainage.[67] CT scan may better demonstrate pancreatic and peripancreatic collections and their relationship to other anatomical structures, especially when there is overlying stomach and bowel.

US-guided percutaneous cholecystostomy tube placement is a commonly performed interventional procedure in the treatment of acute cholecystitis in critically ill patients who are not surgical candidates. A transhepatic approach should be used to reduce complications. Occasionally, US guidance can also be used in the biopsy of gallbladder lesions, also using a transhepatic approach. Complications include hemorrhage, bile leak, and peritonitis.[68]

FUSION GUIDANCE—CT, MR, PET

Image fusion between US imaging and CT, MRI, and PET is a new technology being used for US-guided procedures. Its most common application is liver biopsy ablations but can be used almost anywhere in the body. This technology allows real-time synchronization of CT or any multiplanar reconstructed images with the corresponding US images.[13] It is performed with an image-processing workstation with built-in fusion software and US equipment with a magnetic motion-tracking device. The magnetic sensor attached to the sonographic probe registers and transmits the position and orientation of the probe to the workstation, into which the patient's previously acquired CT, MRI, or PET volume data have been downloaded. Fused images are then created, and images weighted toward either US or to the fused modality, such as CT.

When lesions are difficult to visualize by conventional US, this can lead to increased radiation exposure (because of CT utilization), inadequate biopsy specimens, and increased number of needle insertions (because of insufficient sampling). Fusion imaging, or virtual CT, MRI, or PET-US, ameliorates those problems by targeting lesions depicted by other modalities but not clearly seen on conventional US imaging for biopsy or ablation (**Figs. 24** and **25**). The advantages of incorporating US fusion technology are real-time imaging, ease of image-guided intervention, and lack of radiation exposure.

SUMMARY

US imaging should be the first-line modality for most abdominal diagnostic and therapeutic interventions. The ability to use real-time image guidance to view needle trajectory and placement and to identify blood vessels and other important structures in the needle path without the use of ionizing radiation gives US imaging added benefits compared with CT. Faster procedure times, portability, and decreased cost further increase its utility. Fusion technology allows US imaging to merge with CT, MRI, and PET to better localize lesions. Furthermore, needle-guidance and volume-navigation technology assist in precise targeting of difficult lesions. With steadfast advances in machine and transducer technology, the applications of US will continue to increase.

SUPPLEMENTARY DATA

Video related to this article can be found online at http://dx.doi.org/10.1016/j.cult.2014.07.012.

REFERENCES

1. Sheafor DH, Paulson EK, Simmons CM, et al. Abdominal percutaneous interventional procedures: comparison of CT and US guidance. Radiology 1998;207(3):705–10.
2. Kliewer MA, Sheafor DH, Paulson EK, et al. Percutaneous liver biopsy: a cost-benefit analysis comparing sonographic and CT guidance. AJR Am J Roentgenol 1999;173(5):1199–202.
3. Gerzof SG, Robbins AH, Birkett DH, et al. Percutaneous catheter drainage of abdominal abscesses guided by ultrasound and computed tomography. AJR Am J Roentgenol 1979;133(1):1–8.
4. Nakamoto DA, Haaga JR. Emergent ultrasound interventions. Radiol Clin North Am 2004;42(2): 457–78.
5. Dodd GD 3rd, Esola CC, Memel DS, et al. Sonography: the undiscovered jewel of interventional radiology. Radiographics 1996;16(6):1271–88.
6. Meloni MF, Andreano A, Zimbaro F, et al. Contrast enhanced ultrasound: roles in immediate post-procedural and 24-h evaluation of the effectiveness of thermal ablation of liver tumors. J Ultrasound 2012;15(4):207–14.
7. Furness PN. ACP. Best practice no 160. Renal biopsy specimens. J Clin Pathol 2000;53(6):433–8.
8. Gupta S, Wallace MJ, Cardella JF, et al, Society of Interventional Radiology Standards of Practice Committee. Quality improvement guidelines for percutaneous needle biopsy. J Vasc Interv Radiol 2010;21(7):969–75.
9. Vijayaraghavan GR, David S, Bermudez-Allende M, et al. Imaging-guided parenchymal liver biopsy: how we do it. J Clin Imaging Sci 2011;1:30.

10. Manno C, Strippoli GF, Arnesano L, et al. Predictors of bleeding complications in percutaneous ultrasound-guided renal biopsy. Kidney Int 2004; 66(4):1570–7.

11. Atwell TD, Smith RL, Hesley GK, et al. Incidence of bleeding after 15,181 percutaneous biopsies and the role of aspirin. AJR Am J Roentgenol 2010; 194(3):784–9.

12. Gerzof SG. Percutaneous drainage technique. In: Dondelinger RF, editor. Interventional radiology. Stuttgart (Germany): Georg Thieme; 1990. p. 96–101.

13. Childs DC, Tchelepi H. Ultrasound and abdominal intervention: new luster on an old gem. In: Tchelepi H, editor. Ultrasound clinics: ultrasound-guided procedures, vol. 4. Philadelphia: Saunders; 2009. p. 25–43.

14. Patel IJ, Davidson JC, Nikolic B, et al, Standards of Practice Committee, with Cardiovascular and Interventional Radiological Society of Europe (CIRSE) Endorsement. Consensus guidelines for periprocedural management of coagulation status and hemostasis risk in percutaneous image-guided interventions. J Vasc Interv Radiol 2012;23(6):727–36.

15. Holland LL, Brooks JP. Toward rational fresh frozen plasma transfusion: the effect of plasma transfusion on coagulation test results. Am J Clin Pathol 2006;126(1):133–9.

16. Segal JB, Dzik WH, Transfusion Medicine/Hemostasis Clinical Trials Network. Paucity of studies to support that abnormal coagulation test results predict bleeding in the setting of invasive procedures: an evidence-based review. Transfusion 2005;45(9): 1413–25.

17. Eckman MH, Erban JK, Singh SK, et al. Screening for the risk for bleeding or thrombosis. Ann Intern Med 2003;138(3):W15–24.

18. Smetana GW, Macpherson DS. The case against routine preoperative laboratory testing. Med Clin North Am 2003;87(1):7–40.

19. O'Connor SD, Taylor AJ, Williams EC, et al. Coagulation concepts update. AJR Am J Roentgenol 2009;193(6):1656–64.

20. Greinacher A, Selleng K. Thrombocytopenia in the intensive care unit patient. Hematology Am Soc Hematol Educ Program 2010;135–43.

21. Eisenstein EL, Anstrom KJ, Kong DF, et al. Clopidogrel use and long-term clinical outcomes after drug-eluting stent implantation. JAMA 2007; 297(2):159–68.

22. Iakovou I, Schmidt T, Bonizzoni E, et al. Incidence, predictors, and outcome of thrombosis after successful implantation of drug-eluting stents. JAMA 2005;293(17):2126–30.

23. Dzik W, Rao A. Why do physicians request fresh frozen plasma? Transfusion 2004;44(9):1393–4.

24. Desborough M, Stanworth S. Plasma transfusion for bedside, radiologically guided, and operating room invasive procedures. Transfusion 2012; 52(Suppl 1):20S–9S.

25. Malloy PC, Grassi CJ, Kundu S, et al. Standards of Practice Committee, with Cardiovascular and Interventional Radiological Society of Europe (CIRSE) Endorsement; Standards of Practice Committee of the Society of Interventional Radiology. Consensus Guidelines for Periprocedural Management of Coagulation Status and Hemostasis Risk in Percutaneous Image-guided Interventions. J Vasc Interv Radiol 2009;20:S240–9.

26. Patel IJ, Davidson JC, Nikolic B, et al. Standards of Practice Committee, with Cardiovascular and Interventional Radiological Society of Europe (CIRSE) Endorsement; Standards of Practice Committee of the Society of Interventional Radiology. Consensus Guidelines for Periprocedural Management of Coagulation Status and Hemostasis Risk in Percutaneous Image-guided Interventions. J Vasc Interv Radiol 2012;23:727–36.

27. Patel IJ, Davidson JC, Nikolic B, et al, Standards of Practice Committee, with Cardiovascular and Interventional Radiological Society of Europe (CIRSE) Endorsement; Standards of Practice Committee of the Society of Interventional Radiology. Addendum of newer anticoagulants to the SIR consensus guideline. J Vasc Interv Radiol 2013; 24(5):641–5.

28. Kitchin DR, Munoz del Rio A, Woods M, et al. Percutaneous liver biopsy and relaxed coagulation guidelines: a nine year experience. Radiologic Society of North America, 99th Scientific Assembly and Annual Meeting. Chicago, Illinois, December 1 – 6, 2013.

29. Tyng CJ, Bitencourt AG, Martins EB, et al. Technical note: CT-guided paravertebral adrenal biopsy using hydrodissection – a safe and technically easy approach. Br J Radiol 2012;85:e339–42.

30. Bluvol N, Kornecki A, Shaikh A, et al. Freehand versus guided breast biopsy: comparison of accuracy, needle motion, and biopsy time in a tissue model. Am J Roentgenol 2009;192:1720–5.

31. Shabana W, Kielar A, Vermani V, et al. Accuracy of sonographically guided biopsy using a freehand versus needle-guided technique computed tomographic correlation study. J Ultrasound Med 2013;32(3):535–40.

32. Stewart CJ, Coldewey J, Stewart IS. Comparison of fine needle aspiration cytology and needle core biopsy in the diagnosis of radiologically detected abdominal lesions. J Clin Pathol 2002;55:93–7.

33. Scanga LR, Maygarden SJ. Utility of fine-needle aspiration and core biopsy with touch preparation in the diagnosis of renal lesions. Cancer Cytopathol 2014;122(3):182–90.

34. Appelbaum L, Kane RA, Kruskal JB, et al. Focal hepatic lesions: US-guided biopsy—lessons from

review of cytologic and pathologic examination results. Radiology 2009;250:453–8.

35. Thabet A, Arellano RS. Catheter drainage of abdominal abscesses and fluid collections. In: Kandarpa K, Machan L, editors. Handbook of interventional radiologic procedures. 4th edition. Philadelphia: Wolters Kluwer/Lippincott Williams & Wilkins Health; 2011. p. 527–36.

36. Little AF, Ferris JV, Dodd GD 3rd, et al. Image-guided percutaneous hepatic biopsy: effect of ascites on the complication rate. Radiology 1996;1: 79–83.

37. Winter TC, Lee FT Jr, Hinshaw JL. Ultrasound-guided biopsies in the abdomen and pelvis. Ultrasound Q 2008;24(1):45–68.

38. Senzolo M, Burra P, Cholongitas E, et al. The transjugular route: the key hole to the liver world. Dig Liver Dis 2007;39(2):105–16.

39. Giorgio A, de Stefano G, Di Sarno A, et al. Percutaneous needle aspiration of multiple pyogenic abscesses of the liver: 13-year single-center experience. AJR Am J Roentgenol 2006;187(6): 1585–90.

40. Zerem E, Hadzic A. Sonographically guided percutaneous catheter drainage versus needle aspiration in the management of pyogenic liver abscess. AJR Am J Roentgenol 2007;189(3):W138–42.

41. Rajak CL, Gupta S, Jain S, et al. Percutaneous treatment of liver abscesses: needle aspiration versus catheter drainage. AJR Am J Roentgenol 1998;170:1035–9.

42. Mueller PR, Dawson SL, Ferrucci IT, et al. Hepatic echinococcal cyst: successful percutaneous drainage. Radiology 1985;155:627–8.

43. Ben Amor N, Gargouri M, Gharbi HA, et al. Trial therapy of inoperable abdominal hydatid cysts by puncture. Ann Parasitol Hum Comp 1986;61:689–92.

44. Giorgio A, Tarantino L, Francica G, et al. Unilocular hydatid liver cysts: treatment with US-guided, double percutaneous aspiration and alcohol injection. Radiology 1992;182:705.e10.

45. Giorgio A, de Stefano G, Esposito V, et al. Long term results of percutaneous treatment of hyatid liver cysts: a single centre 17 years experience. Infection 2007;36(3):256–61.

46. Benoist S, Brouquet A, Penna C, et al. Complete response of colorectal liver metastases after chemotherapy: does it mean cure? J Clin Oncol 2006;24(24):3939–45.

47. Giorgio A, Tarantino L, de Stefano G, et al. Complications after interventional sonography of focal liver lesions: a 22-year single-center experience. J Ultrasound Med 2003;22(2):193–205.

48. Ustünsöz B, Akhan O, Kamiloğlu MA, et al. Percutaneous treatment of hydatid cysts of the liver: long-term results. AJR Am J Roentgenol 1999; 172(1):91–6.

49. Mody MK, Kazerooni EA, Korobkin M. Percutaneous CT-guided biopsy of adrenal masses: immediate and delayed complications. J Comput Assist Tomogr 1995;19:434–9.

50. Silverman SG, Gan YU, Mortele KJ, et al. Renal masses in the adult patient: the role of percutaneous biopsy. Radiology 2006;240:6–22.

51. Walker PD. The renal biopsy. Arch Pathol Lab Med 2009;133(2):181–8.

52. Vassiliades VG, Bernardino ME. Percutaneous renal and adrenal biopsies. Cardiovasc Intervent Radiol 1991;14:50–4.

53. Smith EH. Complications of percutaneous abdominal fine-needle biopsy: review. Radiology 1991; 178:253–8.

54. Liang P, Gao Y, Wang Y, et al. US-guided percutaneous needle biopsy of the spleen using 18-gauge versus 21-gauge needles. J Clin Ultrasound 2007; 35(9):477–82.

55. Lucey BC, Boland GW, Maher MM, et al. Percutaneous nonvascular splenic intervention: a 10-year review. AJR Am J Roentgenol 2002; 179(6):1591–6.

56. Tam A, Krishnamurthy S, Pillsbury EP, et al. Percutaneous image-guided splenic biopsy in the oncology patient: an audit of 156 consecutive cases. J Vasc Interv Radiol 2008;19(1):80–7.

57. Muraca S, Chait PG, Connolly BL, et al. US-guided core biopsy of the spleen in children. Radiology 2001;218(1):200–6.

58. Venkataramu NK, Gupta S, Sood BP, et al. Ultrasound guided fine needle aspiration biopsy of splenic lesions. Br J Radiol 1999;72(862):953–6.

59. Tasar M, Ugurel MS, Kocaoglu M, et al. Computed tomography-guided percutaneous drainage of splenic abscesses. Clin Imaging 2004;28:44–8.

60. Walser E, Raza S, Hernandez A, et al. Sonographically guided trangluteal drainage of pelvic abscesses. AJR Am J Roentgenol 2003;181:498–500.

61. Ryan RS, McGrath FP, Haslam PJ, et al. Ultrasound guided endocavitary drainage of pelvic abscesses: technique, results and complications. Clin Radiol 2003;58:75–9.

62. Harisinghani MG, Gervais DA, Hahn PF, et al. CT-guided transgluteal drainage of deep pelvic abscesses: indications, technique, procedure-related complications and clinical outcome. Radiographics 2002;22(6):1353–67.

63. Saokar A, Arellano R, Gervais D, et al. Transvaginal drainage of pelvic fluid collections: results, expectations and experience. AJR Am J Roentgenol 2008;191:1352–8.

64. Lata J, Marecek Z, Fejfar T, et al. The efficacy of terlipressin in comparison with albumin in the prevention of circulatory changes after the paracentesis of tense ascites – a randomized multicentric study. Hepatogastroenterology 2007;54(79):1930–3.

65. Gupta S, Rajak CL, Sood BP, et al. Sonographically guided fine needle aspiration biopsy of abdominal lymph nodes: experience in 102 patients. J Ultrasound Med 1999;18(2):135–9.

66. Fisher AJ, Paulson EK, Sheafor DH, et al. Small lymph nodes of the abdomen, pelvis, and retroperitoneum: usefulness of sonographically guided biopsy. Radiology 1997;205(1):185–90.

67. Nealon WH, Walser E. Main pancreatic ductal anatomy can direct choice of modality for treating pancreatic pseudocysts (surgery versus percutaneous drainage). Ann Surg 2002;235(6): 751–8.

68. Ginat D, Saad WE. Cholecystostomy and transcholecystic biliary access. Tech Vasc Interv Radiol 2008;11(1):2–13.

Index

Note: Page numbers of article titles are in **boldface** type.

A

Abdominal ultrasonography
  for interventions, **793–820**
  of abdominal wall, **775–791**
  of aorta, **723–749**
  of biliary tract, **567–586**
  of bowel, **751–773**
  of gallbladder, **567–586,** 817
  of kidney. *See* Renal ultrasonography.
  of liver. *See* Liver, ultrasonography of.
  of mesenteric arteries, **723–749**
  of retroperitoneum, **697–721**
  of spleen, **557–562**
Abdominal wall, ultrasonography of, **775–791**
  anatomy of, 775–776
  for fluid collections, 780–781
  for hernias, 777–780
  for masses, 781–785, 787
  for vascular abnormalities, 784, 786
  technique for, 777
Ablation therapy, for liver masses, 618
Abscesses
  after liver transplantation, 648–649
  in gallbladder interventions, 575
  in inflammatory bowel disease, 760–761
  of abdominal wall, 780–781
  of kidney, 658, 690
  of liver, 555–556, 611
  of retroperitoneum, 718
  of spleen, 560–561, 810–811
Acalculous cholecystitis, 572–575
Accessory spleen, 558
Acoustic radiation force impulse elastography, 627, 690
ACUSON S3000 system, 627–628
Acute abdomen, 763–770
  left lower quadrant pain in, 768–770
  right lower quadrant pain in, 763–768
Acute tubular necrosis, in kidney transplantation, 688–690
Adenocarcinomas, of pancreas, 633, 707–708, 710
Adenomas
  of adrenal glands, 702
  of liver, 549, 552–553, 611
Adenomyomatosis, of gallbladder, 576–578
Adrenal cortical carcinomas, 703–704
Adrenal glands

  biopsy of, 807–808
  ultrasonography of, 700–704
Amebic abscesses, of liver, 555–556
Aneurysms
  aortic
    diagnostic criteria for, 732–733
    growth rate of, 732
    natural history of, 731
    pathophysiology of, 731–732
    rupture of, 731–732, 734
    screening for, 732
    types of, 732
    ultrasonography for, 733–734
  false, 601–602
  splanchnic arteries, 745–747
Angiolipomas, of abdominal wall, 782
Angiomyolipomas
  of kidney, 672, 674–675
  of retroperitoneum, 714–715
Anticoagulants, interventions and, 797–799
Aorta, ultrasonography of, **723–749**
  anatomy of, 723
  atherosclerosis and, 726–730
  for aneurysms. *See* Aneurysms, aortic.
  for coarctation, 730
  for dissection, 737, 739–740
  for liver transplantation evaluation, 642
  for occlusion, 729
  for stenosis, 727–730
  hemodynamics of, 724–725
  normal sizes of, 729, 731
  protocol for, 726
  technique for, 726
Appendices epiploicae, torsion of, 767
Appendicitis, 763–766
Appendicoliths, 764
Arteriovenous fistulas
  after kidney biopsy, 687–688
  after TIPS procedure, 601–602
  of kidney, 679–680
Ascariasis, cholangitis in, 581
Ascites, after liver transplantation, 648
Asplenia, 558
Atherosclerosis
  of aorta, 726–730
  of mesenteric arteries, 740–744
Atlanta classification, of pancreatitis, 706
Autoimmune pancreatitis, 707

Ultrasound Clin 9 (2014) 821–829
http://dx.doi.org/10.1016/S1556-858X(14)00104-2

B

Bacterial cholangitis, 580
Beak sign, in retroperitoneal ultrasonography, 699
Benign developmental hepatic cysts, 551
Bile leak
    after liver transplantation, 647–648
    in interventions, 575
Biliary colic, 571
Biliary hamartomas, 556
Biliary sludge, 571–572
Biliary tract, ultrasonography of, **567–586**
    anatomy of, 568–570
    for cholangitis, 579–582
    for choledochal cysts, 583–585
    for choledocholithiasis, 577, 579
    for interventional complications, 575
    for malignancies, 582–583
    for obstruction, 646–647
    technique for, 568–570
Bilomas, 575, 647–648
Biopsy
    adrenal gland, 807–808
    kidney, 808–810
    liver, 803–807
    needles for, 795–796
    omentum, 815
    sample types from, 801
    spleen, 810–811
    technique for, 800–801
Bleeding risk and control, in interventions, 797–799
Bolus injection method, for contrast-enhanced
    ultrasound, 608
Bowel
    elastography of, 636
    ischemia of. See Mesenteric arteries.
    ultrasonography of, **761–773**
        for acute abdomen, 763–770
        for blood flow evaluation, 753, 755
        for inflammatory bowel disease, 755–763
        for neoplasms, 753
        for wall thickness, 752
        gut signature in, 751–752, 754
        technique for, 752–753
"Bright liver," in steatosis, 546
Budd-Chiari syndrome, 548
    after liver transplantation, 645
    hepatic vein thrombosis in, 597
    portal hypertension in, 594
"Bull's-eye" appearance
    in liver abscess, 556
    in splenic abscess, 561

C

Calcification
    in gallbladder, 571, 575–576
    in kidney, 662–663
    in liver metastasis, 553–554
    in splenic sarcoidosis, 562
Calcium, in gallbladder, 571
Calculous cholecystitis, 572–575
Candidiasis
    of liver, 556
    of spleen, 561
Caroli disease, 585
Carrel patch, in kidney transplantation, 684
Catheters, for drain placement, 796, 801–802
Caudate-to-right-lobe ratio, in cirrhosis, 548
Cavernous hemangiomas, of liver, 549–551
Cavernous transformation, of portal vein thrombus,
    594–595
Charcot triad, in cholangitis, 580
Child-Turcotte-Pugh scoring system, for liver
    disease, 642
Cholangiocarcinomas, 554–555, 583, 616
Cholangiopancreatography, after liver
    transplantation, 647–648
Cholangiopathy, in HIV infections, 580–581
Cholangitis, 579–582
Cholecystitis, 571–575
Cholecystostomy, percutaneous, 817
Choledochal cysts, 583–585
Choledochoceles, 584–585
Choledocholithiasis, 577, 579–580
Cholelithiasis, 570–571
Cholesterol gallstones, 571
Cholesterol polyps, in gallbladder, 576–578
Cholesterolosis, 576–577
Cirrhosis
    of biliary tract, 594
    of liver, 548–549, 592–593, 611
        elastography for, 628–631
        hepatic vein changes with, 596
Colic
    biliary, 571
    renal, 661
Color Doppler ultrasonography
    for aorta, 726, 729, 733, 736
    for appendicitis, 764–765
    for biliary sludge, 572
    for bowel, 753
    for hepatocellular carcinomas, 550
    for inflammatory bowel disease, 758
    for intervention guidance, 794
    for kidney transplantation, 683, 687–688
    for liver transplantation, 642–643, 645
    for mesenteric arteries, 726, 738, 746
    for splenic abscesses, 560–561
Colorectal cancer, after liver transplantation, 649–650
Columns of Bertin, prominent, 654
Comet tail artifact, in foreign body, 788
Common bile duct, 577, 579
Common hepatic duct, 569

Compartment syndrome, in kidney transplantation, 688
Complex cysts, of liver, 551–552
Compression sonography, for bowel, 752–753
Computed tomography
    for adrenal biopsy, 807–808
    for adrenal pathology, 700–704
    for appendicitis, 763–764, 766
    for cholecystitis, 574
    for hepatocellular carcinoma, 615–616
    for hydronephrosis, 661, 663
    for inflammatory bowel disease, 756
    for liver masses, 614
    for pancreatic disorders, 704–709
    for perirenal pathology, 678
    for porcelain gallbladder, 576
    for pyelonephritis, 659
    for renal cell carcinoma, 672, 674
    for retroperitoneal pathology, 700–719
    for urinary stones, 692
    fusion guidance for, 817
Conn disease, 702
Contrast-enhanced ultrasound
    for inflammatory bowel disease, 758
    for kidney transplantation, 690
    for liver masses, **605–623**
        ablation, 618
        agents for, 606–607
        benign, 609–611
        characterization of, 609
        contraindications to, 607
        detection of, 617
        enhancement phases in, 606–607
        equipment for, 608
        intraoperative, 617–618
        limitations of, 618–619
        malignant, 611–617
        pitfalls in, 619
        preliminary conventional ultrasound for, 609
        procedure for, 608–609
        quantitative, 619
        side effects of, 607
        software for, 608
        targeted, 620
        three- and four-dimensional, 619–620
Core needle biopsy, 801
Crohn disease. See Inflammatory bowel disease.
Crossed renal ectopia, 656
Cushing syndrome, 702
Cyst(s)
    abdominal wall, 783, 785
    adrenal, 700–701
    choledochal, 583–585
    kidney, 666–670
    liver, 551–552, 611, 803–805
    spleen, 560
Cystadenenocarcinomas, of liver, 552

Cystadenomas
    of liver, 552
    of pancreas, 635
Cystic disease, of kidney, 666–670

D

Desmoid tumors, of abdominal wall, 783, 785
Dissection, of aorta and branches, 737, 739–740
Diverticula, of bile duct, 584–585
Diverticulitis
    left-sided, 768–770
    right-sided, 766
Doppler resistive index, in renal ultrasonography, 683
Doppler ultrasonography. See also Color Doppler ultrasonography; Power Doppler ultrasonography.
    for hepatic veins, 595–598
    for hydronephrosis, 661
    for liver, **587–604,** 643–651
    for portal venous system, 588–595
    for renal vein thrombosis, 679
    for transjugular intrahepatic portosystemic shunts, 598–602
"Dotted-line sign," in cirrhosis, 548
Double puncture-aspiration-injection procedure, 806
Drain placement, 801–802
    catheters for, 796, 801–802
    in gallbladder, 817
    in liver, 803
    in pancreas, 815, 817
    in pelvis, 811–814
Dromedary hump, 654–655
Drug toxicity, in kidney transplantation, 688–690
Duplication, in urinary tract, 665
Dysplastic nodules, in liver, 548, 612

E

Echinococcosis, 555–556, 560
Ectopia, kidney, 656
Edema, perirenal, 674–676
Elastography, **625–640**
    indications for, 625–626
    of gastrointestinal tract, 636
    of kidney, 690
    of liver, 628–632, 634
    of pancreas, 633, 635
    principles of, 626–628
    techniques for, 625–628
ElastPQ system, 628
Embedded organ sign, in retroperitoneal ultrasonography, 699
Emphysematous cholecystitis, 571, 573–574
Emphysematous pyelonephritis, 657, 659
Endoleaks, in aortic aneurysm repair, 735–738
Endometriosis, of abdominal wall, 783–784

Endoscopic retrograde cholangiopancreatography, after liver transplantation, 647–648
Endoscopy, for inflammatory bowel disease, 756
Epidermal inclusion cyst, of abdominal wall, 783, 785
Epigastic hernias, 778, 780
Epstein-Barr virus infections, posttransplant lymphoproliferative disease and, 650
Erdheim-Chester disease, 676

F

Fat, inflammatory
    in diverticulitis, 767
    in inflammatory bowel disease, 757
Fat necrosis, of abdominal wall, 782
Fatty infiltration, of liver, 611, 614, 616, 630
Fecaliths, in diverticulitis, 767
Femoral hernias, 778–779
Fibromatosis, of abdominal wall, 783
Fibromuscular dysplasia, renal hypertension in, 676–677
Fibroscan instrument, 629–630
Fibrosis. See also Cirrhosis.
    retroperitoneal, 714–715
Fine needle aspiration biopsy, 801
Fistulas, in inflammatory bowel disease, 762
Fixed acute angulations, in inflammatory bowel disease, 758–759
Fluid collections
    after kidney transplantation, 690–691
    drainage of. See Drain placement.
    of abdominal wall, 780–781
    of pelvis, 811–814
    of retroperitoneum, 717–719
    perirenal, 674–676, 678
    subcutaneous, 815
Focal nodular hyperplasia, of liver, 549, 552, 610
Foreign bodies, in abdominal wall, 788
Four-dimensional imaging, for liver masses, 619–620
Fresh frozen plasma, for interventions, 797–798
Fungal infections
    of liver, 556
    of spleen, 561

G

Gallbladder
    ultrasonography of, **567–586**
        anatomy of, 568
        for adenomyomatosis, 576–578
        for biliary sludge, 571–572
        for cholecystitis, 572–575
        for drain placement, 817
        for gallstones, 570–571
        for interventional complications, 575
        for malignancies, 576

for perforation, 573
for polyps, 576–578
for porcelain gallbladder, 571, 575–576
for wall thickening, 575–576
technique for, 570
wall thickening of, 575–576
Gallstones, 570–573
Ganglioneuroblastomas, of adrenal glands, 703–704
Ganglions, of retroperitoneum, 716
Gangrenous cholecystitis, 573
Gas, in inflammatory bowel disease, 762
Gastrinomas, 708–710
Gastrointestinal tract, elastography of, 636
Giant-cell arteritis, 677
Glomerulocystic disease, 667
Glucagonomas, 709
Graded compression sonography, for appendicitis, 764
Graft rejection, in transplantation
    kidney, 688–690
    liver, 650–651
Granulomas, of kidney, 660
Groin hernias, 777–780
Gut signature, 751–752, 754

H

"Hailstorm sign," in liver abscess, 555
Hamartomas
    of liver, 556
    of spleen, 560
"Hayfork" appearance, in intussusception, 768
Heart failure, 589–590, 596
Hemangiomas
    of kidney, 675
    of liver, 549–551, 609
    of spleen, 561
Hematomas
    after kidney transplantation, 690
    after liver transplantation, 648
    in aortic rupture, 734
    of abdominal wall, 780–781
    of liver, 557
    of retroperitoneum, 717
    of spleen, 558
    perirenal, 678
    retroperitoneal, 700–701
Hemobilia, 582
Hemorrhage
    adrenal, 700–701
    in gallbladder interventions, 575
    perirenal, 675–676
Hemostatic agents, 797–798
Hepatic arteries, 588–589, 643–644
Hepatic steatosis, 546
Hepatic veins, 595–598
Hepatitis, 547

Hepatitis B, elastography for, 630
Hepatitis C, 593, 630–631
Hepatocellular carcinoma, 549–550, 612–616
    after liver transplantation, 650
    elastography for, 631
    thrombosis in, 595
Hepatolithiasis, 580
Hepato-renal syndrome, 592
Hernias, 777–780
Herpes zoster, of abdominal wall, 788–789
Heterotaxy syndrome, 558
Honeycomb appearance, of liver abscess, 611
Horseshoe kidney, 655–656
Human immunodeficiency virus infections
    cholangiopathy in, 580–581
    kidney disease in, 660
Hydatid disease, 555–556, 561, 803–805
Hydronephrosis, 660–666, 691–692
Hydroureter, 661
Hyperemia
    in diverticulitis, 767
    in inflammatory bowel disease, 758
Hypertension
    portal, 589–595, 784, 786
    renovascular, 655, 676–680
Hypogastric hernias, 778, 780

I

Ileitis, terminal, 766–767
Incisional hernias, 780
Indinavir, kidney stones due to, 660
Infarctions
    of kidney, 686
    of liver, 645–646
    of omentum, 767
    of spleen, 558–559
Inferior vena cava, complications of, in liver
    transplantation, 645
Inflammatory bowel disease, 755–763
    appendicitis in, 765–766
    diagnosis of, 756
    elastography for, 636
    epidemiology of, 755–756
    ultrasonography for, 756–757
        classic features in, 757–758
        complications of, 758–763
        contrast agents for, 758
Inflammatory fat
    in diverticulitis, 767
    in inflammatory bowel disease, 757
Inflammatory masses, in inflammatory bowel disease,
    760–761
Infusion injection method, for contrast-enhanced
    ultrasound, 609
Inguinal hernias, 777–780
Insulinomas, 708–710

Interventions, ultrasonography guidance for,
    793–820. *See also* Biopsy; Drain placement.
    adrenal gland, 807–808
    bleeding risk and control in, 797–799
    environment for, 795
    equipment for, 795–797
    hepatic, 802–807
    pain control in, 799–800
    paracentesis, 814
    pelvic, 811–814
    personnel for, 794–795
    renal, 808–810
    splenic, 810–811
Intraductal cholangiocarcinomas, 554–555
Intraductal papillary mucinous neoplasms, 708,
    711
Intrahepatic ducts, anatomy of, 569
Intrahepatic portal hypertension, 593–594
Intraluminal gut masses, 752
Intraoperative ultrasound, for liver masses, 617–618
Intussusception, 768
Iron deposition, in spleen, 562
Ischemia, bowel. *See* Mesenteric arteries.
Islet cell tumors, 708–709

J

Junctional parenchymal defect, of kidney, 655
Juxtaglomerular cell tumors, 675

K

Kaposi sarcoma, 660
Kidney
    biopsy of, 808–810
    infarction of, 686
    ultrasonography of. *See* Renal ultrasonography.
Klatskin tumors, 583

L

Leiomyosarcomas, 713
Lipomas
    of abdominal wall, 782
    of retroperitoneum, 713–714
Liposarcomas, of retroperitoneum, 711, 713
Liquefactive necrosis, in hepatocellular carcinomas,
    549
Lithium, kidney cystic disease due to, 669
Liver
    elastography of, 628–632, 634
    ultrasonography of, **545–557**
        anatomy of, 545–546
        for abscess, 555–556
        for adenomas, 552–553
        for biliary hamartomas, 556
        for biopsy, 803–807

Liver (*continued*)
    for cavernous hemangiomas, 550–551
    for cholangiocarcinoma, 554–555, 613, 616
    for cirrhosis. *See* Cirrhosis.
    for cysts, 551–552, 611, 803–805
    for diffuse disease, 546–547
    for fatty changes, 611, 614, 616
    for focal nodular hyperplasia, 552, 620
    for hemangiomas, 609
    for hepatitis, 547
    for hepatocellular carcinoma, 549–550,
      612–616
    for infarction, 645–646
    for infections, 611
    for lymphomas, 556, 617
    for malignancies, 611–617
    for masses, 549, **605–623**
    for metastasis, 553–554, 613, 617, 628
    for nodules, 612
    for transplantation, **641–652**
    for trauma, 557
Liver fibrosis index, 632
Lymphadenopathy
    in inflammatory bowel disease, 757–758
    in typhlitis, 767
    of retroperitoneum, 716–717
Lymphangiomas, of retroperitoneum, 719
Lymphoceles
    after kidney transplantation, 690
    of retroperitoneum, 718–719
Lymphomas
    of bowel, 754
    of kidney, 660, 673
    of liver, 556, 617
    of spleen, 561

M

Magnetic resonance angiography, for liver
    transplantation evaluation, 642
Magnetic resonance imaging
    for inflammatory bowel disease, 756
    for renal cell carcinoma, 672
    fusion guidance for, 817
Malignancies
    after liver transplantation, 649–650
    in inflammatory bowel disease, 762
    of adrenal glands, 701–704
    of biliary tract, 582–583
    of gallbladder, 576
    of kidney, 670–674, 692–693
Margination, in inflammatory bowel disease, 757
Masses
    in inflammatory bowel disease, 760–761
    of abdominal wall, 781–785, 787
    of bowel, 752–755
    of liver, 549, **605–623**

Mass-forming cholangiocarcinomas, 554–555
Mechanical index imaging, for liver masses, 608
Median arcuate ligament syndrome, 743
Medullary sponge kidney, 669
MELD (Model for End-Stage Liver Disease) scoring
    system, 642
Mesenteric adenitis, 766–767
Mesenteric arteries
    collateral circulation of, 724
    hemodynamics of, 725–726
    ultrasonography of
      anatomy of, 724
      atherosclerosis and, 740–744
      for aneurysms, 745–747
      for dissection, 743
      for occlusion, 743
      for pseudoaneurysms, 745–747
      protocol for, 726
      technique for, 726
Metastasis
    to abdominal wall, 784
    to adrenal glands, 703–704
    to kidney, 673
    to liver, 549, 551, 553–554, 613, 617, 628
    to spleen, 561
Microbubbles. *See* Contrast-enhanced ultrasound.
Middle aortic syndrome, 677
Mirizzi syndrome, 579
Model for End-Stage Liver Disease (MELD) scoring
    system, 642
Mucinous cystadenomas, 708, 711
Multilocular cystic nephromas, 675
Murphy sign, sonographic, 570, 572–575
Myelolipomas, of adrenal glands, 702

N

Necrosis
    in hepatocellular carcinomas, 549
    of gallbladder, 573
Needles, for biopsy, 795–796
Negative beak sign, in retroperitoneal
    ultrasonography, 699
Nephrocalcinosis, 662–663
Nephrolithiasis, 691–692
Nephromas, multilocular cystic, 675
Nephronophthisis, 667
Nephropathy, HIV-associated, 660
Nerve sheath tumors, of retroperitoneum, 716
Neuroblastomas
    of adrenal glands, 703–704
    of retroperitoneum, 716
Neuroendocrine tumors, of pancreas, 708–710
Neurofibromas, of abdominal wall, 785
Neurogenic tumors, of retroperitoneum, 716
Nodules, of liver
    dysplastic, 612

in cirrhosis, 548–549
in hepatocellular carcinomas, 550

O

Obstruction
    after kidney transplantation, 691–692
    in inflammatory bowel disease, 759–760
Obstructive hydronephrosis, 661–665
Omentum
    biopsy of, 815
    infarctions of, 767
Oncocytomas, of kidney, 675
Oriental cholangiohepatitis, 580
Overlying brightness mode, for liver masses, 608

P

Pancreas
    elastography of, 633, 635
    ultrasonography of, 704–709
        anatomy of, 704–705
        for autoimmune disease, 707
        for drain placement, 815, 817
        for pancreatitis, 705–707
        for pseudocysts, 706–707
        for tumors, 707–709
        techniques for, 704–705
Pancreatitis, 635, 705–707
Paracentesis, 788, 814
Paragangliomas, of retroperitoneum, 714–715
Peak systolic velocity, in kidney ultrasonography, 685–686
Pelvic interventions, 811–814
Perforation
    in appendicitis, 765
    in inflammatory bowel disease, 761–762
Perianal disease, in inflammatory bowel disease, 762
Pericholecystic fluid, 572
Periductal infiltrating cholangiocarcinomas, 554–555
Perineal sonography, for inflammatory bowel disease, 762
Persistent fetal lobulation, of kidney, 654
Pheochromocytomas
    extra-adrenal, 715–716
    of adrenal glands, 702–703
Phlegmon, in inflammatory bowel disease, 760–761
Phrygian cap, 568
Piggyback cavocaval anastomosis, in liver transplantation, 645
Platelet transfusion, for interventions, 797
Pleomorphic sarcomas, undifferentiated, of retroperitoneum, 713
Pneumobilia, 579
Polycystic disease
    of kidney, 666–670
    of liver, 551–552

Polyps, gallbladder, 576–578
Polysplenia, 558
Porcelain gallbladder, 571, 575–576
Portal hypertension, 589–595, 784, 786
Portal triad, anatomy of, 568–569
Portal venous system
    gas in, 589, 591
    stenosis of, 589–595
        in heart failure, 589–590
        in liver transplantation, 644–645
        portal hypertension in, 589–595
    thrombosis of, in liver transplantation, 644–645
Positron emission tomography, fusion guidance for, 817
Posterior urethral valves, 665
Posthepatic portal hypertension, 594
Posttransplant lymphoproliferative disease
    after kidney transplantation, 692–693
    after liver transplantation, 650
Power Doppler ultrasonography, for kidney transplantation, 688
Prehepatic portal hypertension, 593
Primary biliary cirrhosis, portal hypertension in, 594
Primary sclerosing cholangitis, 581
Pseudoaneurysms, of kidney, 679–680, 688
Pseudocysts, of pancreas, 706–707
Pseudokidney sign, in thickened gut, 752, 754
Pseudolesions, of retroperitoneum, 699, 719
Pseudotumors, of kidney, 654, 656, 659
Putty kidney, 660
Pyelonephritis, 656–659
Pyogenic abscesses, of liver, 555–556
Pyonephrosis, 660

R

Rejection, in transplantation
    kidney, 688–690
    liver, 650–651
Renal arteries, pathology of, 676–680
Renal colic, 661
Renal ultrasonography, **653–681**
    anatomy of, 653–654
    for biopsy, 807–808
    for cystic disease, 666–670
    for hydronephrosis, 660–666
    for infections and inflammation, 656–660
    for malignancies, 670–674, 692–693
    for masses, 807–808
    for neoplasia, 670–674
    for perirenal pathology, 674–676, 678
    for renal cell carcinoma, 670–674, 692–693
    for transplantation, **683–695,** 807–808
    for trauma, 675–676
    for vascular pathology, 676–680
    normal variants in, 654–656
    technique for, 654

Renal veins, thrombosis of, 679
Renovascular hypertension, 676–680, 685
Respiration, hepatic vein changes with, 596
Response Evaluation Criteria in Solid Tumors, 619
Retroperitoneal fibrosis, 714–715
Retroperitoneum, ultrasonography of, **697–721**
    algorithm for, 699
    anatomy of, 697
    for adrenal disorders, 700–704
    for extraorgan tumors, 709–719
    for fluid collections, 717–719
    for interventions, 814–815
    for pancreas disorders, 704–709
    for pseudolesions, 699, 719
    normal structures in, 698
    technique for, 697–698
"Reverse target sign," in cirrhosis, 548
Rib fractures, 788
Ring-down artifact
    in diverticulitis, 767
    in gallbladder adenomyomatosis, 576–577

S

Sarcoidosis
    of liver, 549
    of spleen, 561–562
Sarcomas, of abdominal wall, 783
Schistosomiasis, 555–556, 593
Sclerosis, biliary, 581
Segmental omental infarction, 767
Seldinger method, for drain placement, 801–802
Self-shadowing, in liver ultrasound, 618
Seromas
    after kidney transplantation, 690
    drainage of, 815
    of abdominal wall, 780–781
Serous cystadenomas, 708, 711
Shear wave elastography
    of liver, 631–632
    of pancreas, 633, 635
    principles of, 627–628
Shingles, of abdominal wall, 788–789
Shock abdomen, 768
Side-by-side mode, for liver masses, 608
Simple cysts, of liver, 551–552
Skin cancer, after liver transplantation, 649–650
Skip lesions, in inflammatory bowel disease, 757
Sludge, biliary, 571–572
Solid pseudopapillary neoplasms, 708, 711
Spectral Doppler ultrasonography
    for aorta, 739
    for biliary sludge, 572
    for hepatocellular carcinomas, 550
    for kidney pathology, 679–680
    for kidney transplantation, 685, 687–688
    for mesenteric arteries, 746

    for renal cell carcinoma, 671–672
Spiculated border, in inflammatory bowel disease,
    757
Spigelian hernias, 780
Splanchnic arteries, aneurysms of, 745–747
Spleen, ultrasonography of, **557–562**
    anatomy of, 557–558
    for abscess, 560–561, 810–811
    for biopsy, 810–811
    for cysts, 560
    for hamartomas, 560
    for hemangiomas, 561
    for infarction, 558–559
    for lymphomas, 561
    for metastasis, 561
    for sarcoidosis, 561–562
    for trauma, 558
    technique for, 558
Splenic artery steal syndrome, 646–647
Splenomegaly, in portal hypertension, 590
"Starry night" appearance, in hepatitis, 547
"Stealth lesions," in focal nodular hyperplasia, 552
Steatosis
    elastography for, 630
    hepatic, 546
Stenosis
    of hepatic artery, 589
    of portal venous system, 589–595, 644–645
    of renal arteries, 685–686
Stents
    aortic, 734–738
    transjugular intrahepatic portosystemic, 598–602
Strain elastography
    of gastrointestinal tract, 636
    of liver, 633–634
    of pancreas, 633
    principles of, 626–627
Strain rate imaging, of gastrointestinal tract, 636
Strictures, in inflammatory bowel disease, 758–759

T

Takayasu arteritis, 677
Tardus-parvus waveform
    in hepatic artery stenosis, 589
    in renal artery stenosis, 677, 679
Target pattern, in thickened gut, 752
Targeted imaging, for liver masses, 620
Teratomas, of retroperitoneum, 714–715
Thickened gut, 752, 757
Three-dimensional imaging, for liver masses,
    619–620
Thrombosis
    of hepatic artery, 643
    of portal venous system, 594–595, 644–645
    of renal arteries, 686
    of renal veins, 679

of transjugular intrahepatic portosystemic shunts, 600–601

TIPS (transjugular intrahepatic portosystemic shunts), 598–602

Todani classification, of choledochal cysts, 583–585

Touch preparation, in biopsy, 801

Transient elastography
  of kidney, 690
  of liver, 629–631

Transitional cell carcinomas, of kidney, 673

Transjugular intrahepatic portosystemic shunts, 598–602

Transplantation
  kidney, **683–695**
    anatomy of, 684–685
    biopsy for, 807–808
    compartment syndrome after, 688
    fluid collections in, 690
    graft dysfunction in, 688–690
    neoplastic complications of, 692–693
    procedure for, 683–684
    urologic complications of, 691–692
    vascular complications of, 658–688
  liver, **641–652**
    anastomosis locations in, 643
    complications of, 643–651
    contraindications for, 642
    indications for, 641
    postoperative assessment for, 642–643
    preoperative assessment for, 642
    statistics on, 641

Transvaginal sonography, 753
  for appendicitis, 765
  for inflammatory bowel disease, 762

Trauma
  to kidney, 675–676
  to liver, 557
  to spleen, 558

Tricuspid valve regurgitation, hepatic vein changes with, 596

Trocar method, for drain placement, 801–802

Tuberculosis
  of colon, 767
  of kidney, 660

Tumefactive sludge, 572

Tumors, adrenal, 701–704

Twinkle artifact, in urinary stones, 692

Typhilitis, 766–767

U

Ulcerations, in inflammatory bowel disease, 762

Ulcerative colitis. *See* Inflammatory bowel disease.

Umbilical hernias, 778, 780

Undifferentiated pleomorphic sarcomas, of retroperitoneum, 713

Ureter(s), strictures of, 663

Ureteral jets, 662

Ureteroceles, 665

Ureteroneocystostomy, 691

Ureteropelvic junction, 664–665

Ureteroureterostomy, 691

Urine leak, after kidney transplantation, 690–691

Urinomas, 690–691, 718

Urolithiasis, 661–662, 691–692

V

Varices, portal hypertension and, 595

Vasculitis, kidney disorders in, 677

Vesicoureteral reflux, 665–666

Virtual Touch Imaging, 627

von Meyerburg complexes, 556

W

Wall layer retention, in inflammatory bowel disease, 757

Wall-echo-shadow (WES) sign, 571

"Water-lily sign"
  in liver abscess, 555
  in splenic abscess, 561

WES sign, for gallstones, 571

"Wheel-within-a-wheel" appearance
  in liver abscess, 556
  in splenic abscess, 561

X

Xanthogranulomatous cholecystitis, 575

Xanthogranulomatous pyelonephritis, 656–657

Y

Yin-yang sign
  in aortic aneurysm, 733
  in false aneurysm, 601–602

United States Postal Service
Statement of Ownership, Management, and Circulation
(All Periodicals Publications Except Requestor Publications)

1. Publication Title	2. Publication Number	3. Filing Date
Ultrasound Clinics	0 0 0 - 7 1 1 1	9/14/14

4. Issue Frequency	5. Number of Issues Published Annually	6. Annual Subscription Price
Jan, Apr, Jul, Oct	4	$270.00

7. Complete Mailing Address of Known Office of Publication (Not printer) (Street, city, county, state, and ZIP+4®)

Elsevier Inc.
360 Park Avenue South
New York, NY 10010-1710

Contact Person
Stephen R. Bushing
Telephone (Include area code)
215-239-3688

8. Complete Mailing Address of Headquarters or General Business Office of Publisher (Not printer)

Elsevier Inc., 360 Park Avenue South, New York, NY 10010-1710

9. Full Names and Complete Mailing Addresses of Publisher, Editor, and Managing Editor (Do not leave blank)

Publisher (Name and complete mailing address)

Linda Belfus, Elsevier, Inc. 1600 John F. Kennedy Blvd. Suite 1800, Philadelphia, PA 19103-2899

Editor (Name and complete mailing address)

John Vassallo, Elsevier, Inc., 1600 John F. Kennedy Blvd. Suite 1800, Philadelphia, PA 19103-2899

Managing Editor (Name and complete mailing address)

Adrianne Brigido, Elsevier, Inc., 1600 John F. Kennedy Blvd. Suite 1800, Philadelphia, PA 19103-2899

10. Owner (Do not leave blank. If the publication is owned by a corporation, give the name and address of the corporation immediately followed by the names and addresses of all stockholders owning or holding 1 percent or more of the total amount of stock. If not owned by a corporation, give the names and addresses of the individual owners. If owned by a partnership or other unincorporated firm, give its name and address as well as those of each individual owner. If the publication is published by a nonprofit organization, give its name and address.)

Full Name	Complete Mailing Address
Wholly owned subsidiary of	1600 John F. Kennedy Blvd. Ste. 1800
Reed/Elsevier, US holdings	Philadelphia, PA 19103-2899

11. Known Bondholders, Mortgagees, and Other Security Holders Owning or Holding 1 Percent or More of Total Amount of Bonds, Mortgages, or Other Securities. If none, check box ☐ None

Full Name	Complete Mailing Address
N/A	

12. Tax Status (For completion by nonprofit organizations authorized to mail at nonprofit rates) (Check one)
The purpose, function, and nonprofit status of this organization and the exempt status for federal income tax purposes:
☐ Has Not Changed During Preceding 12 Months
☐ Has Changed During Preceding 12 Months (Publisher must submit explanation of change with this statement)

PS Form **3526**, August 2012 (Page 1 of 3 (Instructions Page 3)) PSN 7530-01-000-9931 **PRIVACY NOTICE:** See our Privacy policy in www.usps.com

---

13. Publication Title	14. Issue Date for Circulation Data Below
Ultrasound Clinics	July 2014

15. Extent and Nature of Circulation			Average No. Copies Each Issue During Preceding 12 Months	No. Copies of Single Issue Published Nearest to Filing Date
a. Total Number of Copies (Net press run)			330	324
b. Paid Circulation (By Mail and Outside the Mail)	(1)	Mailed Outside-County Paid Subscriptions Stated on PS Form 3541. (Include paid distribution above nominal rate, advertiser's proof copies, and exchange copies)	147	134
	(2)	Mailed In-County Paid Subscriptions Stated on PS Form 3541 (Include paid distribution above nominal rate, advertiser's proof copies, and exchange copies)		
	(3)	Paid Distribution Outside the Mails Including Sales Through Dealers and Carriers, Street Vendors, Counter Sales, and Other Paid Distribution Outside USPS®	34	37
	(4)	Paid Distribution by Other Classes Mailed Through the USPS (e.g. First-Class Mail®)		
c. Total Paid Distribution (Sum of 15b (1), (2), (3), and (4))		▲	181	171
d. Free or Nominal Rate Distribution (By Mail and Outside the Mail)	(1)	Free or Nominal Rate Outside-County Copies Included on PS Form 3541	60	53
	(2)	Free or Nominal Rate In-County Copies Included on PS Form 3541		
	(3)	Free or Nominal Rate Copies Mailed at Other Classes Through the USPS (e.g. First-Class Mail)		
	(4)	Free or Nominal Rate Distribution Outside the Mail (Carriers or other means)		
e. Total Free or Nominal Rate Distribution (Sum of 15d (1), (2), (3) and (4))		▲	60	53
f. Total Distribution (Sum of 15c and 15e)		▲	241	224
g. Copies not Distributed (See Instructions to publishers #4 (page #3))			89	100
h. Total (Sum of 15f and g)		▲	330	324
i. Percent Paid (15c divided by 15f times 100)		▲	75.10%	76.34%

16. Total circulation includes electronic copies. Report circulation on PS Form 3526-X worksheet.

17. Publication of Statement of Ownership
If the publication is a general publication, publication of this statement is required. Will be printed in the October 2014 issue of this publication.

18. Signature and Title of Editor, Publisher, Business Manager, or Owner   Date

Stephen R. Bushing – Inventory Distribution Coordinator   September 14, 2014

I certify that all information furnished on this form is true and complete. I understand that anyone who furnishes false or misleading information on this form or who omits material or information requested on the form may be subject to criminal sanctions (including fines and imprisonment) and/or civil sanctions (including civil penalties).

PS Form **3526**, August 2012 (Page 2 of 3)

Moving?

Make sure your subscription moves with you!

To notify us of your new address, find your **Clinics Account Number** (located on your mailing label above your name), and contact customer service at:

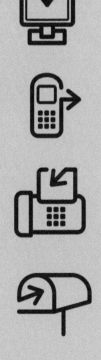

Email: journalscustomerservice-usa@elsevier.com

800-654-2452 (subscribers in the U.S. & Canada)
314-447-8871 (subscribers outside of the U.S. & Canada)

Fax number: 314-447-8029

Elsevier Health Sciences Division
Subscription Customer Service
3251 Riverport Lane
Maryland Heights, MO 63043

ELSEVIER

Printed and bound by CPI Group (UK) Ltd, Croydon, CR0 4YY

03/10/2024

01040379-0004